Clinical PET/CT: Quarter-Century Transformation of Oncology

Editor

RATHAN M. SUBRAMANIAM

PET CLINICS

www.pet.theclinics.com

Consulting Editor
ABASS ALAVI

April 2024 • Volume 19 • Number 2

ELSEVIER

1600 John F. Kennedy Boulevard • Suite 1800 • Philadelphia, Pennsylvania, 19103-2899

http://www.pet.theclinics.com

PET CLINICS Volume 19, Number 2
April 2024 ISSN 1556-8598, ISBN-13: 978-0-443-13069-4

Editor: John Vassallo (j.vassallo@elsevier.com)
Developmental Editor: Varun Gopal

PET Clinics (ISSN 1556-8598) is published quarterly by Elsevier Inc., 360 Park Avenue South, New York, NY 10010-1710. Months of issue are January, April, July, and October. Periodicals postage paid at New York, NY, and additional mailing offices. Subscription prices per year are $288.00 (US individuals), $100.00 (US students), $304.00 (Canadian individuals), $100.00 (Canadian students), $306.00 (foreign individuals), and $140.00 (foreign students). For institutional access pricing please contact Customer Service via the contact information below. To receive student and resident rate, orders must be accompanied by name of affiliated institution, date of term, and the signature of program/residency coordinator on institution letterhead. Orders will be billed at individual rate until proof of status is received. Foreign air speed delivery is included in all Clinics subscription prices. All prices are subject to change without notice. POSTMASTER: Send address changes to PET Clinics, Elsevier Health Sciences Division, Subscription Customer Service, 3251 Riverport Lane, Maryland Heights, MO 63043. **Customer Service: 1-800-654-2452 (U.S. and Canada); 314-447-8871 (outside U.S. and Canada). Fax: 314-447-8029. E-mail: journalscustomerservice-usa@elsevier.com (for print support); journalsonlinesupport-usa@elsevier.com (for online support).**

Reprints. For copies of 100 or more of articles in this publication, please contact the Commercial Reprints Department, Elsevier Inc., 360 Park Avenue South, New York, NY 10010-1710. Tel.: 212-633-3874; Fax: 212-633-3820; E-mail: reprints@elsevier.com.

PET Clinics is covered in MEDLINE/PubMed (Index Medicus).

Contributors

CONSULTING EDITOR

ABASS ALAVI, MD, MD (Hon), PhD (Hon), DSc (Hon)
Professor of Radiology and Neurology, Director of Research Education, Division of Nuclear Medicine, Department of Radiology, Hospital of the University of Pennsylvania, Perelman School of Medicine, University of Pennsylvania, Philadelphia, Pennsylvania

EDITOR

RATHAN M. SUBRAMANIAM, MD, PhD, MPH, MBA, FRSN, FACR, FACNM, FSNMMI, FRANZCR, FAUR, FAANMS
Executive Dean, Faculty of Medicine, Nursing, Midwifery and Health Sciences, Professor of Radiology and Nuclear Medicine, University of Notre Dame Australia, Sydney, Australia; Department of Radiology, Duke University, Durham, North Carolina, USA; Department of Medicine, University of Otago Medical School, Dunedin, New Zealand

AUTHORS

CHANDRASEKHAR BAL, MD
Professor and Head, Department of Nuclear Medicine, AIIMS, New Delhi, India

STEPHEN M. BROSKI, MD
Professor, Department of Radiology, Mayo Clinic, Rochester, Minnesota

JAMES P. BUTEAU, MD
Nuclear Medicine Physician, Prostate Cancer Theranostics and Imaging Centre of Excellence, Molecular Imaging and Therapeutic Nuclear Medicine, Cancer Imaging, Peter MacCallum Cancer Centre, Sir Peter MacCallum Department of Oncology, The University of Melbourne, Melbourne, Victoria, Australia

KUNAL RAMESH CHANDEKAR, MD
Senior Resident, Department of Nuclear Medicine, AIIMS, New Delhi, India

DAVID C. CHEN, BMedSc
Research Fellow, Prostate Cancer Theranostics and Imaging Centre of Excellence, Molecular Imaging and Therapeutic Nuclear Medicine, Cancer Imaging, Peter MacCallum Cancer Centre, Sir Peter MacCallum Department of Oncology, The University of Melbourne, Melbourne, Victoria, Australia

WAN KAM CHIU, MB ChB (HK), FHKAM (Obstetrics and Gynaecology)
Associate Consultant, Department of Obstetrics and Gynaecology, United Christian Hospital, Kowloon, Hong Kong, China

ALIREZA GHODSI, MD
Research Fellow, Department of Radiology, Research Fellow, University of Washington, Seattle, Washington

MICHAEL A. GORIN, MD
Associate Professor, Milton and Carroll Petrie Department of Urology, Icahn School of Medicine at Mount Sinai, New York, New York

DAVID GROHEUX, MD, PhD
Nuclear Medicine Physician, Nuclear Department of Nuclear Medicine, Saint-Louis Hospital, Paris, France; Centre d'Imagerie Radio-Isotopique (CIRI), La Rochelle, France; University Paris-Diderot, Paris, France

RODNEY J. HICKS, MD, FRACP
Professor, Department of Medicine, St Vincent's Hospital, The University of Melbourne, Melbourne, Victoria, Australia; Department of Medicine, Central Clinical School, The Alfred Hospital, Monash University, Melbourne, Australia; The Melbourne Theranostic Innovation Centre, North Melbourne, Australia

GRACE HO, MB ChB (HK), FRCR, FHKCR, FHKAM (Radiology)
Consultant Radiologist, Department of Radiology, Queen Mary Hospital, Hong Kong SAR, China

JEAN HOFFMAN-CENSITS, MD
Associate Professor, Department of Medical Oncology and Urology, Sidney Kimmel Comprehensive Cancer Center, The Johns Hopkins University School of Medicine, Baltimore, Maryland

MICHAEL S. HOFMAN, MBBS
Nuclear Medicine Physician, Prostate Cancer Theranostics and Imaging Centre of Excellence, Molecular Imaging and Therapeutic Nuclear Medicine, Cancer Imaging, Peter MacCallum Cancer Centre, Sir Peter MacCallum Department of Oncology, The University of Melbourne, Melbourne, Victoria, Australia

SIYU HUANG, MD
Department of Surgery, The University of Melbourne, Melbourne, Victoria, Australia

AMIR IRAVANI, MD, FRACP
Associate Professor, Department of Radiology, Nuclear Medicine Physician and Associate Professor, University of Washington, Seattle, Washington

ASHA KANDATHIL, MBBS, DMRD, MD
Associate Professor, Department of Radiology, University of Texas Southwestern Medical Center, Dallas, Texas

RAGHAVA KASHYAP, MD
Nuclear Medicine Physician, Prostate Cancer Theranostics and Imaging Centre of Excellence, Molecular Imaging and Therapeutic Nuclear Medicine, Cancer Imaging, Peter MacCallum Cancer Centre, Sir Peter MacCallum Department of Oncology, The University of Melbourne, Melbourne, Victoria, Australia

DAMIEN KEE, MBBS, FRACP
Olivia Newton-John Cancer Research Institute, La Trobe University, Department of Medical Oncology, Olivia Newton-John Cancer and Wellness Centre, Austin Hospital, Austin Health, Heidelberg, Australia

AMIR H. KHANDANI, MD
Professor, Molecular Imaging and Therapeutics, Department of Radiology, University of North Carolina, Chapel Hill, North Carolina

YOGITA KHANDELWAL, MD
Senior Resident, Department of Nuclear Medicine, All India Institute of Medical Sciences, New Delhi, India

NATALIA KOVALEVA, MBBS
Nuclear Medicine Registrar, Department of Molecular Imaging and Therapy, Austin Health, Heidelberg, Australia

SHUK TAK KWOK, MBBS (HK), MRCOG, FHKCOG
Associate Consultant, Department of Obstetrics and Gynaecology, Queen Mary Hospital, Hong Kong SAR, China

ELAINE YUEN PHIN LEE, BMedSci, BMBS (UK), MD (HK), FRCR
Clinical Associate Professor, Department of Diagnostic Radiology, School of Clinical Medicine, Queen Mary Hospital, University of Hong Kong, Hong Kong SAR, China

SZE-TING LEE, MBBS, PhD, FRACP, FAANMS
Associate Professor, Department of Molecular Imaging and Therapy, Austin Health, Heidelberg, Australia; Department of Medicine, The University of Melbourne, Department of Surgery, The University of Melbourne, School of Health and Biomedical Sciences, RMIT University, Melbourne, Australia; Olivia Newton-John Cancer Research Institute, La Trobe University, Heidelberg, Australia

CHARLES MARCUS, MD
Assistant Professor, Division of Nuclear Medicine, Department of Radiology and Imaging Sciences, Emory University School of Medicine, Atlanta, Georgia

MATTHEW I. MILOWSKY, MD, FASCO
Professor, Lineberger Comprehensive Cancer Center, University of North Carolina, Chapel Hill, North Carolina

SALIKH MURTAZALIEV, MD
Division of Nuclear Medicine and Molecular Imaging, The Russell H. Morgan Department of Radiology and Radiological Science, Johns Hopkins Hospital, Baltimore, Maryland

SAIMA MUZAHIR, MD, FCPS, FRCPE
Assistant Professor, Division of Nuclear Medicine, Department of Radiology and Imaging Sciences, Emory University School of Medicine, Atlanta, Georgia

SRIDHAR NIMMAGADDA, PhD
Professor, The Russell H. Morgan Department of Radiology and Radiological Science, The Johns Hopkins University School of Medicine, Baltimore, Maryland

JORGE D. OLDAN, MD
Associate Professor, Molecular Imaging and Therapeutics, Department of Radiology, University of North Carolina, Chapel Hill, North Carolina

NIHARIKA PANT, MBBS, MD
Clinical Research Coordinator - II, Radiology, Mallinckrodt Institute of Radiology, Washington University School of Medicine, St. Louis, Missouri

ASHWIN SINGH PARIHAR, MBBS, MD
Chief Resident/Fellow, Nuclear Medicine, Mallinckrodt Institute of Radiology, Washington University School of Medicine, St. Louis, Missouri

PUN CHING PHILIP IP, MB ChB (UK), FRCPath, FHKCPath, FHKAM (Pathology)
Clinical Professor, Department of Pathology, School of Clinical Medicine, University of Hong Kong, Hong Kong SAR, China

MARIGDALIA K. RAMIREZ-FORT, MD
President and CEO, BioDefense, BioFort Corp., Guaynabo, Puerto Rico

W. KIMRYN RATHMELL, MD, PhD
Professor, Department of Medicine, Vanderbilt University Medical Center, Nashville, Tennessee

STEVEN P. ROWE, MD, PhD
Professor and Chief, Molecular Imaging and Therapeutics, Department of Radiology, University of North Carolina, Chapel Hill, North Carolina; Professor, Division of Nuclear Medicine and Molecular Imaging, The Russell H. Morgan Department of Radiology and Radiological Science at Johns Hopkins Hospital, Baltimore, Maryland

SWAYAMJEET SATAPATHY, MD
Senior Resident, Department of Nuclear Medicine, AIIMS, New Delhi, India

JENNIFER A. SCHROEDER, MD
Assistant Professor, Molecular Imaging and Therapeutics, Department of Radiology, University of North Carolina, Chapel Hill, North Carolina

ANDREW M. SCOTT, MBBS, MD, FRACP, FAHMS, FAANMS
Associate Professor, Department of Molecular Imaging and Therapy, Austin Health, Heidelberg, Australia; Department of Medicine, The University of Melbourne, Melbourne,

Australia; Olivia Newton-John Cancer Research Institute, and La Trobe University, Heidelberg, Australia

CLARE SENKO, MBBS, FRACP
Olivia Newton-John Cancer Research Institute, La Trobe University, Department of Medical Oncology, Olivia Newton-John Cancer and Wellness Centre, Austin Health, Heidelberg, Australia

SARA SHEIKHBAHAEI, MD, MPH
Assistant Professor, Division of Nuclear Medicine and Molecular Imaging, The Russell H. Morgan Department of Radiology and Radiological Science, Johns Hopkins Hospital, Baltimore, Maryland

GOLMEHR SISTANI, MD
Radiologist and Nuclear Medicine Specialist, Medical Imaging Department, Royal Victoria Regional Health Centre, Barrie, Ontario, Canada

LILJA B. SOLNES, MD, MBA
Director, Division of Nuclear Medicine and Molecular Imaging, Associate Professor, The Russell H. Morgan Department of Radiology and Radiological Science, The Johns Hopkins University School of Medicine, Johns Hopkins Hospital, Baltimore, Maryland

RATHAN M. SUBRAMANIAM, MD, PhD, MPH, MBA, FRSN, FACR, FACNM, FSNMMI, FRANZCR, FAUR, FAANMS
Executive Dean, Faculty of Medicine, Nursing, Midwifery and Health Sciences, Professor of Radiology and Nuclear Medicine, University of Notre Dame Australia, Sydney, Australia; Department of Radiology, Duke University,

Durham, North Carolina, USA; Department of Medicine, University of Otago Medical School, Dunedin, New Zealand

KA YU TSE, MBBS (HK), MMedSc (HK), FHKCOG, FRCOG, Cert RCOG (Gynae Onc), FHKAM (Obstetrics and Gynaecology)
Clinical Associate Professor, Department of Obstetrics and Gynaecology, School of Clinical Medicine, University of Hong Kong, Hong Kong SAR, China

GARY A. ULANER, MD, PhD
Director, Molecular Imaging and Therapy, Hoag Family Cancer Institute, Irvine, California; Departments of Radiology and Translational Genomics, University of Southern California, Los Angeles, California

SOFIA CARRILHO VAZ, MD, FEBNM
Nuclear Medicine Physician, Nuclear Medicine-Radiopharmacology, Champalimaud Clinical Center, Champalimaud Foundation, Lisbon, Portugal; Department of Radiology, Leiden University Medical Center, Leiden, The Netherlands

RUDOLF A. WERNER, MD
Senior Physician, Division of Nuclear Medicine and Molecular Imaging, The Russell H. Morgan Department of Radiology and Radiological Science, Johns Hopkins Hospital, Baltimore, Maryland; Department of Nuclear Medicine, University Hospital Würzburg, Würzburg, Germany

KATHERINE ZUKOTYNSKI, MD, PhD
Professor, Department of Radiology, McMaster University, Hamilton, Ontario, Canada

Contents

During the last 2 decades, f-18 fluorodeoxyglucose positron emission tomography/computed tomography (^{18}F FDG PET/CT) has transformed the clinical head and neck cancer imaging for patient management and predicting survival outcomes. It is now widely used for staging, radiotherapy planning, posttherapy assessment, and for detecting recurrence in head and neck cancers and is widely included in NCCN and other evidence based clinical practice guidelines. Future directions would include evaluating the potential value of FAPI PET/CT for head and neck cancers, opportunity to use volumetric and tumor heterogeneity parameters and deploying AI in diagnostic and therapeutic assessments.

PET/computed tomography (CT) is a valuable hybrid imaging modality for the evaluation of thyroid cancer, potentially impacting management decisions. ^{18}F-fluorodeoxyglucose (FDG) PET/CT has proven utility for recurrence evaluation in differentiated thyroid cancer (DTC) patients having thyroglobulin elevation with negative iodine scintigraphy. Aggressive histologic subtypes such as anaplastic thyroid cancer shower higher FDG uptake. ^{18}F-FDOPA is the preferred PET tracer for medullary thyroid cancer. Fibroblast activation protein inhibitor and arginylglycylaspartic acid -based radiotracers have emerged as promising PET agents for radioiodine refractory DTC patients with the potential for theranostic application.

PET radiotracers have become indispensable in the care of patients with breast cancer. ^{18}F-fluorodeoxyglucose has become the preferred method of many oncologists for systemic staging of breast cancer at initial diagnosis, detecting recurrent disease, and for measuring treatment response after therapy. ^{18}F-Sodium Fluoride is valuable for detection of osseous metastases. ^{18}F-fluoroestradiol is now FDA-approved with multiple appropriate clinical uses. There are multiple PET radiotracers in clinical trials, which may add utility of PET imaging for patients with breast cancer in the future. This article will describe the advances during the last quarter century in PET for patients with breast cancer.

[18F] Fluorodeoxyglucose (^{18}F-FDG) PET/CT can improve the staging accuracy and clinical management of patients with hepatobiliary and pancreatic cancers, by detection of unsuspected metastases. ^{18}F-FDG PET/CT metabolic parameters are valuable in predicting treatment response and survival. Metabolic response on ^{18}F-FDG PET/CT can predict preoperative pathologic response to neoadjuvant therapy in patients with pancreatic cancer and determine prognosis. Several novel non-FDG tracers, such as ^{68}Ga prostate-specific membrane antigen (PSMA) and ^{68}Ga-fibroblast activation protein inhibitor (FAPI) PET/CT, show promise for imaging hepatobiliary and pancreatic cancers with potential for radioligand therapy.

This article focuses on the role of PET/computed tomography in evaluating and managing gastric cancer and colorectal cancer. The authors start with describing the common aspects of imaging with 2-deoxy-2-^{18}F-D-glucose, followed by tumor-specific discussions of gastric and colorectal malignancies. Finally, the authors provide a brief overview of non-FDG tracers including their potential clinical applications, and describe future directions in imaging these malignancies.

Significant improvement in molecular imaging and theranostics in the management of neuroendocrine tumors (NETs) has been made in the last few decades. Somatostatin receptor–targeted PET imaging outperforms conventional, planar, and single-photon emission computed tomography imaging and is indicated in the evaluation of these patients when available, resulting in a significant impact on staging, treatment response assessment, and restaging of these patients. Radionuclide therapy can have an impact on patient outcome in metastatic disease when not many treatment options are available.

Renal cell carcinoma (RCC) and urothelial carcinoma (UC) are two of the most common genitourinary malignancies. 2-deoxy-2-[18F]fluoro-d-glucose (^{18}F-FDG) can play an important role in the evaluation of patients with RCC and UC. In addition to the clinical utility of ^{18}F-FDG PET to evaluate for metastatic RCC or UC, the shift in molecular imaging to focus on specific ligand-receptor interactions should provide novel diagnostic and therapeutic opportunities in genitourinary malignancies. In combination with the rise of artificial intelligence, our ability to derive imaging biomarkers that are associated with treatment selection, response assessment, and overall patient prognostication will only improve.

Over the last quarter of a century, fluorine-18-fluorodeoxyglucose (FDG) PET/computed tomography (CT) has revolutionized the diagnostic algorithm of ovarian cancer, impacting on the initial disease evaluation including staging and surgical planning, treatment response assessment and prognostication, to the most important role in detection of recurrent disease. The role of FDG PET/CT is expanding with the adoption of new therapeutic agents. Other non-FDG tracers have been explored with fibroblast activation protein inhibitor being promising. Novel tracers may provide the basis for future theragnostic work. This article will review the evolution and impact of PET/CT in ovarian cancer management.

The past 25 years have seen significant growth in the role of positron emission tomography/computed tomography (PET/CT) in musculoskeletal oncology. Substantiative advances in technical capability and image quality have been paralleled by increasingly widespread clinical adoption and implementation. It is now recognized that PET/CT is useful in diagnosis, staging, prognostication, response assessment, and surveillance of bone and soft tissue sarcomas, often providing critical information in addition to conventional imaging assessment. As individualized, precision medicine continues to evolve for patients with sarcoma, PET/CT is uniquely positioned to offer additional insight into the biology and management of these tumors.

Skin cancers are the most common cancers, with melanoma resulting in the highest cause of death in this category. Accurate clinical, histologic, and imaging staging with fludeoxyglucose positron emission tomography (FDG PET) is most important to guide patient management. Whilst surgical excision with clear margins is the gold-standard treatment for primary cutaneous melanoma, targeted therapies have generated remarkable and rapid clinical responses in melanoma, for which FDG PET also plays an important role in assessment of treatment response and post-therapy surveillance. Non-FDG PET tracers, advanced PET technology, and PET radiomics may potentially change the landscape of the utilization of PET in the imaging of patients with cutaneous malignancies.

This article provides a comprehensive review of the role of 2-deoxy-2-[18F]fluoro-D-glucose (^{18}F FDG) positron emission tomography/computed tomography (PET/CT) in multiple myeloma (MM) and related plasma cell disorders. MM is a hematologic malignancy characterized by the neoplastic proliferation of plasma cells. ^{18}F FDG PET/CT integrates metabolic and anatomic information, allowing for accurate localization of metabolically active disease. The article discusses the use of ^{18}F FDG PET/CT in initial diagnosis, staging, prognostication, and assessing treatment response. Additionally, it provides valuable insights into the novel imaging targets including chemokine receptor C-X-C motif 4 and CD38.

Although positron emission tomography/computed tomography (PET/CT) underwent rapid growth during the last quarter-century, becoming a new standard-of-
care for imaging most cancer types, CT and bone scan remained the gold standard
for patients with prostate cancer. This occurred as 2-fluorine-18-fluoro-2-deoxy-D-
glucose was perceived to have a limited role owing to low sensitivity in many patients. A resurgence of interest occurred with the use of fluorine-18-sodium-fluoride
PET/CT as a replacement for bone scintigraphy, and then choline, fluciclovine, and
dihydrotestosterone (DHT) PET/CT as prostate "specific" radiotracers. The last decade, however, has seen a true revolution with the meteoric rise of prostate-specific
membrane antigen PET/CT.

The clinical landscape of lymphomas has changed dramatically over the last 2 decades, including significant progress made in the understanding and utilization of
imaging modalities and the available treatment options for both indolent and aggressive lymphomas. Since the introduction of hybrid PET/CT scanners in 2001, the indications of ^{18}F-fluorodeoxyglucose (FDG) PET/CT in the management of
lymphomas have grown rapidly. In today's clinical practice, FDG PET/CT is used
in successful management of the vast majority patients with lymphomas.

Immunotherapy approaches have changed the treatment landscape in a variety of
malignancies with a high anti-tumor response. Immunotherapy may be associated
with novel response and progression patterns that pose a substantial challenge to
the conventional criteria for assessing treatment response, including response evaluation criteria in solid tumors (RECIST) 1.1. In addition to the morphologic details
provided by computed tomography (CT) and MRI, hybrid molecular imaging
emerges as a comprehensive imaging modality with the capacity to interrogate
pathophysiological mechanisms like glucose metabolism. This review highlights
the current status of 2-deoxy-2-[18F]fluoro-D-glucose positron emission tomogra-
phy/computed tomography (^{18}F-FDG PET/CT) in prognostication, response monitoring, and identifying immune-related adverse events. Furthermore, it investigates
the potential role of novel immuno-PET tracers that could complement the utilization
of ^{18}F-FDG PET/CT by imaging the specific pathways involved in immunotherapeutic strategies.

PET CLINICS

SERIES OF RELATED INTEREST

Advances in Clinical Radiology
Available at: Advancesinclinicalradiology.com
MRI Clinics of North America
Available at: MRI.theclinics.com
Neuroimaging Clinics of North America
Available at: Neuroimaging.theclinics.com
Radiologic Clinics of North America
Available at: Radiologic.theclinics.com

THE CLINICS ARE AVAILABLE ONLINE!
Access your subscription at:
www.theclinics.com

PROGRAM OBJECTIVE
The goal of the *PET Clinics* is to keep practicing radiologists and radiology residents up to date with current clinical practice in positron emission tomography by providing timely articles reviewing the state of the art in patient care.

TARGET AUDIENCE
Practicing radiologists, radiology residents, and other health care professionals who provide patient care utilizing radiologic findings.

LEARNING OBJECTIVES
Upon completion of this activity, participants will be able to:
1. Review why multiphase CT or MRI is the mainstay in diagnosis, staging, and surveillance of patients with cancer.
2. Discuss the indispensable role of PET/CT in oncology.
3. Recognize immunotherapeutic strategies have substantially transformed the treatment landscape of various cancers.

ACCREDITATION
The Elsevier Office of Continuing Medical Education (EOCME) is accredited by the Accreditation Council for Continuing Medical Education (ACCME) to provide continuing medical education for physicians.

The EOCME designates this journal-based CME activity for a maximum of 14 *AMA PRA Category 1 Credit*(s)™. Physicians should claim only the credit commensurate with the extent of their participation in the activity.

All other health care professionals requesting continuing education credit for this enduring material will be issued a certificate of participation.

DISCLOSURE OF CONFLICTS OF INTEREST
The EOCME assesses conflict of interest with its instructors, faculty, planners, and other individuals who are in a position to control the content of CME activities. All relevant conflicts of interest that are identified are thoroughly vetted by EOCME for fair balance, scientific objectivity, and patient care recommendations. EOCME is committed to providing its learners with CME activities that promote improvements or quality in healthcare and not a specific proprietary business or a commercial interest.

The planning committee, staff, authors, and editors listed below have identified no financial relationships or relationships to products or devices they or their spouse/life partner have with commercial interest related to the content of this CME activity:
Chandrasekhar Bal, MD; Stephen M. Broski, MD; James P. Buteau, MD; Kunal Ramesh Chandekar, MD; David C. Chen, BMedSc; Wan Kam Chiu, MB ChB (HK), FHKAM; Alireza Ghodsi, MD; David Groheux, MD, PhD; Rodney J. Hicks, MD, FRACP; Grace Ho, MB ChB (HK), FRCR, FHKCR, FHKAM; Jean Hoffman-Censits, MD; Siyu Huang, MD; Pun Ching Philip Ip, MB ChB (UK), FRCPath, FHKCPath, FHKAM; Amir Iravani, MD, FRACP; Asha Kandathil, MBBS, DMRD, MD; Raghava Kashyap, MD; Amir H. Khandani, MD; Yogita Khandelwal, MD; Natalia Kovaleva, MBBS; Kothainayaki Kulanthaivelu, BCA, MBA; Shuk Tak Kwok, MBBS (HK), MRCOG, FHKCOG; Elaine Yuen Phin Lee, BMedSci, BMBS (UK), MD (HK), FRCR; Sze-Ting Lee, MBBS, PhD, FRACP, FAANMS; Michelle Littlejohn; Charles Marcus, MD; Matthew I. Milowsky, MD, FASCO; Salikh Murtazaliev, MD; Saima Muzahir, MD, FCPS, FRCPE; Niharika Pant, MBBS, MD, PGDHHM; Ashwin Singh Parihar, MBBS, MD; Marigdalia Ramirez-Fort, MD; W. Kimryn Rathmell, MD, PhD; Swayamjeet Satapathy, MD; Jennifer A. Schroeder, MD; Andrew M. Scott, MBBS, MD; Clare Senko, MBBS; Sara Sheikhbahaei, MD, MPH; Golmehr Sistani, MD; Lilja B. Solnes, MD; Rathan M. Subramaniam, MBBS, BMedSci, MPH, MClinEd, PhD, MBA; Ka Yu Tse, MBBS (HK), MMedSc (HK), FHKCOG, FRCOG, Cert RCOG, FHKAM; Sofia Carrilho Vaz, MD, FEBNM; Katherine Zukotynski, MD, PhD

The planning committee, staff, authors, and editors listed below have identified financial relationships or relationships to products or devices they or their spouse/life partner have with commercial interest related to the content of this CME activity:
Michael A. Gorin, MD: Speaker: Lantheus Medical Imaging; Consultant: Lantheus Medical Imaging, Telix Pharmaceuticals

Michael S. Hofman, MBBS: Researcher: Novartis AG, Bayer, Isotopia; Consultant: Astellas, AstraZeneca

Damien Kee, MBBS, FRACP: Advisor: Bristol-Myers Squibb, Merck Sharpe & Dohme, Medison Pharma

Sridhar Nimmagadda, PhD: Royalties/patent beneficiary/consultant/researcher/ownership interest: Precision Molecular, Inc

Jorge D. Oldan, MD: Advisor: Telix Pharmaceuticals

Steven P. Rowe, MD, PhD: Consultant: Progenics Pharmaceuticals; Precision Molecular; Ownership Interest: Precision Molecular

Lilja B. Sólnes, MD, MBA: Researcher: Novartis AG, Cellectar, Inc., Precision Molecular, Inc.; Consultant: Progenics Pharmaceuticals

Gary A. Ulaner, MD, PhD: Researcher, Consultant, Speaker: Curium, GE Heathcare, Lantheus, Nuclidium, POINT Biopharma, RayzeBio, Briacell, and ImaginAb

Rudolf A. Werner, MD: Speaker: Novartis AG, PentixaPharma; Advisor: Novartis AG, Bayer

UNAPPROVED/OFF-LABEL USE DISCLOSURE
The EOCME requires CME faculty to disclose to the participants:
1. When products or procedures being discussed are off-label, unlabelled, experimental, and/or investigational (not US Food and Drug Administration [FDA] approved); and
2. Any limitations on the information presented, such as data that are preliminary or that represent ongoing research, interim analyses, and/or unsupported opinions. Faculty may discuss information about pharmaceutical agents that is outside of FDA-approved labelling. This information is intended solely for CME and is not intended to promote off-label use of these medications. If you have any questions, contact the medical affairs department of the manufacturer for the most recent pre-scribing information.

TO ENROLL
To enroll in the *PET Clinics* Continuing Medical Education program, call customer service at 1-800-654-2452 or sign up online at http://www.theclinics.com/home/cme. The CME program is available to subscribers for an additional annual fee of USD 254.00.

METHOD OF PARTICIPATION
In order to claim credit, participants must complete the following:
1. Complete enrolment as indicated above.
2. Read the activity.
3. Complete the CME Test and Evaluation. Participants must achieve a score of 70% on the test. All CME Tests and Evaluations must be completed online.

CME INQUIRIES/SPECIAL NEEDS
For all CME inquiries or special needs, please contact elsevierCME@elsevier.com.

Preface

Quarter Century Clinical PET/ Computed Tomography: Transforming Medical Oncology Practice

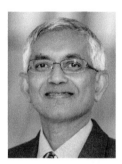

Rathan M. Subramaniam, MD, PhD, MPH, MBA
Editor

It is nearly 100 years since basic scientific research led to advances in PET and over a quarter century since the US Centers for Medicare and Medicaid Services (CMS) approved reimbursement for PET for clinical investigation of pulmonary nodule. A prototype hybrid PET/computed tomographic (CT) scanner was developed, and clinical evaluation commenced in 1998. Hybrid PET/CT scanners were introduced to the clinical practice in 2001 and more recently the hybrid PET/MRI scanners. Evolution of PET in clinical use and in medical oncology has been an iterative process of incorporating tremendous advances in technology, radiochemistry, and validation and application through clinical trials and practice. Technology advancements allowed PET spatial resolution to improve more than a factor of 10 and sensitivity by a factor more than 40, compared with the early designs of scanners to the current modern PET/CT scanners, including whole-body PET/CT scanners. PET/MRI allows combining of the high sensitivity of PET and high soft tissue resolution and functional components of MRI.

The National Oncologic PET Registry (NOPR) I and II developed the evidence over a decade that resulted in reimbursement for most of ^{18}F-FDG-PET indications in clinical oncology and led to widespread use of PET in clinical practice in the United States. Advances in radiochemistry allowed production and distribution of novel radiotracers, both cyclotron and generator produced, which led to many new phase II and III clinical trials resulting in a record number of new radiotracers approved by the Food and Drug Administration and reimbursement by the CMS for oncologic applications in the last two decades. One important noteworthy evolution is that, unlike most of the technological and PET radiochemistry developments in the last century that were from the United States, most of the successful new diagnostic and theranostic radiotracers development, early human clinical trials and early clinical applications in the last quarter century were from countries outside the United States. This is a tremendous achievement for the field of PET and nuclear medicine and the trend is likely to continue for the foreseeable future.

PET Clin 19 (2024) xv–xvi
https://doi.org/10.1016/j.cpet.2024.01.001
1556-8598/24/© 2024 Published by Elsevier Inc.

These innovations in basic biological, technological, radiochemistry, and clinical PET advancements led to PET transforming many of the diagnostic and therapeutic clinical applications in medical oncology today. We are ever grateful for all those individuals, teams, and institutions who made these advancements possible for humanity. This has been a tremendous journey for the field and for all those who championed the field. This issue of *PET Clinics* summarizes the numerous advancements made in the field of PET and their contributions to improving patient outcomes in the first quarter of this century. It is reasonable to predict that PET advancement and contributions to patient care in the next quarter century will be multiple-folds greater than what has been achieved in the last quarter century.

Rathan M. Subramaniam, MD, PhD, MPH, MBA
Faculty of Medicine, Nursing
Midwifery and Health Sciences
University of Notre Dame Australia
Sydney, Australia

E-mail address:
rathan.subramaniam@nd.edu.au

Quarter Century Positron Emission Tomography/ Computed Tomography Transformation of Oncology
Head and Neck Cancer

Rathan M. Subramaniam, MD, PhD, MPH, MBA[a,b,c,*]

KEYWORDS

- [18]F FDG PET/CT • Head and neck cancer • NCCN • Cancer-associated fibroblasts

KEY POINTS

- F-18 fluorodeoxyglucose positron emission tomography/computed tomography (^{18}F FDG PET/CT) has transformed the diagnosis, staging, therapy planning, and therapy response assessment of head and neck cancers during the last quarter century.
- National Comprehensive Cancer Network (NCCN) head and neck squamous cell carcinoma guideline recommends ^{18}F FDG PET/CT for the detection of unknown primary, staging disease with focus on detecting neck nodal and distant metastases and for assessing therapy response.
- For nasopharyngeal carcinoma, ^{18}F FDG PET/CT demonstrates superiority for detecting distant metastases and similar performance in detecting neck nodal metastases compared with MR imaging and CT. NCCN guidelines recommend ^{18}F FDG PET/CT for detecting distant metastases.
- Future directions include potential value of FAPI PET/CT in diagnosis, staging, and theranostic applications in head and neck cancers, opportunity to use FDG volumetric and tumor heterogeneity parameters in clinical practice and deploy deep learning and artificial intelligence algorithms for diagnostic and therapeutic assessments in head and neck cancers.

INTRODUCTION

In July 2001, the United States Center for Medicare and Medicaid Services approved reimbursement for PET imaging for evaluating diagnosis, initial staging, and restaging for 6 cancer types—non-small cell lung, esophageal, colorectal, and head and neck cancers, lymphoma and melanoma.[1] During the last 2 decades, F-18 fluorodeoxyglucose positron emission tomography/computed tomography (^{18}F FDG PET/CT) has transformed the clinical head and neck cancer imaging for patient management and predicting survival outcomes. It is now widely used for staging, radiotherapy planning, posttherapy assessment, and for detecting recurrence in head and neck cancers.[2–6] The 2022 National Comprehensive Cancer Network (NCCN) guideline for head and neck cancer recommends ^{18}F FDG PET/CT for detecting unknown primary tumors, initial staging focusing on detecting neck nodal and distant metastases and for therapy assessment.

[a] Faculty of Medicine, Nursing & Midwifery and Health Sciences, University of Notre Dame Australia, Sydney, Australia; [b] Department of Radiology, Duke University, Durham, NC, USA; [c] Department of Medicine, University of Otago Medical School, Dunedin, New Zealand
* Faculty of Medicine, Nursing & Midwifery and Health Sciences, University of Notre Dame Australia, Sydney, Australia.
E-mail address: rathan.subramaniam@nd.edu.au

PET Clin 19 (2024) 125–129
https://doi.org/10.1016/j.cpet.2023.12.013

EVIDENTIAL CLINICAL PRACTICE
Head and Neck Squamous Cell Carcinoma

Detection: unknown head and neck primary

[18]F FDG PET/CT is recommended after neck CT or MR imaging failed to identify a primary site in the context of neck nodal metastases because ^{18}F FDG PET/CT detects the primary site in 25% to 40% of these patients, before any invasive procedures. A meta-analysis, including 7 studies showed that ^{18}F FDG PET/CT primary tumor detection rate, sensitivity, and specificity were 0.44 (95% CI = 0.31–0.58), 0.97 (95% CI = 0.63–0.99), and 0.68 (95% CI = 0.49–0.83), respectively. Area under the curve was 0.83 (95% CI = 0.80–0.86).[7] [18]F FDG PET/CT will direct the clinician to a potential head and neck primary site in situations where other imaging modalities have failed.[8]

Staging: detection of neck nodal and distant metastases

[18]F FDG PET/CT is superior to CT/MR imaging in detecting neck nodal and distant metastases. In a meta-analysis including 18 studies (1044 patients), the pooled sensitivity for ^{18}F FDG PET or PET/CT for the detection of lymph node (LN) metastasis was 0.58 and a pooled specificity of 0.87 for patient-based analysis. However, the negative predictive value (NPV) was 0.96 (95% CI 0.95–0.97) in the level-based analysis.[9] This is further confirmed by the prospective, multicenter ACRIN 6685 clinical trial, which included patients with T2-T4 head and neck squamous cell carcinoma (HNSCCs), and showed an NPV of 0.94 (95% CI, 0.93–0.95) for clinical N0 neck, and the findings from the ^{18}F FDG PET/CT changed surgical plan in 22% of patients[10] and predicted outcomes.[11] Hence, in patients who are considered for primary surgical approach, ^{18}F FDG PET/CT can be performed, especially for tumors approaching midline to decide on the surgical approach to the contralateral neck. Patients who are planned for definite radiation therapy approach for contralateral neck also benefit from high-sensitive detection of neck nodal metastases by ^{18}F FDG PET/CT. Recent single-center study, including cT1-2N0 tongue SCC, has reported a low rate of contralateral neck failure in patients with ^{18}F FDG PET/CT-directed management of contralateral neck compared with elective contralateral neck dissection. The 5-year regional control was 86% and 87% and 5-year disease specific survival was 93% and 90% in ^{18}F FDG PET/CT-directed management group versus elective contralateral neck dissection group, respectively.[12] For locally advanced disease with T2-T4 primary or > N1 nodal stage, ^{18}F FDG PET/CT is recommended for the detection of distant metastases. [18]F FDG PET/CT detects more synchronous primary cancers and distant metastases compared with conventional imaging.[13,14]

Therapy response assessment and survival outcomes

[18]F FDG PET/CT-based posttherapy surveillance approach led to fewer planned neck dissections and considerable cost saving compared with routine planned neck dissection posttherapy in a phase III randomized multicenter clinical trial of patients with HNSCC with N2-N3 nodal disease who received definitive radiation therapy (RT) treatments.[15] [18]F FDG PET/CT should be performed between 3 and 6 months after definite RT or combined systemic therapy/RT to assess therapy response and detect any residual disease.[16] A posttherapy ^{18}F FDG PET/CT scan is performed after 12 weeks from completion of therapy to minimize radiation therapy-induced inflammatory FDG uptake. Patients who have a negative posttherapy ^{18}F FDG PET/CT has better survival outcomes.[17,18]

Posttherapy scans are commonly interpreted with standardized, qualitative methods[17,19–21] with quantitative maximum standardized uptake value (SUVmax) values are also provided in clinical practice. There is no significant difference in standardized qualitative versus semiquantitative interpretation in accuracy of therapy assessment or predicting survival outcomes. Hopkins criteria posttherapy assessment with FDG PET/CT (**Fig. 1**) is routinely used in clinical interpretations and has been validated by phase III multicenter clinical trials including posttherapy assessment of standard chemoradiation therapy in HPV-positive and HPV-negative population[18] and deintensified therapy in HPV-positive population.[22]

Posttherapy follow-up

There are no consensus guidelines or evidence for using imaging for surveillance in asymptomatic patients after therapy, which improves patient survival.[23,24] The majority of recurrences, particularly in patients with advanced disease, occur within the first 2 posttreatment years. The chances of detecting occult recurrences by ^{18}F FDG PET/CT at 12 months and 24 months after therapy are approximately 9% and 4%, respectively.[25] This study further confirmed that if the 3-month posttherapy ^{18}F FDG PET/CT scan was negative, there was no significant difference in 3-year disease-free survival in patients undergoing imaging surveillance versus those only receiving clinical surveillance. Hence, there is no evidential basis to perform ^{18}F FDG PET/CT scan or any imaging studies in patients who are symptomatic in follow-up period,

Hopkins Criteria: ^{18}F FDG PET/CT Post therapy Assessment Interpretation

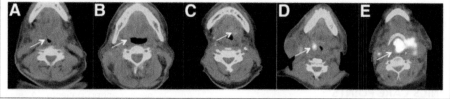

Primary Tumor Assessment

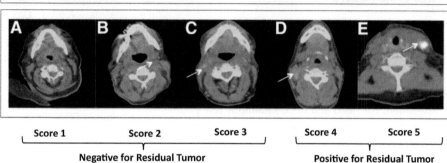

Neck Nodal Assessment

| Score 1 | Score 2 | Score 3 | Score 4 | Score 5 |

Negative for Residual Tumor   Positive for Residual Tumor

Fig. 1. Hopkins criteria interpretation of posttherapy. ^{18}F FDG PET/CT Score I: FDG uptake is less than or equal to the uptake at IJV. Score 2: Focal FDG uptake is greater than the uptake in IJV but less than liver. Score 3: Diffuse FDG uptake greater than IJV or liver (likely radiation induced uptake). Score 4: Focal FDG uptake equal or greater than liver. Score 5: Focal intense FDG uptake greater than liver (2–3 times). IJV, internal jugular vein. *Arrows* point to FDG avidity in primary tumor and neck nodal sites.

especially with a negative 3-month posttherapy assessment ^{18}F FDG PET/CT scan.

NASOPHARYNGEAL CANCER

For nasopharyngeal SCC, NCCN recommends ^{18}F FDG PET/CT for detecting distant metastases. A meta analysis including 23 studies demonstrated superiority of ^{18}F FDG PET/CT for detecting distant metastases and similar performance in detecting neck nodal metastases compared with MR imaging and CT.[26] ^{18}F FDG PET/CT is more effective in detecting smaller (5–10 mm) neck nodal metastases and improving staging than MR imaging.[27] Due to proximity to the primary site, some retropharyngeal nodes may be missed by ^{18}F FDG PET/CT. ^{18}F FDG PET/MR imaging may have the best diagnostic/staging effectiveness in NPC for primary tumor, neck nodal, and distant metastases[28] but more robust evidence is needed.

FUTURE DIRECTIONS
FAPI PET/CT and Head and Neck Cancers

Cancer-associated fibroblasts (CAFs) are known as important drivers of stromal interactions in tumor microenvironment. The fibroblast activation protein (FAP) is a serine proteinase that is highly expressed on the cell surface of activated fibroblasts but not of resting fibroblasts.[29] FAP-positive CAFs were found in more than 90% of epithelial tumors, and this makes FAP a potential

target for imaging and therapy of a large variety of malignancies.[30] There is low FAP inhibitor (FAPI) background uptake in normal tissues—in brain, sublingual glands, lingual tonsil, submandibular glands, and other head and neck tissues.[31] This low FAPI uptake provides a distinct advantage in identifying unknown primary tumors, especially in lingual and palatine tonsil, salivary glands, oral mucosa, and brain and skull metastases.[32–34] Primary tumors and nodal metastases demonstrated more intense ^{18}F FDG PET uptake than ^{68}Ga FAPI uptake, regardless of histologic diagnosis of HNSCC or nasopharyngeal carcinoma (NPC). However, the tumor to background uptake ratio was higher in ^{68}Ga FAPI studies than ^{18}F FDG studies due to low background uptake.[31–36] FAPI PET/CT is a promising new tool that has potential to offer both diagnostic and therapeutic options for HNSCC and NPC in the future.

FDG Volumetric and Tumor Heterogeneity Parameters

FDG volumetric parameters such as metabolic tumor volume, total lesion glycolysis, and tumor heterogeneity parameters may provide more tumor biologic information, therapy response prediction, and better prediction of survival outcomes than simple parameters such as SUVmax or peak standardized uptake value (SUVpeak).[37–41] However, use of these parameters in clinical practice are currently limited due to variability in standardization of image acquisition, varied segmentation methods, inadequate automated measurement options, and lack of prospective multicenter validation. With improved image processing and deep learning and artificial algorithms, these barriers could be overcome in the future.

CLINICS CARE POINTS

- FDG PET/CT is recommended for initial staging (for locoregional nodal metastasis and distant metastasis), detection of unknown primary, and post-chemoradation therapy assessment for head and neck squamous cell cancers.
- FDG PET/CT is recommended for locoregional nodal metastasis and distant metastasis detection and post therapy assessment for nasopharyngeal carcinoma.

DISCLOSURE

No conflict of interest.

REFERENCES

1. Hillner BE, Tosteson AN, Song Y, et al. Growth in the use of PET for six cancer types after coverage by medicare: additive or replacement? J Am Coll Radiol 2012;9(1):33–41.
2. Sanli Y, Zukotynski K, Mittra E, et al. Update 2018: 18F-FDG PET/CT and PET/MRI in head and neck cancer. Clin Nucl Med 2018;43(12):e439–52.
3. Goel R, Moore W, Sumer B, et al. Clinical practice in PET/CT for the management of head and neck squamous cell cancer. AJR Am J Roentgenol 2017; 209(2):289–303.
4. Hadiprodjo D, Ryan T, Truong MT, et al. Parotid gland tumors: preliminary data for the value of FDG PET/CT diagnostic parameters. AJR Am J Roentgenol 2012;198(2):W185–90.
5. Mohandas A, Marcus C, Kang H, et al. FDG PET/CT in the management of nasopharyngeal carcinoma. AJR Am J Roentgenol 2014;203(2):W146–57.
6. Davison JM, Ozonoff A, Imsande HM, et al. Squamous cell carcinoma of the palatine tonsils: FDG standardized uptake value ratio as a biomarker to differentiate tonsillar carcinoma from physiologic uptake. Radiology 2010;255(2):578–85.
7. Zhu L, Wang N. 18F-fluorodeoxyglucose positron emission tomography-computed tomography as a diagnostic tool in patients with cervical nodal metastases of unknown primary site: a meta-analysis. Surg Oncol 2013;22(3):190–4.
8. Civantos FJ, Vermorken JB, Shah JP, et al. Metastatic squamous cell carcinoma to the cervical lymph nodes from an unknown primary cancer: management in the HPV era. Front Oncol 2020; 10:593164.
9. Kim SJ, Pak K, Kim K. Diagnostic accuracy of F-18 FDG PET or PET/CT for detection of lymph node metastasis in clinically node negative head and neck cancer patients; A systematic review and meta-analysis. Am J Otolaryngol 2019;40(2): 297–305.
10. Lowe VJ, Duan F, Subramaniam RM, et al. Multicenter trial of [(18)F]fluorodeoxyglucose positron emission tomography/computed tomography staging of head and neck cancer and negative predictive value and surgical impact in the N0 neck: results from ACRIN 6685. J Clin Oncol 2019; 37(20):1704–12.
11. Stack BC Jr, Duan F, Romanoff J, et al. Impact of neck PET/CT positivity on survival outcomes-visual and quantitative assessment: results from ACRIN 6685. Clin Nucl Med 2023;48(2):126–31.
12. Zhu F, Sun S, Ba K. Comparison between PET-CT-guided neck dissection and elective neck dissection in cT1-2N0 tongue squamous cell carcinoma. Front Oncol 2020;10:720.
13. Rohde M, Nielsen AL, Johansen J, et al. Head-to-Head comparison of chest X-ray/head and neck MRI, chest CT/head and neck MRI, and (18)F-FDG PET/CT for detection of distant metastases and synchronous cancer in oral, pharyngeal, and laryngeal cancer. J Nucl Med 2017;58(12): 1919–24.
14. Kim Y, Roh JL, Kim JS, et al. Chest radiography or chest CT plus head and neck CT versus (18)F-FDG PET/CT for detection of distant metastasis and synchronous cancer in patients with head and neck cancer. Oral Oncol 2019;88:109–14.
15. Mehanna H, Wong WL, McConkey CC, et al. PET-CT surveillance versus neck dissection in advanced head and neck cancer. N Engl J Med 2016; 374(15):1444–54.
16. Expert Panel on Neurological, I.. ACR appropriateness criteria(R) staging and post-therapy assessment of head and neck cancer. J Am Coll Radiol 2023;20(11S):S521–64.
17. Marcus C, Ciarallo A, Tahari AK, et al. Head and neck PET/CT: therapy response interpretation criteria (Hopkins Criteria)-interreader reliability, accuracy, and survival outcomes. J Nucl Med 2014; 55(9):1411–6.
18. Van den Wyngaert T, Helsen N, Carp L, et al. Fluorodeoxyglucose-Positron emission tomography/computed tomography after concurrent chemoradiotherapy in locally advanced head-and-neck squamous cell cancer: the ECLYPS study. J Clin Oncol 2017;35(30):3458–64.

19. Porceddu SV, Pryor DI, Burmeister E, et al. Results of a prospective study of positron emission tomography-directed management of residual nodal abnormalities in node-positive head and neck cancer after definitive radiotherapy with or without systemic therapy. Head Neck 2011;33(12):1675–82.

20. Koksel Y, Gencturk M, Spano A, et al. Utility of Likert scale (Deauville criteria) in assessment of Chemoradiotherapy response of primary oropharyngeal squamous cell Cancer site. Clin Imag 2019;55:89–94.

21. Zhong J, Sundersingh M, Dyker K, et al. Post-treatment FDG PET-CT in head and neck carcinoma: comparative analysis of 4 qualitative interpretative criteria in a large patient cohort. Sci Rep 2020;10(1):4086.

22. Subramaniam RM, DeMora L, Yao M, et al. (18)F-FDG PET/CT prediction of treatment outcomes in human papillomavirus-positive, locally advanced oropharyngeal cancer patients receiving deintensified therapy: results from NRG-HN002. J Nucl Med 2023;64(3):362–7.

23. You H, Subramaniam RM. PET/Computed tomography: post-therapy follow-up in head and neck cancer. Pet Clin 2022;17(2):319–26.

24. You H, Xi Y, Moore W, et al. Timing and impact of posttreatment PET/CT after first 6 Months on patient management and outcomes in oropharyngeal squamous cell carcinoma. AJR Am J Roentgenol 2019;1–6.

25. Ho AS, Tsao GJ, Chen FW, et al. Impact of positron emission tomography/computed tomography surveillance at 12 and 24 months for detecting head and neck cancer recurrence. Cancer 2013;119(7):1349–56.

26. Chen WS, Li JJ, Hong L, et al. Comparison of MRI, CT and 18F-FDG PET/CT in the diagnosis of local and metastatic of nasopharyngeal carcinomas: an updated meta analysis of clinical studies. Am J Transl Res 2016;8(11):4532–47.

27. Peng H, Chen L, Tang LL, et al. Significant value of (18)F-FDG-PET/CT in diagnosing small cervical lymph node metastases in patients with nasopharyngeal carcinoma treated with intensity-modulated radiotherapy. Chin J Cancer 2017;36(1):95.

28. Chan SC, Yeh CH, Yen TC, et al. Clinical utility of simultaneous whole-body (18)F-FDG PET/MRI as a single-step imaging modality in the staging of primary nasopharyngeal carcinoma. Eur J Nucl Med Mol Imag 2018;45(8):1297–308.

29. Kuyumcu S, Sanli Y, Subramaniam RM. Fibroblast-activated protein inhibitor PET/CT: cancer diagnosis and management. Front Oncol 2021;11:758958.

30. Jiang GM, Xu W, Du J, et al. The application of the fibroblast activation protein alpha-targeted immunotherapy strategy. Oncotarget 2016;7(22):33472–82.

31. Syed M, Flechsig P, Liermann J, et al. Fibroblast activation protein inhibitor (FAPI) PET for diagnostics and advanced targeted radiotherapy in head and neck cancers. Eur J Nucl Med Mol Imag 2020;47(12):2836–45.

32. Gu B, Xu X, Zhang J, et al. The added value of (68)Ga-FAPI-04 PET/CT in patients with head and neck cancer of unknown primary with (18)F-FDG negative findings. J Nucl Med 2021.

33. Serfling S, Zhi Y, Schirbel A, et al. Improved cancer detection in Waldeyer's tonsillar ring by (68)Ga-FAPI PET/CT imaging. Eur J Nucl Med Mol Imag 2021;48(4):1178–87.

34. Qin C, Liu F, Huang J, et al. A head-to-head comparison of (68)Ga-DOTA-FAPI-04 and (18)F-FDG PET/MR in patients with nasopharyngeal carcinoma: a prospective study. Eur J Nucl Med Mol Imag 2021;48(10):3228–37.

35. Linz C, Brands RC, Kertels O, et al. Targeting fibroblast activation protein in newly diagnosed squamous cell carcinoma of the oral cavity - initial experience and comparison to [(18)F]FDG PET/CT and MRI. Eur J Nucl Med Mol Imag 2021;48(12):3951–60.

36. Zhao L, Pang Y, Zheng H, et al. Clinical utility of [(68)Ga]Ga-labeled fibroblast activation protein inhibitor (FAPI) positron emission tomography/computed tomography for primary staging and recurrence detection in nasopharyngeal carcinoma. Eur J Nucl Med Mol Imag 2021;48(11):3606–17.

37. Alluri KC, Tahari AK, Wahl RL, et al. Prognostic value of FDG PET metabolic tumor volume in human papillomavirus-positive stage III and IV oropharyngeal squamous cell carcinoma. AJR Am J Roentgenol 2014;203(4):897–903.

38. Paidpally V, Chirindel A, Chung CH, et al. FDG volumetric parameters and survival outcomes after definitive chemoradiotherapy in patients with recurrent head and neck squamous cell carcinoma. AJR Am J Roentgenol 2014;203(2):W139–45.

39. Yu J, Cooley T, Truong MT, et al. Head and neck squamous cell cancer (stages III and IV) induction chemotherapy assessment: value of FDG volumetric imaging parameters. J Med Imaging Radiat Oncol 2014;58(1):18–24.

40. Paidpally V, Chirindel A, Lam S, et al. FDG-PET/CT imaging biomarkers in head and neck squamous cell carcinoma. Imaging Med 2012;4(6):633–47.

41. Sanli Y, Leake J, Odu A, et al. Tumor heterogeneity on FDG PET/CT and immunotherapy: an imaging biomarker for predicting treatment response in patients with metastatic melanoma. AJR Am J Roentgenol 2019;212(6):1318–26.

Positron Emission Tomography/Computed Tomography in Thyroid Cancer
An Updated Review

Kunal Ramesh Chandekar, MD, Swayamjeet Satapathy, MD,
Chandrasekhar Bal, MD*

KEYWORDS

• PET/CT • Thyroid cancer • Differentiated thyroid cancer • FDG • FAPI • TENIS

KEY POINTS

- The histologic subtype and tumor de-differentiation are the key factors driving ^{18}F-fluorodeoxyglucose (FDG) uptake in thyroid cancer.
- FDG PET/CT is an extremely useful tool in differentiated thyroid cancer (DTC), particularly for recurrence evaluation in patients with thyroglobulin elevation with negative iodine scintigraphy and for prognostication.
- Fibroblast activation protein inhibitor and arginylglycylaspartic acid -based radiotracers have emerged as promising PET agents for radioiodine-refractory-DTC patients with the potential for theranostic application.
- Understanding the utility of different radiotracers in specific clinical scenarios is key to realizing the full potential of PET/CT in patients with thyroid cancer.

INTRODUCTION

Thyroid cancer is the most common endocrine malignancy, with rising trends in global incidence, amounting to more than half a million new cases each year as per recent estimates.[1] Most of thyroid cancer burden is noted in South East Asia.[2] Owing to distinct biologic and clinical characteristics, primary thyroid cancer is commonly classified based on its histology into papillary thyroid carcinoma (PTC), follicular thyroid carcinoma (FTC), medullary thyroid carcinoma (MTC), and anaplastic thyroid carcinoma (ATC). Differentiated thyroid cancer (DTC), which includes PTC and FTC, accounts for ~90% of all thyroid cancers.[3] DTC has an excellent long-term prognosis and a 10-year overall survival (OS) rate of more than 90% following standard treatment including surgery and radio active iodine (RAI) therapy.[4] Despite advances in diagnostic modalities

and the emergence of newer therapeutic options, radioiodine-refractory DTC (RR-DTC), poorly DTC (PDTC), MTC, and ATC have a more aggressive disease course and significantly worse outcomes.[5,6] PET/computed tomography (CT) is a hybrid imaging tool that has revolutionized oncological imaging.[7] This review aims to summarize the evolving role of PET/CT imaging in thyroid cancer subtypes in different clinical scenarios.

Imaging in Thyroid Cancer

Neck ultrasonography (USG) is the first-line imaging tool for patients with thyroid cancer. Neck USG has multifold utility including the detection and characterization of thyroid nodules, evaluation of cervical lymph nodes, and guiding cytologic/tissue sampling.[8] Whole-body scintigraphy with ^{131}I or ^{123}I is a time-tested functional imaging modality

Department of Nuclear Medicine, AIIMS, New Delhi 110029, India
* Corresponding author.
E-mail address: drcsbal@gmail.com

PET Clin 19 (2024) 131–145
https://doi.org/10.1016/j.cpet.2023.12.001
1556-8598/24/© 2023 Elsevier Inc. All rights reserved.

in DTC. DTC cells concentrate iodine owing to their usually maintained sodium–iodide symporter (NIS) protein expression. This allows the recognition and treatment of recurrent/metastatic DTC with radioactive iodine.[9]

^{18}F-fluorodeoxyglucose PET/Computed Tomography

^{18}F-fluorodeoxyglucose (FDG) PET/CT is a hybrid imaging modality with established clinical utility for a variety of oncological conditions.[7] Human glucose transporters (GLUTs), particularly GLUT-1 and GLUT-3, mediate the transport of FDG into thyroid tumor cells.[10] Molecular mechanisms causing the upregulation of glucose metabolism in thyroid cancer are not completely understood at present. However, oncogene-mediated activation of intracellular signal transduction cascades such as the adenylate cyclase and RAS-PI3K-AKT pathways are involved.[11]

Interpretation of Incidental ^{18}F-fluorodeoxyglucose Uptake by the Thyroid

The normal thyroid gland shows negligible FDG uptake. Incidental FDG uptake by the thyroid has been reported in ~1% to 4% of patients undergoing FDG PET/CT and can be characterized as diffuse or focal.[12] Diffusely increased FDG uptake within the thyroid is usually suggestive of a benign pathology (**Fig. 1**). Are and colleagues reported incidental diffuse thyroid uptake in 162 of 8800 (1.8%) patients who underwent FDG PET/CT for non-thyroid-related indications, of whom only 2 of 162 (1.2%) were found to have thyroid malignancy.[13] Similarly,

Karantanis and colleagues reported incidental diffuse FDG uptake in the thyroid in 138 of 4732 (2.9%) patients. Common causes of diffuse thyroid uptake were subclinical/overt hypothyroidism or autoimmune thyroiditis. Diffuse FDG uptake in thyroiditis is usually attributed to intra-thyroidal activated lymphoid tissue.[14]

Incidental focal FDG uptake by a thyroid nodule may be associated with malignancy. A recent meta-analysis of 50 research studies (including 640,616 PET/CTs) by de Leijer and colleagues reported incidental focal FDG uptake by the thyroid in 2.22% of patients with pooled risk of malignancy being 30.8%. PTC was the most commonly reported histology (83%) among those with proven malignancy.[15] Hence, incidental focal FDG uptake by the thyroid warrants further USG and cytologic evaluation (**Fig. 2**). The analysis of PET-based volumetric parameters, such as metabolic tumor volume (MTV), total lesion glycolysis (TLG), and radiomic features, offers a promising approach to further characterize thyroid incidentalomas.[16,17]

Thyroid Nodules with Indeterminate Cytology: Can ^{18}F-fluorodeoxyglucose PET/Computed Tomography Predict Malignancy?

The Bethesda system is a standardized reporting system for thyroid cytopathology consisting of six diagnostic categories.[18] Approximately 20% to 30% of all thyroid fine needle aspiration specimens are characterized as indeterminate for malignancy (Bethesda categories III–V). This presents a diagnostic challenge as surgery (usually hemithyroidectomy) with postoperative histopathological analysis remains the only way to clinch a definitive diagnosis.

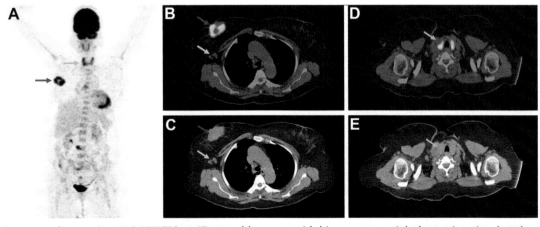

Fig. 1. Baseline staging FDG PET/CT in a 47-year-old woman with biopsy-proven right breast invasive ductal carcinoma. In addition to the tracer avid right breast primary (*red arrows: A, B, C*) and a few mildly tracer avid right axillary lymph nodes (*yellow arrows: A, B, C*), PET/CT revealed incidental diffuse FDG uptake in both lobes of the thyroid (*green arrows: A, D, E*). A subsequent review of the patient's records revealed that she is a known case of Hashimoto's thyroiditis on treatment with levothyroxine, 25 mcg daily.

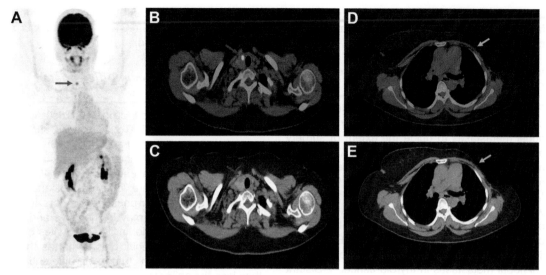

Fig. 2. FDG PET/CT done for surveillance in a 43-year-old woman with left breast invasive ductal carcinoma post left-modified radical mastectomy and adjuvant chemoradiotherapy. No abnormality was detected in the left chest wall or axillary region (*green arrows*: D, E) to suggest breast cancer residual/recurrence. However, PET/CT revealed incidental focal FDG uptake (*red arrows*: A, B, C) in a hypodense nodule (measuring ~1.2 × 1.0 cm) in the right thyroid lobe. Fine needle aspiration cytology (FNAC) correlation was advised. FNAC from this nodule was reported as Bethesda category V (suspicious for malignancy).

However, a vast majority (~70–80%) of such patients have a benign diagnosis postsurgery.[19] Particularly, given the high costs and limited availability of mutation testing, gene expression, and micro-RNA analyses, FDG PET/CT could help in further characterization of thyroid nodules with indeterminate cytology and reduce the number of inappropriate surgeries and their associated complications.

Early studies reported a high (~80–100%) negative predictive value (NPV) of FDG PET/CT in detecting malignancy in the preoperative evaluation of thyroid nodules, suggesting that FDG PET/CT could potentially reduce futile hemithyroidectomies.[20,21] Kim and colleagues evaluated FDG PET/CT in 36 patients who had cytologically indeterminate thyroid nodules (size >1 cm). FDG PET was positive in all 36 nodules. There was no significant difference between the mean SUVmax of malignant and benign nodules. Contrary to the previously published results, the investigators concluded that FDG PET had a limited role in this setting.[22] The 2015 American Thyroid Association (ATA) guidelines for thyroid nodules and DTC do not routinely recommend FDG PET for the evaluation of thyroid nodules with indeterminate cytology.[23] However, this is a weak recommendation with moderate-quality evidence.

Castellana and colleagues consolidated existing literature on this topic, and eight studies (overall 431 nodules) were included in their meta-analysis.

The pooled sensitivity, specificity, positive predictive value (PPV), and NPV of FDG PET/CT to predict malignancy were reported as 74%, 58%, 34%, and 74%, respectively. The investigators concluded that FDG PET/CT can discriminate between benign and malignant thyroid nodules given its moderately high NPV.[24] EfFECTS trial was the first randomized controlled multicenter trial to assess the impact of an FDGPET/CT-driven approach to rule out malignancy in Bethesda III or IV thyroid nodules. A total of 132 patients were randomly assigned to the FDG PET group or diagnostic surgery group in a 2:1 ratio. After 1 year of follow-up, the number of futile surgeries was significantly lower (*P* < .001) in the FDG PET/CT-driven group (38/91, 42%) when compared with the diagnostic surgery group (34/41, 83%). FDG PET/CT-driven management avoided surgery for 25/63 (40%) benign nodules. The sensitivity, specificity, NPV, and PPV of FDG PET/CT were 94.1%, 39.8%, 95.1%, and 35.2%, respectively.[25] Subsequently, the investigators also published a cost-utility analysis concluding that the FDG PET/CT-based approach reduced the 1-year thyroid nodule related and societal costs while sustaining the quality of life in these patients. The results of this study established that FDG PET/CT-driven diagnostic workup of indeterminate thyroid nodules alters patient management and reduces futile surgeries.[26] However, one must bear in mind that in a real-world clinical scenario, the results of FDG PET/CT are never considered in isolation and are corroborated with individual risk factors, family history, USG findings, and patient preference.

Initial Staging in Differentiated Thyroid Cancer

Preoperative workup in DTC should include an accurate assessment of the primary tumor stage and nodal metastases to guide the extent of surgery and reduce the risk of recurrence. The ATA recommends neck USG in all patients planned for thyroidectomy. The guidelines also state that CT or MR imaging may be used as adjunct imaging tools when there is clinical suspicion of invasive primary or multiple/bulky lymph nodes.[23] A meta-analysis of nine studies reported that FDG PET/CT has limited sensitivity (30%) for the detection of cervical nodal metastases in thyroid cancer.[27] Distant metastases are seen in only 1% to 4% of DTC patients at baseline. Also, distant metastases do not preclude surgery of the primary tumor in DTC, unlike many other malignancies.[28] Hence, the current ATA guidelines do not recommend the routine use of FDG PET/CT for initial staging in DTC.[23]

Postoperative Evaluation in Differentiated Thyroid Cancer

Postoperative treatment in DTC is guided by a dynamic risk stratification system which includes clinicopathological, biochemical, and imaging findings.[23] Several studies have established that FDG PET/CT performed at the time of initial ^{131}I treatment can predict response to therapy. Patients with negative FDG PET/CT are more frequently observed to have a favorable response to RAI therapy and longer survival.[29–31] Lee and colleagues reported that FDG PET/CT done at the time of ^{131}I ablation identified additional recurrent/metastatic lesions in 14% of intermediate and high-risk DTC patients that were not seen on ^{131}I post-therapy scans. On subgroup analysis, FDG PET/CT was particularly useful in stage T3-T4N1 with tumor size greater than 2.0 cm.[32] Rosenbaum-Krumme and colleagues studied 90 high-risk DTC patients in whom FDG PET/CT was done about 1 week after the first RAI treatment. A total of 26 of 90 (29%) patients had positive findings on FDG PET/CT. In 8 of 90 (8.9%) patients tumor node metastasis (TNM) staging was changed due to PET findings compared with ^{131}I post-therapy scans. PET impacted management in 19 of 90 (21%) patients, mostly limited to patients with FDG+ve RAI−ve status (15/90, 16.6%) and only 4 patients with RAI+ve status.[33] Therefore, given that the change in stage and management was seen in a relatively low proportion of patients, especially in those with iodine concentration, the clinical significance of routine postoperative FDG PET-CT in such patients remains to be ascertained.

Recurrence Evaluation in Differentiated Thyroid Cancer

After initial therapy, follow-up in DTC is usually done with serum thyroglobulin (Tg), neck USG, and diagnostic whole-body scintigraphy (DxWBS). Despite a good prognosis overall, recurrence is noted in up to 35% of DTC patients more than 40 years, two-thirds of which are loco-regional and one-third at distant sites.[34] In patients with more aggressive disease, DxWBS may be negative and FDG PET/CT may be superior in detecting sites of disease. The rationale behind this is that as thyroid cancer cells undergo tumor de-differentiation, they lose the ability to concentrate RAI secondary to reduced NIS expression, and probably membrane translocation of the NIS protein. In contrast, GLUT1 is upregulated accompanied by increased proliferative rates. This inverse relationship between RAI and FDG uptake during the de-differentiation process is described as a "flip-flop" phenomenon.[35] A meta-analysis by Schütz and colleagues reported higher sensitivity of FDG PET (89.7%) and FDG PET/CT (94.3%) compared with conventional whole-body imaging (65.4%) in detecting DTC recurrence with similar results for specificity.[36]

As per the ATA guidelines, the most important indication for FDG PET/CT is Tg elevation with negative iodine scintigraphy (TENIS).[23] Based on a meta-analysis of 18 studies, Caetano and colleagues reported high sensitivity (93%), specificity (81%), and diagnostic accuracy (93%) of FDG PET/CT in detecting DTC recurrence in patients with negative DxWBS.[37] PET/CT positivity is strongly and positively correlated with serum Tg levels.[38] ATA usually recommends FDG PET/CT when the thyroid stimulating hormone (TSH)-stimulated Tg levels are greater than 10 ng/mL because at lower values it has limited sensitivity ranging from less than 10% to 30%.[23]

Several authors have tried to assess if FDG PET/CT with TSH stimulation (sPET/CT) offers any potential advantage over one without TSH stimulation (nsPET/CT). Leboulleux and colleagues conducted a prospective study in 63 DTC patients with TENIS. They reported that sPET/CT detected a significantly higher number of lesions compared with nsPET/CT but the number of patients in whom any lesion was detected was not different between the two states.[39] A meta-analysis by Ma and colleagues revealed a statistically significant difference in the number of PET-detected lesions (odds ratio [OR]

4.92) and the number of patients with PET true-positive lesions (OR 2.45) when comparing sPET/CT with nsPET/CT.[40] However, in contrast, a recent meta-analysis by Qichang and colleagues found no significant difference between sPET/CT and nsPET/CT for all the diagnostic estimate indexes during pair-wise comparison (All $P > .05$).[41] To date, there is no definite consensus on the actual clinical benefit accrued by performing sPET/CT.

Kinetic parameters such as Tg-doubling time (TgDT) and Tg-velocity (Tg-vel) may help to predict FDG PET/CT results in DTC patients with TENIS. Based on a retrospective study including 139 patients, Albano and colleagues reported that Tg-vel was significantly higher (mean Tg-vel 4.2 vs 1.7 ng/mL/y, $P < .001$) and TgDT was significantly shorter (mean TgDT 1.4 vs 4.4 years, $P < .001$) in patients with a positive PET/CT scan compared with those with a negative scan. Receiver operating curve analysis revealed that stimulated Tg, TgDT, and Tg-vel thresholds of 18 ng/mL, 1.36 years, and 1.95 ng/mL/y, respectively, were best able to predict FDG PET positivity.[42]

The presence of anti-thyroglobulin antibodies (TgAbs) interferes with laboratory measurements of serum Tg levels posing challenges to biochemical monitoring in DTC.[43] Persistent or rising serum TgAb levels may indicate persistent, recurrent, or progressive DTC despite undetectable Tg levels. A meta-analysis of nine studies reported that FDG PET/CT had a pooled sensitivity, specificity, and diagnostic OR of 84%, 78%, and 18, respectively, for the detection of recurrent DTC in patients with progressively and/or persistently elevated TgAb levels and negative DxWBS.[44]

Existing literature emphasizes that FDG PET/CT is extremely useful for recurrence evaluation in DTC patients, particularly for intermediate and high-risk categories with negative DxWBS (**Fig. 3**).

Prognostic Role in Differentiated Thyroid Cancer

Wang and colleagues.evaluated the prognostic role of FDG PET/CT in 125 DTC patients. Univariate analysis revealed that age greater than 45 years, presence of distant metastases, PET positivity, higher FDG uptake, and high volume of FDG avid disease were associated with reduced survival. The volume of FDG avid disease was the single strongest predictor of reduced survival on multivariate analysis.[45] Later, the same group retrospectively reviewed FDG PET/CT in 400 DTC patients (median follow-up duration 7.9 years) and assessed the prognostic value of clinical and PET parameters. On multivariate analysis, only FDG PET positivity (relative risk [RR] 7.69) and

age (RR 1.33) were strong predictors of survival. The intensity of FDG uptake and the number of FDG-avid lesions showed significant inverse relationships with survival.[46] Subsequent studies have consistently reported FDG PET positivity to be strongly associated with reduced survival in DTC patients.[47,48]

Vural and colleagues prospectively evaluated the prognostic role of FDG PET/CT in 105 DTC patients with TENIS. Negative FDG PET/CT predicted a favorable prognosis and lack of recurrence on follow-up in patients with Tg level less than 1 ng/mL under TSH suppression despite the significant elevation of Tg in the off-therapy state.[49] Albano and colleagues evaluated the prognostic role of PET-based semi-quantitative parameters in 122 DTC patients with TENIS. Total MTV (hazard ratio [HR] 2.54) and total TLG (HR 2.48) were the only independent prognostic indicators for OS.[50] Bogsrud and colleagues retrospectively evaluated the prognostic role of FDG PET/CT in RAI-negative DTC patients with elevated circulating TgAb. They reported that negative PET results were associated with the absence of active disease and declining TgAb over time.[51]

Role in Radioiodine Refractory Thyroid Cancer

As previously mentioned, FDG PET/CT can detect additional recurrent or metastatic lesions that are not seen on I-131 post-therapy scans, particularly in high-risk DTC patients.[32,33] Given their high costs and serious toxicity profiles, the use of tyrosine kinase inhibitors (TKIs) should be reserved for RR-DTC patients with rapidly progressive, symptomatic, and/or imminently threatening disease which is not otherwise amenable to local therapeutic options.[23] In this context, FDG PET/CT may help in earlier treatment response assessment compared with anatomic imaging with CT as metabolic changes usually precede structural change (**Fig. 4**).

As a part of a phase II trial evaluating the efficacy of sunitinib in RR patients with thyroid cancer, Carr and colleagues analyzed the role of early PET/CT-based response assessment. They found that patients with disease control (DC) had a significantly greater decline in standardized uptake value (SUV) compared with patients with progressive disease.[52] Ahmaddy and colleagues evaluated the role of FDG PET/CT to assess response in RR-DTC patients treated with lenvatinib. Tumor responses based on a modified Positron Emission Tomography Response Criteria In Solid Tumors (mPERCIST) and the widely accepted Response Evaluation Criteria in Solid Tumors (RECIST) 1.1 were compared. All responders (by RECIST)

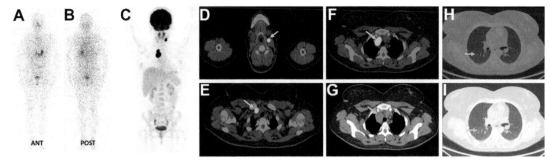

Fig. 3. A 26-year-old woman, a known case of PTC (tall cell variant), post total thyroidectomy and selective neck nodal dissection had elevated serum thyroglobulin of 89.1 ng/mL and negative DxWBS (*A, B*), that is, TENIS (*C*). FDG PET/CT done for recurrence evaluation revealed metabolically active left level II cervical (*D*), right supraclavicular (*E*), and enlarged right upper paratracheal (*F, G*) lymph nodes, and rounded parenchymal nodule in right lung lower lobe (*H, I*) suggestive of nodal and lung metastases (*yellow arrows*).

showed a decline in PET parameters such as SUVmax, MTV, and TLG. Nonresponders according to mPERCIST showed significantly lower median progression-free survival (PFS) and disease-specific survival (DSS), whereas RECIST nonresponders had only a significantly lower DSS.[53] Rendl and colleagues retrospectively evaluated PET-based response assessment in RR-DTC patients treated with lenvatinib. They reported that patients classified as DC exhibited a longer median PFS than patients classified as disease progression based on PERCIST and mPERCIST criteria (*P* = .037).[54] FDG PET/CT has a promising role in the response assessment of RR-DTC patients receiving TKIs (**Fig. 5**).

PET in Medullary Thyroid Cancer

MTC accounts for ∼1 to 4% of all thyroid malignancies. MTC originates from neuroendocrine parafollicular C cells. MTC is usually sporadic (75% of cases). Hereditary forms of MTC may be associated with multiple endocrine neoplasia syndromes. Serum calcitonin and carcinoembryonic antigen (CEA) are used as tumor markers in MTC.[55] Overall tumor stage is a critical prognostic factor in MTC as 10-year survival rates decrease from greater than 95% for intra-thyroidal disease to approximately 40% in the presence of distant metastases.[56] Hence, an accurate assessment of disease extent is important. The mainstay of

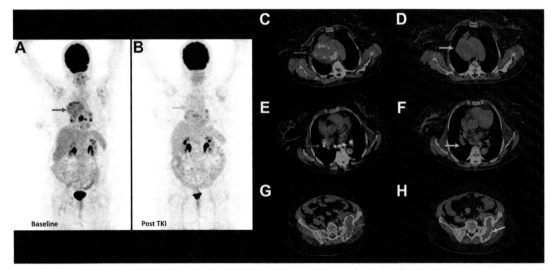

Fig. 4. A 50-year-old woman with metastatic RR-DTC (*A,B*). FDG PET/CT done before starting lenvatinib showed tracer avid subcentimetric and enlarged mediastinal lymph nodes (*red arrows: C, E*) and lytic lesion with associated soft tissue component in the left iliac bone (*red arrow: G*). FDG PET/CT done after 6 months of lenvatinib therapy showed a significant reduction of tracer avidity in the mediastinal lymph nodal (*green arrows: D, F*) and skeletal metastases (*green arrow: H*) with no significant structural change suggestive of a partial metabolic response as per PET-based response criteria. In contrast, RECIST 1.1 criteria based on CT imaging only would classify this patient as having a stable disease suggesting that PET-based response assessment may be more appropriate.

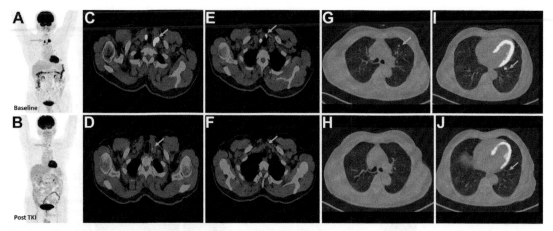

Fig. 5. A 63-year-old man with metastatic RR-DTC. FDG PET/CT done before starting lenvatinib (MIP: *A*) showed tracer avid multiple pre- and paratracheal (*green arrows*: *C, E*) lymph nodes and bilateral lung nodules (*green arrows*: *G, I*). FDG PET/CT done after 6 months of lenvatinib therapy (MIP: *B*) showed a significant decrease in size, number, and tracer avidity of the nodal (*green arrows*: *D, F*) and lung (*green arrows*: *J*) metastases suggestive of a partial response to therapy.

treatment is surgery, that is, total thyroidectomy with risk-adapted nodal dissection.[55]

Upregulation of L-type amino acid transporters and aromatic L-amino acid decarboxylase by MTC permits its imaging with 6-^{18}F-fluoro-L-3,4-dihydroxyphenylalanine (^{18}F-FDOPA) PET/CT.[57] In addition to the USG neck, cross-sectional imaging of the neck, chest, and abdomen is recommended if there is suspicion of invasive/metastatic disease and when serum calcitonin levels are greater than 500 pg/mL. Neither FDG PET/CT nor ^{18}F-FDOPA PET/CT is currently recommended by the 2015 ATA guidelines for initial staging in MTC.[58] However, a retrospective study by Rasul and colleagues published in 2018 evaluated the role of preoperative ^{18}F-FDOPA PET with contrast-enhanced CT in 32 MTC patients; 28/32 patients had DOPA PET-positive primary tumors (sensitivity of 88%). DOPA PET was more sensitive than neck USG for the detection of central (53% vs 20%) and lateral (73% vs 39%, respectively) metastatic neck nodes.[59] These single-center results need further validation in larger prospective studies.

In the postoperative setting, PET/CT may have a role in detecting recurrent disease, particularly when serum calcitonin levels are greater than 150 pg/mL and anatomic imaging is negative or inconclusive.[58] In a meta-analysis of nine studies, the detection rates (DRs) of ^{18}F-FDOPA PET and PET/CT were 66% (per patient) and 71% (per-lesion analysis).[60] Early acquisition of ^{18}F-FDOPA PET (at 15 minutes post-injection) may be more appropriate than delayed acquisition due to tracer washout with time.[57]

A meta-analysis by Treglia and colleagues found that on a patient-based analysis, the DR of FDG PET/CT in recurrent MTC was modest at best (59%). The DRs improved in patients with higher calcitonin and CEA values and lower calcitonin and CEA doubling times.[61] Neuroendocrine cells in MTC may show overexpression of somatostatin receptors (SSTRs). The DR of SSTR PET or PET/CT in recurrent MTC is suboptimal, ranging from 25% to 86.7% (per patient) as reported by a meta-analysis of nine heterogeneous studies.[62] However, it may be used in selected cases (**Fig. 6**). In addition, one can assess the feasibility of peptide receptor radionuclide therapy (PRRT) in patients with metastatic MTC having limited therapeutic options.[63] In conclusion, ^{18}F-FDOPA PET/CT should be preferred in MTC patients with suspected recurrence based on evidence from a recent network meta-analysis in which ^{18}F-FDOPA performed better than other radiotracers in both patient- and lesion-based analyses.[64]

PET in Poorly Differentiated Thyroid Cancer

PDTC represents an intermediary clinicopathological state between DTC and ATC. The 2022 World Health Organization (WHO) classification of thyroid neoplasms defines PDTC as per the Turin criteria.[3] PDTC typically shows higher GLUT1 expression and FDG uptake compared with DTC.[65] PDTC cells show higher FDG uptake under TSH stimulation.[66] FDG PET/CT is potentially useful for restaging PDTC in the post-thyroidectomy setting, particularly for patients stratified as high risk.[67] Civan and colleagues reported a case of a 55-year-old man with metastatic PDTC which showed different patterns of tracer avidity on ^{18}F-FDG, ^{68}Ga-DOTA-TATE, and ^{68}Ga-PSMA PET/CT highlighting tumor

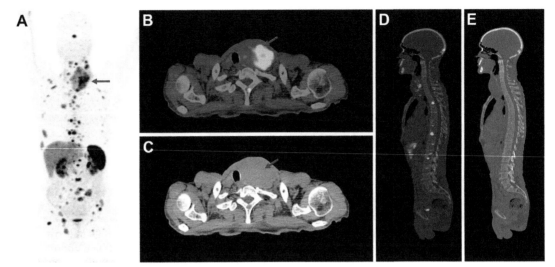

Fig. 6. A 61-year-old man with thyroid FNAC suggestive of MTC and serum calcitonin levels of 2970 pg/mL.[68]Ga-DOTANOC PET/CT done for metastatic evaluation revealed a large, ill-defined mass in the left thyroid lobe with heterogeneous increased tracer avidity (*red arrows: A, B, C*) and multiple tracer avid lytic skeletal metastases (*D, E*). As most lesions show tracer avidity equal to or higher than the liver, the patient may be considered for PRRT with ^{177}Lu-labelled SSTR analogs.

heterogeneity.[68] Owing to the dearth of literature at present, further studies are needed to define the precise role and clinical impact of PET/CT imaging in PDTC.

PET in Anaplastic Thyroid Cancer

ATC is a rare malignancy accounting for less than 1% of all thyroid cancer cases. ATC is typically seen in older individuals and is more common in areas with endemic goiter. ATC may originate de novo or as a result of de-differentiation of DTC cells wherein they lose the ability to concentrate iodine and produce Tg.[69] ATC cells have higher proliferative rates and GLUT1 expression compared with DTC and PDTC.[65] This could potentially explain their highly aggressive tendency to produce local invasion and distant metastases. ATC has a dismal prognosis with 1-year survival rates being less than 20%.[70]

Bosgrud and colleagues assessed the role of FDG PET/CT in 16 ATC patients and compared it with other diagnostic modalities such as USG, CT, and MR imaging. All primary tumors were positive on FDG PET with high lesional tracer uptake. FDG PET/CT directly impacted treatment decisions in 8 of 16 (50%) of patients.[71] In another study from France, FDG PET/CT was evaluated in 20 ATC patients. Functional tumor volume and lesion SUV-max were significant predictors of survival. PET/CT led to treatment modifications in 25% of the patients. PET/CT enabled earlier treatment response evaluation in 4 of 11 patients compared with

stand-alone CT.[72] Kim and colleagues evaluated the role of pretreatment FDG PET/CT in 40 ATC patients. In 37.5% of patients, distant metastases were detected exclusively on FDG PET/CT. On multivariate analysis, tumor SUVmax was found to be the most important predictor of OS with an HR of 5.105 (*P* = .010).[73] The studies concluded that FDG PET/CT impacts clinical management in ATC patients by potential upstaging of disease and providing reliable prognostic information. The 2021 ATA guidelines for the management of ATC patients recognize the utility of FDG PET/CT and recommend it for initial radiological staging and further evaluation of metastases when clinically indicated.[74]

PET in Hürthle Cell Carcinoma

Hürthle cell thyroid carcinoma (HCTC) is currently recognized as a distinct histologic subtype of follicular cell-derived neoplasms. It is important to note that the 2022 WHO classification of thyroid neoplasms discourages the use of the term "Hürthle Cell" as it is a historical misnomer. The revised and accepted terminology is oncocytic carcinoma of thyroid (OCA). OCA has a different oncogene expression and a more aggressive clinical course compared with DTC.[3] OCA lesions do not concentrate iodine and are typically FDG avid. To date, very few studies have evaluated the role of FDG PET/CT in HCTC or OCA exclusively. Pryma and colleagues retrospectively evaluated the role of FDG PET/CT in HCTC in 44 patients with heterogeneous clinical indications and reported an overall sensitivity of 95.8% and specificity of 95%. FDG avidity also provided prognostic information as patients with SUVmax $\geq$ 10 had a 5-year all-cause mortality of 36% compared with 8% in those with SUVmax less than 10 ($P <$ .01).[75] Few other studies have also reported similar findings of FDG PET/CT being a highly sensitive imaging modality for HCTC, potentially impacting treatment decisions.[76,77]

Non-^{18}F-fluorodeoxyglucose Radiotracers

I-124 PET/computed tomography

PET imaging with [124]I is feasible and has shown superior sensitivity and spatial resolution compared with diagnostic ^{123}I and ^{131}I planar imaging.[78] A meta-analysis of five studies reported that [124]I PET/CT had excellent pooled sensitivity (94.2%) and low specificity (49%) in detecting DTC lesions.[79] The long half-life of [124]I ($t_{1/2}$ 4.2 days) allows imaging at delayed time points, thereby facilitating dosimetric studies. Optimum therapeutic activity can be personalized for each patient by the dosimetric approach. This may be particularly useful in patients with metastatic DTC where toxicity to organs at risk such as bone marrow and lungs needs to be considered. A recent retrospective study found that [124]I PET/CT-based lesional dosimetry in DTC patients correlated with treatment response to ^{131}I therapy. Among lesions that showed an objective response, a significant majority (82%) had absorbed dose (AD) and biological equivalent dose (BED) greater than 75 Gy. Stable or progressive lesions had AD and BED less than 75 Gy.[80] Feasibility issues and lack of procedural standardization are major limitations to the routine clinical use of dosimetry. Overall, limitations of [124]I PET/CT include a relatively low positron yield, high positron energy, complex decay involving multiple high-energy gamma photons, limited availability, and high costs of the radiotracer.[81]

Fibroblast activation protein inhibitor PET/computed tomography

Fibroblast activation protein (FAP) is a transmembrane glycoprotein belonging to the dipeptidyl peptidase family. Owing to its negligible expression in normal adult tissues and significant overexpression in cancer-associated fibroblasts (CAFs) of various tumor types, FAP has emerged as a promising theranostic target. CAFs in tumor stroma form a major component of the overall tumor burden.[82] Several radiolabeled small molecule FAP inhibitors (FAPIs) have been evaluated as PET tracers for various tumors in early clinical studies.[83]

Fu and colleagues reported the first case of DTC with TENIS demonstrating intensely tracer avid local recurrence and distant metastases on ^{68}Ga-FAPI PET/CT.[84] Subsequently, in another case with RR-DTC, ^{68}Ga-FAPI PET/CT picked up additional metastatic lesions not seen on FDG PET/CT due to its better signal-to-background ratio.[85] Prompted by these encouraging findings, Fu and colleagues conducted a prospective study to evaluate the clinical utility of ^{68}Ga-FAPI-04 PET/CT in 35 metastatic DTC patients and compared its performance with FDG PET/CT. Overall, tracer avidity (SUVmax) in most metastatic DTC lesions was higher on FAPI PET/CT than FDG PET/CT (7.03 vs 4.15; $P <$ .001). On a lesion-based analysis, FAPI PET/CT was found to have higher sensitivity than FDG PET/CT for detecting cervical lesions (83% vs 65%; $P =$ .01) and distant metastases (79% vs 59%; $P <$ .001)[86] (Fig. 7). From a theranostic point of view, radiolabeled homodimer of squaramide-conjugated FAPI, ^{177}Lu-DOTAGA. (SA.FAPi)$_2$, has shown promising results based on a pilot study in 15 RR-DTC patients who had prior progression on sorafenib/lenvatinib.[87]

Somatostatin receptor PET/computed tomography

DTC cells may show expression of SSTRs, particularly SSTR 1. In a prospective study by Kundu and colleagues ^{68}Ga-DOTANOC PET/CT demonstrated disease in 40 of 62 (65%) and FDG PET/CT in 45/62 (72%) DTC patients with TENIS. Per-patient sensitivity and specificity of ^{68}Ga-DOTANOC PET/CT were 78.4% and 100%, compared with 86.3% and 90.9%, respectively, for FDG PET/CT. FDG PET/CT demonstrated significantly more lesions than ^{68}Ga-DOTANOC PET/CT (168 vs 121; $P<$.0001).[88] Overall, the sensitivity of SSTR PET/CT is typically lower than FDG PET/CT. SSTR PET/CT may be performed to assess suitability for ^{177}Lu-based PRRT in RR-DTC patients with no alternative treatment options. Few studies have explored ^{177}Lu-DOTATATE therapy in RR-DTC and MTC patients but have reported only modest response rates.[63,89]

Arginylglycylaspartic acid PET/computed tomography

Integrins are a group of transmembrane glycoproteins with two nonidentical subunits. Owing to its overexpression in the neovasculature of various malignancies, integrin $\alpha v \beta 3$ has emerged as a promising target for diagnostic and therapeutic applications.[90] More specifically in thyroid cancer, integrin $\alpha v \beta 3$ overexpression has been reported on both the endothelial cells of tumor vasculature and tumor cells themselves.[91] Arginylglycylaspartic acid (RGD) tripeptide sequence has shown high affinity and specificity toward the integrin $\alpha v \beta 3$.

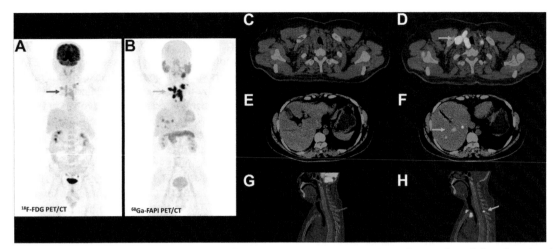

Fig. 7. A 44-year-old man with radioiodine refractory thyroid cancer (mixed papillary and medullary histology) post total thyroidectomy with biochemical recurrence. FDG PET/CT (MIP: *A*) done for recurrence evaluation revealed mildly tracer avid multiple cervical (*red arrow* in *C*), upper mediastinal lymph nodes, and a faint tracer avid liver lesion (*red arrow*) suggestive of metastatic disease. Subsequently, 68 Ga-DOTA.SA.FAPI PET/CT (MIP: *B*) was done. The MIP and cross-sectional images revealed intensely tracer avid multiple cervical (*green arrow* in *D*), upper mediastinal lymph nodes, a few liverlesions in the right lobe (*green arrow* in *F*), and a skeletal lesion in the spinous process of D2 vertebra (*green arrow* in *H*) which was not seen on FDG PET/CT (*red arrow* in *G*). Overall, FAPI PET/CT revealed more number of lesions than FDG PET/CT, with higher tracer avidity and lesion-to-background ratios.

Hence, radiolabeled RGD analogs have been evaluated as theranostic agents. A single-center, prospective study by Parihar and colleagues reported that ^{68}Ga-DOTA-RGD2 PET/CT showed similar sensitivity (82.3% vs 82.3%), but higher specificity (100% vs 50%) and overall accuracy (86.4% vs 75%) than ^{18}F-FDG PET/CT in the detection of lesions in RR-DTC patients. Interestingly, 82.1% of patients positive on ^{68}Ga-DOTA-RGD2 PET/CT showed lesional radiotracer uptake higher than the liver suggesting that they may be suitable for therapy with novel ^{177}Lu-based therapeutic agents.[92] Prompted by these results, the same group also reported the first-in-human use of ^{177}Lu-DOTA-RGD2 therapy (single cycle, 5.5 GBq) in a 54-year-old woman having metastatic DTC with TENIS. The post-therapy scan showed significant tracer accumulation in DTC lesions. Follow-up assessment revealed clinical and radiological improvement.[93] This warrants evaluation of potential clinical feasibility and toxicity in larger prospective studies.

OTHERS

Expression of prostate-specific membrane antigen (PSMA) has been reported in the neovasculature of several non-prostatic tumors including DTC.[94] Based on this rationale, few exploratory studies have evaluated the potential utility of ^{68}Ga-PSMA and ^{18}F-DCFPyL PET/CT in DTC, PDTC, and ATC.[95–97] PSMA-ligand avidity offers the promise

of theranostic strategies. Few studies have also tried using the novel PET tracer, ^{18}F-tetrafluoroborate (^{18}F-TFB), a radiolabeled iodide analog, for imaging the NIS. ^{18}F-TFB has a similar biodistribution to [124]I sodium iodide (NaI), but it does not undergo organification (like ^{99m}Tc-pertechnetate).[98] A German group compared ^{18}F-TFB and [124]I PET/CT in nine DTC patients post-total thyroidectomy. Both tracers detected thyroid remnant tissue in all patients. On a lesion-based analysis, the overall agreement between the two tracers was 91%. Of note, in two patients, additional cervical lymph nodal metastases were detected exclusively by ^{18}F-TFB.[99] Dittmann and colleagues compared ^{18}F-TFB PET/CT and DxWBS in 25 patients with recurrent DTC. ^{18}F-TFB PET/CT detected recurrent/metastatic disease in a significantly higher proportion of patients than DxWBS with SPECT-CT (52% vs 12%, $P = .002$).[100] Further studies are needed to define the clinical utility of such novel radiotracers.

SUMMARY

Based on this review of current literature, PET/CT is an indispensable tool in the evaluation of patients with thyroid cancer, potentially impacting management decisions. FDG PET/CT is particularly useful in the evaluation of DTC recurrence with TENIS and aggressive histologic subtypes such as PDTC and ATC. The prognostic role of FDG PET/CT in predicting response to therapy and OS has been established by multiple studies. ^{18}F-FDOPA is the most useful PET radiotracer for the evaluation of MTC with higher sensitivity in patients with higher serum calcitonin and CEA levels. FAPI and RGD-based radiotracers have emerged as promising PET agents for RR-DTC patients with potential for theranostic application. Understanding the utility of different radiotracers in specific clinical scenarios is key to realizing the full potential of PET/CT in patients with thyroid cancer.

CLINICS CARE POINTS

- There is an inverse relationship between radioiodine and ^{18}F-fluorodeoxyglucose (FDG) uptake during the de-differentiation process in differentiated thyroid cancer.

- FDG PET/CT is recommended in thyroglobulin elevation with negative iodine scintigraphy when the TSH-stimulated Tg levels are greater than 10 ng/mL because at lower values it has limited sensitivity.

- Using kinetic parameters of biochemical tumor markers (eg, Tg-doubling time and calcitonin doubling time) to judiciously guide PET/CT imaging in thyroid cancer leads to improved detection rates.

- Large-scale, prospective studies are needed to further validate the utility of novel fibroblast activation protein inhibitor and arginylglycylaspartic acid-based radiotracers for both PET imaging and therapeutic applications.

DISCLOSURE

All authors declare that they have no relevant disclosures. There is no source of funding.

REFERENCES

1. Sung H, Ferlay J, Siegel RL, et al. Global cancer statistics 2020: GLOBOCAN estimates of incidence and mortality worldwide for 36 cancers in 185 countries. CA Cancer J Clin 2021;71:209–49.

2. Deng Y, Li H, Wang M, et al. Global burden of thyroid cancer from 1990 to 2017. JAMA Netw Open 2020;3:e208759.

3. Baloch ZW, Asa SL, Barletta JA, et al. Overview of the 2022 WHO classification of thyroid neoplasms. Endocr Pathol 2022;33:27–63.

4. Davies L, Welch HG. Thyroid cancer survival in the United States: observational data from 1973 to 2005. Arch Otolaryngol Head Neck Surg 2010;136:440–4.

5. Rendl G, Manzl M, Hitzl W, et al. Long-term prognosis of medullary thyroid carcinoma. Clin Endocrinol 2008;69:497–505.

6. Maniakas A, Dadu R, Busaidy NL, et al. Evaluation of overall survival in patients with anaplastic thyroid carcinoma, 2000-2019. JAMA Oncol 2020;6:1397–404.

7. Basu S, Alavi A. Unparalleled contribution of 18F-FDG PET to medicine over 3 decades. J Nucl Med 2008;49:17N–37N.

8. Lew JI, Solorzano CC. Use of ultrasound in the management of thyroid cancer. Oncol 2010;15:253–8.

9. Avram AM. Radioiodine scintigraphy with SPECT/CT: an important diagnostic tool for thyroid cancer staging and risk stratification. J Nucl Med 2012;53:754–64.

10. Matsuzu K, Segade F, Wong M, et al. Glucose transporters in the thyroid. Thyroid 2005;15:545–50.

11. Heydarzadeh S, Moshtaghie AA, Daneshpoor M, et al. Regulators of glucose uptake in thyroid cancer cell lines. Cell Commun Signal 2020;18:83.

12. Pagano L, Samà MT, Morani F, et al. Thyroid incidentaloma identified by ^{18}F-fluorodeoxyglucose positron emission tomography with CT (FDG-PET/CT): clinical and pathological relevance. Clin Endocrinol 2011;75:528–34.

13. Are C, Hsu JF, Schoder H, et al. FDG-PET detected thyroid incidentalomas: need for further investigation? Ann Surg Oncol 2006;14:239–47.

14. Karantanis D, Bogsrud TV, Wiseman GA, et al. Clinical significance of diffusely increased 18F-FDG uptake in the thyroid gland. J Nucl Med 2007;48:896–901.

15. de Leijer JF, Metman MJH, van der Hoorn A, et al. Focal thyroid incidentalomas on 18F-FDG PET/CT: a systematic review and meta-analysis on prevalence, risk of malignancy and inconclusive fine needle aspiration. Front Endocrinol 2021;12:723394.

16. Gherghe M, Lazar AM, Mutuleanu MD, et al. Radiomics analysis of [18F]FDG PET/CT thyroid incidentalomas: how can it improve patients' clinical management? a systematic review from the literature. Diagnostics 2022;12:471.

17. Sollini M, Cozzi L, Pepe G, et al. [18F]FDG-PET/CT texture analysis in thyroid incidentalomas: preliminary results. Eur J Hybrid Imaging 2017;1:3.

18. Cibas ES, Ali SZ. The 2017 Bethesda system for reporting thyroid cytopathology. Thyroid 2017;27:1341–6.

19. Keutgen XM, Filicori F, Fahey TJ 3rd. Molecular diagnosis for indeterminate thyroid nodules on fine needle aspiration: advances and limitations. Expert Rev Mol Diagn 2013;13:613–23.

20. Mitchell JC, Grant F, Evenson AR, et al. Preoperative evaluation of thyroid nodules with 18FDG-PET/CT. Surgery 2005;138:1166–75.

21. de Geus-Oei LF, Pieters GF, Bonenkamp JJ, et al. 18F-FDG PET reduces unnecessary hemithyroidectomies for thyroid nodules with inconclusive cytologic results. J Nucl Med 2006;47:770–5.

22. Kim JM, Ryu JS, Kim TY, et al. 18F-fluorodeoxyglucose positron emission tomography does not predict malignancy in thyroid nodules cytologically diagnosed as follicular neoplasm. J Clin Endocrinol Metab 2007;92:1630–4.

23. Haugen BR, Alexander EK, Bible KC, et al. 2015 American thyroid association management guidelines for adult patients with thyroid nodules and differentiated thyroid cancer: the American thyroid association guidelines task force on thyroid nodules and differentiated thyroid cancer. Thyroid 2016;26:1–133.

24. Castellana M, Trimboli P, Piccardo A, et al. Performance of 18F-FDG PET/CT in selecting thyroid nodules with indeterminate fine-needle aspiration cytology for surgery. a systematic review and a meta-analysis. J Clin Med 2019;8:1333.

25. de Koster EJ, de Geus-Oei LF, Brouwers AH, et al. [18F]FDG-PET/CT to prevent futile surgery in indeterminate thyroid nodules: a blinded, randomized controlled multicentre trial. Eur J Nucl Med Mol Imag 2022;49:1970–84.

26. de Koster EJ, Vriens D, van Aken MO, et al. FDG-PET/CT in indeterminate thyroid nodules: cost-utility analysis alongside a randomized controlled trial. Eur J Nucl Med Mol Imag 2022;49:3452–69.

27. Kim DH, Kim SJ. Diagnostic role of F-18 FDG PET/CT for preoperative lymph node staging in thyroid cancer patients; A systematic review and meta-analysis. Clin Imag 2020;65:100–7.

28. Sampson E, Brierley JD, Le LW, et al. Clinical management and outcome of papillary and follicular (differentiated) thyroid cancer presenting with distant metastasis at diagnosis. Cancer 2007;110:1451–6.

29. Alzahrani AS, Abouzied ME, Salam SA, et al. The role of F-18-fluorodeoxyglucose positron emission tomography in the postoperative evaluation of differentiated thyroid cancer. Eur J Endocrinol 2008;158:683–9.

30. Gaertner FC, Okamoto S, Shiga T, et al. FDG PET performed at thyroid remnant ablation has a higher predictive value for the long-term survival of high-risk patients with well-differentiated thyroid cancer than radioiodine uptake. Clin Nucl Med 2015;40:378–83.

31. Pace L, Klain M, Salvatore B, et al. Prognostic role of 18F-FDG PET/CT in the postoperative evaluation of differentiated thyroid cancer patients. Clin Nucl Med 2015;40:111–5.

32. Lee JW, Lee SM, Lee DH, et al. Clinical utility of 18F-FDG PET/CT concurrent with 131I therapy in intermediate-to-high-risk patients with differentiated thyroid cancer: dual-center experience with 286 patients. J Nucl Med 2013;54:1230–6.

33. Rosenbaum-Krumme SJ, Görges R, Bockisch A, et al. 18F-FDG PET/CT changes therapy management in high-risk DTC after first radioiodine therapy. Eur J Nucl Med Mol Imag 2012;39:1373–80.

34. Mazzaferri EL, Kloos RT. Clinical review 128: current approaches to primary therapy for papillary and follicular thyroid cancer. J Clin Endocrinol Metab 2001;86:1447–63.

35. Schönberger J, Rüschoff J, Grimm D, et al. Glucose transporter 1 gene expression is related to thyroid neoplasms with an unfavorable prognosis: an immunohistochemical study. Thyroid 2002;12:747–54.

36. Schütz F, Lautenschläger C, Lorenz K, et al. Positron emission tomography (PET) and PET/CT in thyroid cancer: a systematic review and meta-analysis. Eur Thyroid J 2018;7:13–20.

37. Caetano R, Bastos CR, de Oliveira IA, et al. Accuracy of positron emission tomography and positron emission tomography-CT in the detection of differentiated thyroid cancer recurrence with negative (131) I whole-body scan results: a meta-analysis. Head Neck 2016;38:316–27.

38. Özdemir E, Yildirim Poyraz N, Polat SB, et al. Diagnostic value of 18F-FDG PET/CT in patients with TENIS syndrome: correlation with thyroglobulin levels. Ann Nucl Med 2014;28:241–7.

39. Leboulleux S, Schroeder PR, Busaidy NL, et al. Assessment of the incremental value of recombinant thyrotropin stimulation before 2-[18F]-Fluoro-2-deoxy-D-glucose positron emission tomography/computed tomography imaging to localize residual differentiated thyroid cancer. J Clin Endocrinol Metab 2009;94:1310–6.

40. Ma C, Xie J, Lou Y, et al. The role of TSH for 18F-FDG-PET in the diagnosis of recurrence and metastases of differentiated thyroid carcinoma with elevated thyroglobulin and negative scan: a meta-analysis. Eur J Endocrinol 2010;163:177–83.

41. Qichang W, Lin B, Gege Z, et al. Diagnostic performance of 18F-FDG-PET/CT in DTC patients with thyroglobulin elevation and negative iodine scintigraphy: a meta-analysis. Eur J Endocrinol 2019;181:93–102.

42. Albano D, Tulchinsky M, Dondi F, et al. The role of Tg kinetics in predicting 2-[18F]-FDG PET/CT results and overall survival in patients affected by differentiated thyroid carcinoma with detectable Tg and negative 131I-scan. Endocrine 2021;74:332–9.

43. Ringel MD, Nabhan F. Approach to follow-up of the patient with differentiated thyroid cancer and positive

anti-thyroglobulin antibodies. J Clin Endocrinol Metab 2013;98:3104–10.

44. Kim SJ, Lee SW, Pak K, et al. Diagnostic performance of PET in thyroid cancer with elevated anti-Tg Ab. Endocr Relat Cancer 2018;25:643–52.

45. Wang W, Larson SM, Fazzari M, et al. Prognostic value of [18F]fluorodeoxyglucose positron emission tomographic scanning in patients with thyroid cancer. J Clin Endocrinol Metab 2000;85:1107–13.

46. Robbins RJ, Wan Q, Grewal RK, et al. Real-time prognosis for metastatic thyroid carcinoma based on 2-[18F]fluoro-2-deoxy-D-glucose-positron emission tomography scanning. J Clin Endocrinol Metab 2006;91:498–505.

47. Nagamachi S, Wakamatsu H, Kiyohara S, et al. Comparison of diagnostic and prognostic capabilities of ¹⁸F-FDG-PET/CT, ¹³¹I-scintigraphy, and diffusion-weighted magnetic resonance imaging for postoperative thyroid cancer. Jpn J Radiol 2011;29:413–22.

48. Deandreis D, Al Ghuzlan A, Leboulleux S, et al. Do histological, immunohistochemical, and metabolic (radioiodine and fluorodeoxyglucose uptakes) patterns of metastatic thyroid cancer correlate with patient outcome? Endocr Relat Cancer 2011;18: 159–69.

49. Vural GU, Akkas BE, Ercakmak N, et al. Prognostic significance of FDG PET/CT on the follow-up of patients of differentiated thyroid carcinoma with negative 131I whole-body scan and elevated thyroglobulin levels: correlation with clinical and histopathologic characteristics and long-term follow-up data. Clin Nucl Med 2012;37:953–9.

50. Albano D, Dondi F, Mazzoletti A, et al. Prognostic role of 2-[18F]FDG PET/CT metabolic volume parameters in patients affected by differentiated thyroid carcinoma with high thyroglobulin level, negative 131I WBS and positive 2-[18F]-FDG PET/CT. Diagnostics 2021;11:2189.

51. Bogsrud TV, Hay ID, Karantanis D, et al. Prognostic value of 18F-fluorodeoxyglucose-positron emission tomography in patients with differentiated thyroid carcinoma and circulating antithyroglobulin autoantibodies. Nucl Med Commun 2011;32:245–51.

52. Carr LL, Mankoff DA, Goulart BH, et al. Phase II study of daily sunitinib in FDG-PET-positive, iodine-refractory differentiated thyroid cancer and metastatic medullary carcinoma of the thyroid with functional imaging correlation. Clin Cancer Res 2010;16:5260–8.

53. Ahmaddy F, Burgard C, Beyer L, et al. 18F-FDG-PET/CT in patients with advanced, radioiodine refractory thyroid cancer treated with lenvatinib. Cancers 2021; 13:317.

54. Rendl G, Schweighofer-Zwink G, Sorko S, et al. Assessment of treatment response to lenvatinib in thyroid cancer monitored by F-18 FDG PET/CT

Using PERCIST 1.0, Modified PERCIST and EORTC criteria-which one is most suitable? Cancers 2022; 14:1868.

55. Kaliszewski K, Ludwig M, Ludwig B, et al. Update on the diagnosis and management of medullary thyroid cancer: what has changed in recent years? Cancers 2022;14:3643.

56. Roman S, Lin R, Sosa JA. Prognosis of medullary thyroid carcinoma: demographic, clinical, and pathologic predictors of survival in 1252 cases. Cancer 2006;107:2134–42.

57. Giovanella L, Treglia G, Iakovou I, et al. EANM practice guideline for PET/CT imaging in medullary thyroid carcinoma. Eur J Nucl Med Mol Imag 2020; 47:61–77.

58. Wells SA Jr, Asa SL, Dralle H, et al. Revised American thyroid association guidelines for the management of medullary thyroid carcinoma. Thyroid 2015;25:567–610.

59. Rasul S, Hartenbach S, Rebhan K, et al. [18F] DOPA PET/CECT in diagnosis and staging of primary medullary thyroid carcinoma prior to surgery. Eur J Nucl Med Mol Imag 2018;45:2159–69.

60. Treglia G, Cocciolillo F, Di Nardo F, et al. The detection rate of recurrent medullary thyroid carcinoma using fluorine-18 dihydroxyphenylalanine positron emission tomography: a meta-analysis. Acad Radiol 2012;19:1290–9.

61. Treglia G, Villani MF, Giordano A, et al. Detection rate of recurrent medullary thyroid carcinoma using fluorine-18 fluorodeoxyglucose positron emission tomography: a meta-analysis. Endocrine 2012;42: 535–45.

62. Treglia G, Tamburello A, Giovanella L. Detection rate of somatostatin receptor PET in patients with recurrent medullary thyroid carcinoma: a systematic review and a meta-analysis. Hormones (Basel) 2017;16:362–72.

63. Parghane RV, Naik C, Talole S, et al. Clinical utility of 177 Lu-DOTATATE PRRT in somatostatin receptor-positive metastatic medullary carcinoma of thyroid patients with the assessment of efficacy, survival analysis, prognostic variables, and toxicity. Head Neck 2020;42:401–16.

64. Lee SW, Shim SR, Jeong SY, et al. Comparison of 5 different PET radiopharmaceuticals for the detection of recurrent medullary thyroid carcinoma: a network meta-analysis. Clin Nucl Med 2020;45: 341–8.

65. Grabellus F, Nagarajah J, Bockisch A, et al. Glucose transporter 1 expression, tumor proliferation, and iodine/glucose uptake in thyroid cancer with emphasis on poorly differentiated thyroid carcinoma. Clin Nucl Med 2012;37:121–7.

66. Kim CH, Yoo IeR, Chung YA, et al. Influence of thyroid-stimulating hormone on 18F-fluorodeoxyglucose and 99mTc-methoxyisobutylisonitrile uptake in

human poorly differentiated thyroid cancer cells in vitro. Ann Nucl Med 2009;23:131–6.

67. Abraham T, Schöder H. Thyroid cancer–indications and opportunities for positron emission tomography/computed tomography imaging. Semin Nucl Med 2011;41:121–38.

68. Civan C, Isik EG, Simsek DH. Metastatic poorly differentiated thyroid cancer with heterogeneous distribution of 18F-FDG, 68Ga-DOTATATE, and 68Ga-PSMA on PET/CT. Clin Nucl Med 2021;46:e212–3.

69. Perri F, Lorenzo GD, Scarpati GD, et al. Anaplastic thyroid carcinoma: a comprehensive review of current and future therapeutic options. World J Clin Oncol 2011;2:150–7.

70. Corrigan KL, Williamson H, Elliott Range D, et al. Treatment outcomes in anaplastic thyroid cancer. J Thyroid Res 2019;2019:8218949.

71. Bogsrud TV, Karantanis D, Nathan MA, et al. 18F-FDG PET in the management of patients with anaplastic thyroid carcinoma. Thyroid 2008;18:713–9.

72. Poisson T, Deandreis D, Leboulleux S, et al. 18F-fluorodeoxyglucose positron emission tomography and computed tomography in anaplastic thyroid cancer. Eur J Nucl Med Mol Imag 2010;37:2277–85.

73. Kim HJ, Chang HS, Ryu YH. Prognostic role of pretreatment [18F]FDG PET/CT in patients with anaplastic thyroid cancer. Cancers 2021;13:4228.

74. Bible KC, Kebebew E, Brierley J, et al. 2021 American thyroid association guidelines for management of patients with anaplastic thyroid cancer. Thyroid 2021;31:337–86.

75. Pryma DA, Schöder H, Gönen M, et al. Diagnostic accuracy and prognostic value of 18F-FDG PET in Hürthle cell thyroid cancer patients. J Nucl Med 2006;47:1260–6.

76. Lowe VJ, Mullan BP, Hay ID, et al. 18F-FDG PET of patients with Hürthle cell carcinoma. J Nucl Med 2003;44:1402–6.

77. Plotkin M, Hautzel H, Krause BJ, et al. Implication of 2-18fluor-2-deoxyglucose positron emission tomography in the follow-up of Hürthle cell thyroid cancer. Thyroid 2002;12:155–61.

78. Van Nostrand D, Moreau S, Bandaru VV, et al. 124I positron emission tomography versus (131)I planar imaging in the identification of residual thyroid tissue and/or metastasis in patients who have well-differentiated thyroid cancer. Thyroid 2010;20:879–83.

79. Santhanam P, Taieb D, Solnes L, et al. Utility of I-124 PET/CT in identifying radioiodine avid lesions in differentiated thyroid cancer: a systematic review and meta-analysis. Clin Endocrinol 2017;86:645–51.

80. Plyku D, Hobbs RF, Wu D, et al. I-124 PET/CT image-based dosimetry in patients with differentiated thyroid cancer treated with I-131: correlation of patient-specific lesional dosimetry to treatment response. Ann Nucl Med 2022;36:213–23.

81. Kuker R, Sztejnberg M, Gulec S. I-124 imaging and dosimetry. I-124 Görüntüleme ve Dozimetri. Mol Imaging Radionucl Ther 2017;26:66–73.

82. Hicks RJ, Roselt PJ, Kallur KG, et al. Fapi PET/CT: will it end the hegemony of 18F-FDG in oncology? J Nucl Med 2021;62:296–302.

83. Kratochwil C, Flechsig P, Lindner T, et al. 68Ga-FAPI PET/CT: tracer uptake in 28 different kinds of cancer. J Nucl Med 2019;60:801–5.

84. Fu H, Fu J, Huang J, et al. 68Ga-FAPI PET/CT in thyroid cancer with thyroglobulin elevation and negative iodine scintigraphy. Clin Nucl Med 2021;46:427–30.

85. Fu H, Fu J, Huang J, et al. 68Ga-FAPI PET/CT versus 18F-FDG PET/CT for detecting metastatic lesions in a case of radioiodine-refractory differentiated thyroid cancer. Clin Nucl Med 2021;46:940–2.

86. Fu H, Wu J, Huang J, et al. 68Ga Fibroblast activation protein inhibitor pet/ct in the detection of metastatic thyroid cancer: comparison with 18F-FDG PET/CT. Radiology 2022;304:397–405.

87. Ballal S, Yadav MP, Moon ES, et al. First-in-human results on the biodistribution, pharmacokinetics, and dosimetry of [177Lu]Lu-DOTA.SA.FAPi and [177Lu]Lu-DOTAGA.(SA.FAPi)2. Pharmaceuticals 2021;14:1212.

88. Kundu P, Lata S, Sharma P, et al. Prospective evaluation of (68)Ga-DOTANOC PET-CT in differentiated thyroid cancer patients with raised thyroglobulin and negative (131)I-whole body scan: comparison with (18)F-FDG PET-CT. Eur J Nucl Med Mol Imag 2014;41:1354–62.

89. Roll W, Riemann B, Schäfers M, et al. 177Lu-DOTATATE Therapy in radioiodine-refractory differentiated thyroid cancer: a single center experience. Clin Nucl Med 2018;43:e346–51.

90. Chen X. Multimodality imaging of tumor integrin alphavbeta3 expression. Mini Rev Med Chem 2006;6:227–34.

91. Hoffmann S, Maschuw K, Hassan I, et al. Differential pattern of integrin receptor expression in differentiated and anaplastic thyroid cancer cell lines. Thyroid 2005;15:1011–20.

92. Parihar AS, Mittal BR, Kumar R, et al. 68Ga-DOTA-RGD2 positron emission tomography/computed tomography in radioiodine refractory thyroid cancer: prospective comparison of diagnostic accuracy with 18F-FDG positron emission tomography/computed tomography and evaluation toward potential theranostics. Thyroid 2020;30:557–67.

93. Parihar AS, Sood A, Kumar R, et al. Novel use of 177Lu-DOTA-RGD2 in treatment of 68Ga-DOTA-RGD2-avid lesions in papillary thyroid cancer with TENIS. Eur J Nucl Med Mol Imag 2018;45:1836–7.

94. Salas Fragomeni RA, Amir T, Sheikhbahaei S, et al. Imaging of nonprostate cancers using PSMA-targeted radiotracers: rationale, current state of the field, and a call to arms. J Nucl Med 2018;59: 871–7.

95. Taywade SK, Damle NA, Bal C. PSMA expression in papillary thyroid carcinoma: opening a new horizon in management of thyroid cancer? Clin Nucl Med 2016;41:e263–5.

96. de Vries LH, Lodewijk L, Braat AJAT, et al. 68Ga-PSMA PET/CT in radioactive iodine-refractory differentiated thyroid cancer and first treatment results with 177Lu-PSMA-617. EJNMMI Res 2020;10:18.

97. Subudhi TK, Damle NA, Arora G, et al. Ga-68 prostate-specific membrane antigen-HBED-CC positron emission tomography/computed tomography in anaplastic thyroid carcinoma. Indian J Nucl Med 2022;37:310–7.

98. Jiang H, DeGrado TR. [18F]Tetrafluoroborate ([18F]TFB) and its analogs for PET imaging of the sodium/iodide symporter. Theranostics 2018;8: 3918–31.

99. Samnick S, Al-Momani E, Schmid JS, et al. Initial clinical investigation of [18F]tetrafluoroborate PET/CT in comparison to [124I]iodine PET/CT for imaging thyroid cancer. Clin Nucl Med 2018;43:162–7.

100. Dittmann M, Gonzalez Carvalho JM, Rahbar K, et al. Incremental diagnostic value of [18F]tetrafluoroborate PET-CT compared to [131I]iodine scintigraphy in recurrent differentiated thyroid cancer. Eur J Nucl Med Mol Imag 2020;47:2639–46.

Quarter-Century Transformation of Oncology
Positron Emission Tomography for Patients with Breast Cancer

Gary A. Ulaner, MD, PhD[a,b,]*, Sofia Carrilho Vaz, MD, FEBNM[c,d],
David Groheux, MD, PhD[e,f,g]

KEYWORDS

• Position emission tomography • Breast cancer • ^{18}F-FDG • ^{18}F-FES • ^{18}F-NaF

KEY POINTS

- ^{18}F-fluorodeoxyglucose (^{18}F-FDG) PET allows measurement of glucose metabolism and has become widely used in patients with breast cancer. Recent evidence now supports clinical applications including systemic staging of patients with newly diagnosed large or locally advanced disease (stages IIB–IIIC), detecting sites of recurrence, and monitoring treatment response. ^{18}F-FDG PET is mostly recommended for the invasive ductal carcinoma histology because invasive lobular carcinoma (ILC) histology has lower FDG-avidity and less supporting data.
- ^{18}F-FES PET allows assessment of estrogen receptor and was approved by the US Food and Drug Administration in 2020. Clinical applications include assisting in selection of endocrine therapies either at initial diagnosis of metastatic breast cancer or after progression of metastatic disease on endocrine therapy, assessing lesions that are difficult or dangerous to biopsy, and assessing lesions when other tests are inconclusive.
- There are many PET radiotracers under investigation for additional clinical applications in patients with breast cancer, including radiotracers targeting progesterone receptor, human epidermal growth factor receptors 2 and 3, and fibroblast activation protein inhibitor.

MOLECULAR CLASSIFICATION OF BREAST CANCER

A quarter century ago, breast cancer was predominantly evaluated by morphology. However, with the advancement of molecular technologies, breast cancer is now better characterized at the genomic level. Perou and colleagues[1] revolutionized classification of breast cancer into "molecular portraits" in 2000. This genomic analysis grouped breast cancer based on 5 gene expression patterns: luminal A, luminal B, ERBB2 (human epidermal growth factor receptor 2 [HER2]-enriched), basal-like, and normal-breast-like.[1,2] These molecular subtypes of breast cancer demonstrate distinct clinical and pathologic features, responses to systemic therapies,[3] and impact on application of PET radioisotopes.[4,5]

[a] Molecular Imaging and Therapy, Hoag Family Cancer Institute, Irvine, CA, USA; [b] Departments of Radiology and Translational Genomics, University of Southern California, Los Angeles, CA, USA; [c] Nuclear Medicine-Radiopharmacology, Champalimaud Clinical Center, Champalimaud Foundation, Lisbon, Portugal; [d] Department of Radiology, Leiden University Medical Center, Leiden, the Netherlands; [e] Nuclear Department of Nuclear Medicine, Saint-Louis Hospital, Paris, France; [f] Centre d'Imagerie Radio-Isotopique (CIRI), La Rochelle, France; [g] University Paris-Diderot, INSERM U976, HIPI, Paris, France
* Corresponding author. Molecular Imaging and Therapy, Hoag Family Cancer Institute, 16105 Sand Canyon, Irvine, CA.
E-mail address: gary.ulaner@hoag.org

PET Clin 19 (2024) 147–162
https://doi.org/10.1016/j.cpet.2023.12.002
1556-8598/24/© 2023 Elsevier Inc. All rights reserved.

pet.theclinics.com

For instance, HER2-enriched and basal-like breast cancers commonly demonstrate greater ^{18}F-fluorodeoxyglucose (FDG)-avidity than luminal A malignancies.[4] All applications for estrogen receptor (ER)-targeted imaging with16α-^{18}F-fluoro-17β-fluoroestradiol (^{18}F-FES) are dependent on ER expression in tumor cells.[6] Similarly, novel HER2-targeted agents in clinical trials are dependent on HER2 expression.[7] Recent reviews are available with detailed narratives.[8,9]

The most common histologic subtype of breast cancer is invasive ductal breast cancer (invasive ductal carcinoma [IDC]), also known as no special type in the recent classification. Invasive lobular breast cancer (invasive lobular carcinoma [ILC]) is a histologic subtype that has been shown to be a distinct genetic and molecular disease from the more common IDC.[10] ILC lacks expression of the CDH1 gene, which encodes E-cadherin, a cell adhesion molecule. The loss of E-cadherin results in a discohesive morphology of ILC tumors and fewer tumor cells per volume of tissue than IDC tumors with intact cell adhesion. These molecular and morphologic differences make ILC more difficult to detect on many imaging modalities, including mammography, ultrasound, breast magnetic resonance imaging (MR), and ^{18}F-FDG PET.[11–13]

^{18}F-FLUORODEOXYGLUCOSE

The greatest impact of PET imaging in the care of patients with breast cancer has been made with the metabolic radiotracer ^{18}F-fluorodeoxyglucose (^{18}F-FDG). Malignant tumor cells often demonstrate higher metabolism, and thus accumulate more glucose as compared with their normal counterparts. FDG, a radiolabeled glucose analog, accumulates in cells by mechanisms similar to glucose.[14] After intravenous administration, FDG is transported into cells by glucose transporter type 1 or 3. Subsequent intracellular phosphorylation by hexokinase, leads to the formation of FDG-6-phosphate. Both glucose-6-phosphate and FDG-6-phosphate are impermeable to the cell membrane, unable to be used in further glycolysis pathways, and are trapped within the cell.[15] The accumulation of FDG within highly metabolic cells allows for their visualization on FDG-PET imaging.

Minn and Soini were the first to study the utility of ^{18}F-FDG imaging in breast cancer in 1989.[16] At the time, it was likely underappreciated how ^{18}F-FDG would transform systemic imaging of breast cancer. During the last quarter century, systemic imaging of breast cancer focused on anatomic imaging with computed tomography (CT) and nuclear osseous imaging by means of bone scan.[17] However, extensive evidence now demonstrates that ^{18}F-FDG PET/CT is valuable for many patients with breast cancer.[4,18,19] Prospective trials have demonstrated that ^{18}F-FDG PET/CT is often superior to CT/bone scan for systemic staging of newly diagnosed large and locally advanced disease (anatomic stage IIB–IIIC),[20–22] detection of disease recurrence,[23] and measurement of treatment response.[24–28]

Systemic Staging of Newly Diagnosed Large or Locally Advanced Disease

Clinical staging of breast cancer is based on the American Joint Committee on Cancer's Tumor, Node, Metastasis (TNM) staging system (primary breast tumor: T, nodal: N, and distant metastases: M; **Table 1**). T staging of breast tumors remains the domain of dedicated breast imaging, including mammography, ultrasound, and breast MR.[29] Whole-body FDG PET/CT has lower sensitivity than these imaging methods for the primary breast malignancy.[17,30] There are dedicated PET systems to evaluate the breast with higher resolution positron emission mamography (PEM),[31] and in specific situations[32]; however, MR still maintains a higher sensitivity.[33] ^{18}F-FDG PET/MR may provide incremental value over MR for primary breast lesions.[34]

For the utility of ^{18}F-FDG for N staging of breast cancer, it is useful to distinguish axillary nodes from extra-axillary nodes. Although larger nodal metastases may be identified by imaging, smaller and still clinically relevant nodal metastases are only detected by tissue sampling; thus, sentinel node biopsy remains the mainstay for axillary nodal staging.[18,35] Indeed, sentinel node sampling has greater than 95% prediction of axillary nodal disease.[36] ^{18}F-FDG PET is inferior to sentinel node evaluation for axillary nodes, likely because small subcentimeter lesions are better detected by the later.[37,38] Sensitivity of ^{18}F-FDG for axillar nodal metastases may be as low as 40%.[39] For extra-axillary nodal staging, imaging plays a far greater role. Internal mammary, infraclavicular, and supraclavicular nodes are locoregional sites of disease spread, which are usually outside the detection of sentinel node biopsy, yet have important influence of patient stage and therapy.[20] CT has been used for the detection of extra-axillary nodal metastases but accuracy is low.[17,40] ^{18}F-FDG PET/CT detects previously unsuspected extra-axillary nodal metastases with greater success than anatomic imaging,[20,22,41–46] thus altering patient stage, prognosis, and imaging. Recent study with ^{18}F-FDG PET/MR demonstrates similar to slightly better nodal detection rates as compared with PET/CT.[47,48]

Table 1
TNM anatomic stage grouping for breast cancer according to the American Joint Committee on Cancer (AJCC) cancer staging manual

AJCC	TNM		
Stage I	T1	N0	M0
Stage IIA	T0	N1	M0
	T1	N1	M0
	T2	N0	M0
Stage IIB	T2	N1	M0
	T3	N0	M0
Stage IIIA	T3	N1	M0
	T0	N2	M0
	T1	N2	M0
	T2	N2	M0
	T3	N2	M0
Stage IIIB	T4	N0	M0
	T4	N1	M0
	T4	N2	M0
Stage IIIC	any T	N3	M0
Stage IV	any T	any N	M1

M staging is of critical importance in patients with locally advanced breast cancer. The detection of previously unsuspected distant metastases will change a patient's stage from locoregional to stage IV, converting patient management from curative-intent therapy by surgery to palliative systemic therapies. ^{18}F-FDG PET/CT has demonstrated profound impact in M staging. Extensive and increasing evidence suggests that ^{18}F-FDG PET/CT identifies previously unsuspected distant metastases particularly in patients with large primary operable or locally advanced breast cancer (anatomic stages IIB–III; **Fig. 1**).[20,22,41–46,49–55] PET/MR may have better sensitivity for distant liver and osseous metastases[56,57] but worse detection of pulmonary metastases.[58]

Recently, a multicenter prospective trial demonstrated ^{18}F-FDG PET/CT upstaged more than twice as many patients with large or locally advanced invasive ductal breast cancer (IDC) as patients staged with CT of the chest/abdomen/pelvis and bone scan.[21] Among 369 patients randomly assigned to ^{18}F-FDG PET/CT or CT/bone scan, 43 of 184 (23%) of patients who underwent ^{18}F-FDG PET/CT were upstaged to stage IV, compared with 21 of 185 (11%) of patients who underwent CT/bone scan. Because the detection of stage IV disease radically alters optimal treatment strategies, this trial provides outstanding evidence that systemic staging with ^{18}F-FDG PET/CT is more valuable for patients with locally advanced IDC than a strategy using CT/bone scan.

Of note, this mutlicenter prospective trial only included patients with IDC, the most common histology of breast cancer but excluded patients with invasive lobular breast cancer (ILC), the second most common histology. Metastases from ILC are less FDG-avid than comparable IDC metastases,[59,60] making detection of clinically relevant ILC distant metastases more difficult on ^{18}F-FDG PET/CT.

Overall, there is now strong prospective evidence that ^{18}F-FDG PET/CT provides the most sensitive method of detection for potential stage IV disease in patients with newly diagnosed locally advanced IDC. Comparable evidence is still lacking for ILC. This is an area of substantial progress during the last quarter century, with the paradigm for systemic staging of newly diagnosed locally advanced IDC changing from CT/bone scan to ^{18}F-FDG PET/CT. National Comprehensive Cancer Network (NCCN) guidelines, which once discouraged the use of ^{18}F-FDG PET/CT in patients with breast cancer, now solidly place ^{18}F-FDG PET/CT as a test to consider for workup of newly diagnosed locally advanced disease, stating that "FDG PET/CT may also be helpful in identifying unsuspected regional nodal disease and/or distant metastases."[61,62] A developing joint European Association of Nuclear Medicine (EANM) and Society of Nuclear Medicine and Molecular Imaging (SNMMI) guideline for the role of ^{18}F-FDG PET/CT in patients with IDC recommends ^{18}F-FDG PET/CT for initial staging of patients with large or locally advanced (stage IIB to IIIC) IDC.

Detection of Disease Recurrence

Disease recurrence after therapy may be suspected by clinical symptoms, finding on physical examination, and/or elevation of tumor markers. Because the confirmation and localization of disease recurrence is essential to optimal application of therapies, imaging is often performed. Multiple imaging modalities have been evaluated for this purpose, from dedicated breast imaging such as mammography, ultrasound, and breast MR, to systemic modalities such as CT, bone scan, whole-body MR, and ^{18}F-FDG PET/CT. Studies of ^{18}F-FDG PET/CT for the detection of disease recurrence have demonstrated high detection rates,[63,64] benefit over anatomic imaging,[65–67] and impacted clinical management in these patients.[68] Integrated contrast-enhanced whole-body PET/CT provided higher sensitivity for the detection of recurrence than ^{18}F-FDG PET or CT alone.[69]

Two meta-analyses on breast cancer recurrences detection were published in 2010.[70,71]

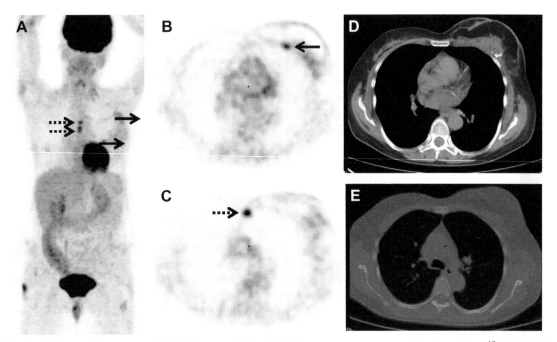

Fig. 1. A 52-year-old woman with initial stage IIB ER+/HER2-breast cancer upstaged to stage IV on ^{18}F-FDG-PET/CT. (*A*) ^{18}F-FDG MIP image demonstrates FDG avidity in the right breast and axilla (*arrow*), as well as overlying the midline chest (*dashed arrow*). (*B*) Axial CT on soft tissue window and (*C*) axial FDG PET through the level of the right breast and axilla demonstrate postsurgical changes from lumpectomy and nodal dissection performed 3 weeks previously (*arrows*). (*D*) Axial CT image on bone window and (*E*) axial FDG PET localize the FDG focus in the midline chest to the sternum (*dashed arrows*), subsequently biopsy-proven to be an osseous metastasis. (Ulaner G.A., Castillo R., Wills J. et al. 18F–FDG-PET/CT for systemic staging of patients with newly diagnosed ER-positive and HER2-positive breast cancer. Eur J Nucl Med Mol Imaging 44, 1420–1427 (2017). https://doi.org/10.1007/s00259-017-3709-1.)

These meta-analyses pooled studies using PET alone and studies using hybrid PET/CT instruments. In the first meta-analysis, MRI and PET (and/or PET/CT) were more effective than ultrasound and CT. No difference was observed between MRI and PET but PET and PET/CT were not separated in the analysis.[70] In the second meta-analysis, PET and PET/CT modalities were evaluated separately.[71] Hybrid PET/CT imaging had significantly higher sensitivity than CT but the difference in specificity was not significant. PET/CT also had higher sensitivity than PET alone, with no significant difference in specificity. No significant difference was noted between PET/CT and MRI (for sensitivity and for specificity) but only one study with whole-body MRI was included.[66]

In a more recent meta-analysis published in 2016, 26 trials evaluating ^{18}F-FDG PET for suspected breast cancer recurrence demonstrated a pooled sensitivity of 0.9 (95% CI 0.88–0.90).[72] The strongest evidence for the value of ^{18}F-FDG PET/CT for the detection of suspected breast cancer recurrence is likely a prospective trial of 100 women with suspected recurrence of breast cancer who underwent bone scan, contrast enhanced CT, and ^{18}F-FDG PET/CT within 10 days, and each imaging modality was interpreted by readers blinded to the others.[23] Twenty-two of 100 patients (22%) were verified with distant recurrence. The area under the receiver operating curve for detection of the sites of recurrence was 0.99 (95% confidence interval [CI] 0.97–1) for ^{18}F-FDG PET/CT but only 0.84 (95% CI 0.73–0.94) for contrast-enhanced CT, and 0.86 (95% CI 0.77–0.94) for combined CT/bone scan.[23] The accuracy of ^{18}F-FDG PET/CT was better than CT/bone scan for local recurrences as well as distant recurrences. This trial provides evidence that ^{18}F-FDG PET/CT is superior to CT/bone scan for the detection of suspected recurrence in patients with breast cancer. NCCN guidelines suggest using ^{18}F-FDG PET/CT to localize IDC recurrence when other imaging methods are equivocal.[61,73,74] A developing joint EANM and SNMMI guideline suggests using ^{18}F-FDG PET/CT to detect the site and extent of suspected recurrent IDC.

Measurement of Treatment Response

Reductions in FDG-avidity have been proposed to correlate with decreased levels of malignancy following effective therapy. Investigators have taken advantage of the availability of pathology from surgical resections following neoadjuvant therapy (NAT) to demonstrate a strong correlation between changes in ^{18}F-FDG SUV (notably early changes after 1 or 2 cycles of NAT) and NAT response on pathology.[75,76] Having pathology for the gold standard has allowed for definition of histologic and molecular markers predicting NAT response, with ^{18}F-FDG PET best for predicting response in HER2+ and triple-negative tumors.[77–83] A meta-analysis of 17 trials evaluating ^{18}F-FDG PET for NAT response suggested that ^{18}F-FDG PET was prognostic for survival.[84]

In 2 multicenter studies, FDG PET findings were used to change treatment early in patients treated in the neoadjuvant setting. The multicenter randomized phase 2 study AVATAXHER included 142 patients who initially received standard therapy combining docetaxel and trastuzumab and evaluated the role of ^{18}F-FDG PET in modulating neoadjuvant treatment according to the metabolic response after one cycle.[85] In the case of poor response after one cycle (low or absence of SUV decrease), a randomization was performed: arm A received bevacizumab in addition to the initial treatment starting from cycle-3, whereas arm B continued the initial treatment. At treatment completion, the pathologic complete response (pCR) rates were, respectively, 37 out of 69 (53.6%) for responding patients (high SUV decrease after one cycle), 21 out of 48 (43.8%) for arm A and 6/25 (24.0%) for arm B. Thus, a change in treatment led to increase in pCR rate in poor responders. Unfortunately, long-term follow-up of this patient cohort showed that the improvement of pCR did not modify disease-free survival.[85] More recently, in the PHERGain multicenter, randomized, open-label, noncomparative, phase 2 study, 356 patients with HER2-positive early-stage BC were included 2-[^{18}F]FDG PET identified patients who were likely to benefit from chemotherapy-free dual HER2 blockade with trastuzumab and pertuzumab, and a reduced negative impact on global health status.[86,87]

Optimal PET parameters to use to define response in the neoadjuvant setting are uncertain.[88] Moreover, no imaging modality, including ^{18}F-FDG PET, has yet demonstrated the ability to discern a complete response from a partial response as defined by pathology, likely because low volume residual disease may be present on pathology without evidence on imaging.[35] As

pathology remains the gold standard for determine NAT response, the clinical value of ^{18}F-FDG PET in predicting NAT response is yet to be defined. Further study may define an adaptive strategy for altering NAT regimens in the middle of therapy based on FDG PET results, such as strategies currently used for patients with lymphoma.[89]

Accurate measurements of treatment response in metastatic breast cancer suffer from the lack of a histologic gold standard in most cases. Allowing for this limitation, studies of ^{18}F-FDG PET in the evaluation treatment response for metastatic disease have demonstrated that FDG PET could assess response versus nonresponse after only 1 to 3 cycles of therapy.[90,91] This provides a basis to consider metabolic changes on ^{18}F-FDG PET, as an alternative to anatomic changes such as changes in size on CT or MR, for measuring treatment response in metastatic breast cancer.[92] Indeed, metabolic changes better predict treatment response than anatomic changes in lymphoma, leading to widespread adoption of ^{18}F-FDG PET Lugano criteria for monitoring lymphoma treatment response.[93] For solid tumors, ^{18}F-FDG PET response criteria in solid tumors (PERCIST) criteria have been proposed.[94] During the past several years, multiple clinical trials have demonstrated the ability of ^{18}F-FDG PET to determine therapy response in metastatic breast cancer when using endocrine-targeted therapies[95] and HER2-targeted therapies.[96] Metabolic response using ^{18}F-FDG has been shown to be particularly superior to anatomic imaging when evaluating osseous metastases[97,98] because sclerotic osseous lesions appearing after therapy may represent osseous healing or new metastases, preventing accurate therapy response assessment by CT (**Fig. 2**). The first head-to-head comparison CT and ^{18}F-FDG PET for measuring treatment response in patients with metastatic breast cancer was a retrospective analysis of 65 patients demonstrating metabolic assessment by FDG PET/CT was a better predictor of both progression-free survival and disease-specific survival than RECIST evaluation on CT.[99] Now, there are several prospective trials with a head-to-head comparison of CT and ^{18}F-FDG PET for breast cancer treatment response. In a prospective trial of 81 patients undergoing Neratinib therapy, ^{18}F-FDG PET allowed assessment of response in patients with RECIST nonmeasurable disease and allowed an earlier detection of progression (see **Fig. 2**).[24] In another prospective trial of 87 evaluable women with biopsy-proven metastatic breast cancer, subjects underwent ^{18}F-FDG PET/CT and contrast-enhanced CT every 9 to 12 weeks and used the contrast-enhanced CT

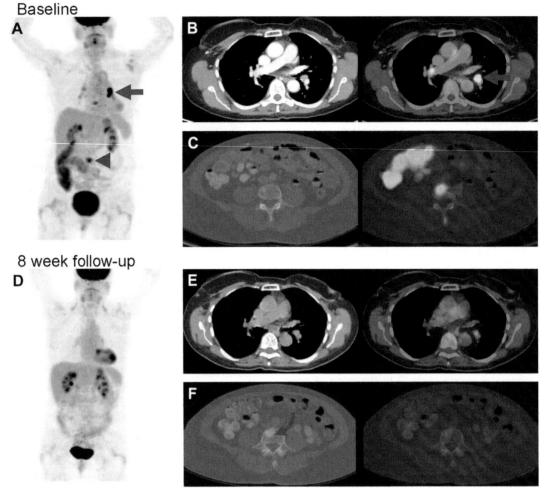

Fig. 2. Example demonstrating measurable disease on ^{18}F-FDG PET but not by RECIST, as well as advantage of measuring response in osseous lesions with ^{18}F-FDG PET. This is a 70-year-old woman with HER2-mutant breast cancer. (*A*) PET MIP image at baseline demonstrates FDG-avid lesions in the chest (*arrow*) and abdomen (*arrow-head*). (*B*) Corresponding axial contrast-enhanced CT and fused PET/CT images of the chest demonstrate a thoracic FDG focus localized to a left hilar node (*arrow*) 8 mm in short axis on CT. This node was measurable by ^{18}F-FDG PET but not by RECIST. (*C*) Corresponding axial CT and fused PET/CT images of the abdomen demonstrate an abdominal FDG focus localized to a vertebral body (*arrowhead*) without clear correlate on CT. This osseous lesion was measurable by ^{18}F-FDG PET but not by RECIST. (*D*) PET MIP at 8-week follow-up demonstrates decrease of all FDG foci to background, representing a complete metabolic response. Corresponding axial images in the chest (*E*) and abdomen (*F*) confirm decrease to background FDG avidity. There was a sclerotic lesion at the prior FDG-avid osseous metastasis (*curved arrow*), which could have been mistaken for a new osseous metastasis without the corresponding PET. (Gary A. Ulaner et al., Impact of FDG PET Imaging for Expanding Patient Eligibility and Measuring Treatment Response in a Genome-Driven Basket Trial of the Pan-HER Kinase Inhibitor, Neratinib. Clin Cancer Res 15 December 2019; 25 (24): 7381–7387. https://doi.org/10.1158/1078-0432.CCR-19-1658.)

with RECIST for clinical decision-making. After the trial was completed, ^{18}F-FDG PET/CT studies were unmasked and analyzed according to PER-CIST.[27] ^{18}F-FDG PET/CT was able to detect progression earlier than contrast-enhanced CT in 43 of 87 (49%) of patients, whereas contrast-enhanced CT detected progression earlier than ^{18}F-FDG PET/CT in only 1 of 87 (1%).[27]

A second analysis of this cohort confirmed response or progression on ^{18}F-FDG PET/CT was a better predictor of survival than contrast-enhanced CT.[28] A separate single-center analysis of 300 patients with biopsy proven metastatic breast cancer that were followed for treatment response by ^{18}F-FDG PET/CT, contrast-enhanced CT, or both, demonstrated a 5-year survival rate of greater than 40% in the groups using ^{18}F-FDG PET/CT but only 16% in the group using CT alone.[100] Thus, the ability to detect disease response and progression earlier using ^{18}F-FDG PET/CT has clinically relevant impact for optimal therapy decisions and outcomes. Overall, there is growing evidence that ^{18}F-FDG PET/CT provides better evaluation of response assessment than CT in patients with metastatic breast cancer.[101] A developing joint EANM and SNMMI guideline suggests ^{18}F-FDG PET/CT may be used for monitoring treatment response in metastatic breast cancer.

SODIUM FLUORIDE

Although ^{18}F-FDG is by far the most widely used PET radiotracer in patients with breast cancer, several other agents are Food and Drug Administration (FDA)-approved and clinically available. Sodium fluoride (^{18}F-NaF) was used for skeletal scintigraphy as early as the 1960s but use at that time was limited by suboptimal features for the conventional gamma imaging that was available at the time.[102] ^{18}F-NaF was replaced by ^{99m}Tc-methylene diphosphonate (MDP) in the 1970s, whose physical characteristics were better for conventional gamma cameras.[103] The development of PET camera renewed interest in the use of ^{18}F-NaF, particularly for malignancies with common osseous involvement. In patients with metastatic breast cancer, ^{18}F-NaF PET/CT has demonstrated superior sensitivity for osseous metastases than ^{99m}Tc-MDP or CT.[104,105] Data from the National Oncology PET Registry demonstrated ^{18}F-NaF PET resulted in a change in clinical management for 24% of 781 patients with breast cancer[106] and a change in the management in 39% of 476 patients using ^{18}F-NaF PET for evaluation of treatment response.[107]

Both ^{18}F-NaF and ^{99m}Tc-MDP function by radiotracer deposition hydroxyl ion exchange in hydroxyapatite crystals during bone mineralization.[108] Thus, these agents detect bone mineralization caused by the presence of tumor, rather than detection of the tumor itself. This leads to a potential problem known as "flare," where increasing number or intensity of lesions on ^{18}F-NaF following therapy may represent increasing bone turnover during successful tumor treatment, rather than increasing disease.[109]

Less data are available comparing ^{18}F-FDG and ^{18}F-NaF. A prospective study of patients with bone-dominant metastatic breast cancer concluded that ^{18}F-FDG parameters predicted time to skeletal-related events (tSRE) and time to progression (TTP) but not overall survival (OS), whereas ^{18}F-NaF parameters were better associated with OS but not with TTP or tSRE.[110]

Given the "flare" limitation of ^{18}F-NaF, and the ability of ^{18}F-FDG to successfully visualize both osseous and nonosseous sites of disease, there may be limited use of ^{18}F-NaF for patients with breast cancer in the near future. However, further studies are needed to compare both radiopharmaceuticals.

16α-^{18}F-FLUORO-17β-FLUOROESTRADIOL

Modern molecular imaging and therapy concepts emphasize targeting specific molecules with specific biding agents. The ER is a molecular target expressed in 80% of breast malignancies,[111] and ER expression acts as a prognostic (distinguishing tumors with favorable and unfavorable prognosis) and predictive (determining efficacy of endocrine therapies) biomarker in breast cancer[112–114] ER status on immunohistochemistry (IHC) is widely used to help predict which patients will respond to endocrine therapy, yet its predictive value is still limited, with up to 50% of ER-positive breast cancers not responding to endocrine therapy.[115] Thus, while ER IHC is highly useful, better biomarkers for selecting patients for endocrine therapy are still needed.

^{18}F-FES is composed of 17-beta estradiol, a hormone which is physiologically expressed in all humans, radiolabeled with Fluorine-18, a positron emitter. ^{18}F-FES is used as a PET radiotracer, allowing for whole body in vivo localization of ER, which is available for ligand binding.[116] ^{18}F-FES PET allows sensitive whole-body, noninvasive detection of ER-positive malignancy[6] with a positive predictive value of 90% (95% CI 83%–94%) and a negative predictive value of 71% (95% CI 55%–83%).[117] The success of ^{18}F-FES has led to it becoming the first FDA-approved ER-targeting PET agent in 2020, under the brand name Cerianna (GE Healthcare, Chicago, IL).

Recently, the Society of Nuclear Medicine and Molecular Imaging has published Appropriate Use Criteria (AUC) for ^{18}F-FES PET.[118] It is important to note that the clinical scenarios appropriate for use of ^{18}F-FES differ from the clinical scenarios most commonly used for ^{18}F-FDG. Although ^{18}F-FDG has demonstrated value for systemic staging of newly diagnosed locally advanced disease, detection of disease recurrence, and measurement of treatment response, ^{18}F-FES has not yet been demonstrated to be highly effective in these situations.[118] Rather, substantial evidence has accumulated that ^{18}F-FES has value in its own unique clinical scenarios.[6,119]

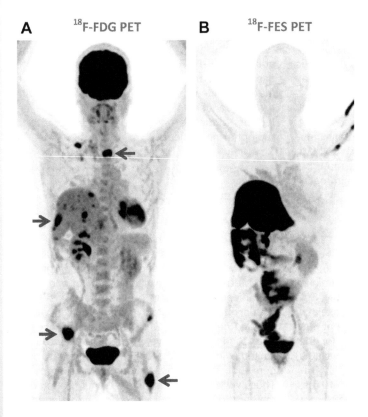

A ^{18}F-FDG PET **B** ^{18}F-FES PET

Fig. 3. Using ^{18}F-FES PET to identify a patient with metastatic ER-positive breast cancer that will likely not respond to endocrine therapy. (*A*) MIP image from an ^{18}F-FDG PET/CT in a 60-year-old woman with ER-positive, HER2-negative metastatic breast cancer with disease progression on first-line endocrine therapy, demonstrates multiple ^{18}F-FDG-avid osseous (*arrows*) and hepatic metastases. A clinical decision was to be made whether to start a second-line endocrine therapy agent or defer to chemotherapy. To help with this decision, an ^{18}F-FES PET/CT was performed. (*B*) MIP image from the ^{18}F-FES PET/CT demonstrates the known osseous disease on the ^{18}F-FDG PET is not ^{18}F-FES-avid. This suggests ER is not able to bind its estrogen ligand and subsequent endocrine-based therapy will not be efficacious. Treatment was shifted to chemotherapy. (37270377Gary A. Ulaner, Amy M. Fowler, Amy S. Clark, Hannah Linden, Estrogen Receptor-Targeted and Progesterone Receptor-Targeted PET for Patients with Breast Cancer,PET Clinics, 18 (4), 2023, 531-542, https://doi.org/10.1016/j.cpet.2023.04.008.)

First, ^{18}F-FES has been demonstrated as a highly successful predictive biomarker, identifying tumors that while ER-positive on IHC, are still unlikely to respond to endocrine therapies (**Fig. 3**). This may be due to the fact that not all ER visualized by IHC is available or functional for binding to its estrogen ligand.[6,116,120] At least 18 prospective trials, including 603 subjects, have demonstrated patients with metastatic breast cancer that are ER-positive on IHC, but are not ^{18}F-FES-avid, are highly unlikely to respond to endocrine-targeted therapies[121–125] (reviewed in[5]). This has led to the SNMMI AUC stating ^{18}F-FES is appropriate for assisting in selection of endocrine therapy in patient initial diagnosis of metastatic disease or after progression of metastatic disease.[118] This is a remarkable clinical indication for ^{18}F-FES PET. Although medical imaging for patients with breast cancer has primarily been used to detect malignancy, assess extent of disease, and evaluate therapy response,[35] imaging was not previously valuable in assisting in the selection of appropriate therapies for patients with breast cancer.[116] Because more than 100,000 patients currently struggle with ER-positive metastatic breast cancer,[126] the use of ^{18}F-FES may help the selection of appropriate therapy, and prevent futile endocrine therapies, in large numbers of patients.

Other clinical scenarios appropriate for utilization of ^{18}F-FES PET include assessing lesions that are difficult or dangerous to biopsy[6] and assessing lesions when other tests are inconclusive.[127–130] ^{18}F-FES PET has also demonstrated use as a pharmacodynamic biomarker in early clinical trials of new ER-targeting therapies, able to determine the biological effective dose of these drugs and assist in the selection of appropriate drug dosages for higher phase clinical trials. This has been successfully accomplished with both FDA-approved drugs such as fulvestrant[124] and elacestrant,[131] as well as novel ER-targeted drugs that are in clinical development.[132,133]

Substantial research is ongoing for additional applications of ER-targeted PET imaging. One such area of investigation is ILC tumors, discussed above as less FDG-avid than IDC tumor. As nearly all ILC are ER-positive,[1,10] several clinical trials have investigated ^{18}F-FES as an alternative radiotracer for this histology of breast cancer. Data are still growing, but some encouraging trials suggest ^{18}F-FES may be valuable for imaging ILC.[134–136] A developing joint SNMMI and EANM guideline recommends using ^{18}F-FES PET/CT in the above-mentioned clinical scenarios.

NOVEL POSITRON EMISSION TOMOGRAPHY RADIOTRACERS IN CLINICAL TRIALS

The next quarter century of PET for patients with breast cancer is likely to be as exciting and productive as the one earlier. Next generating endocrine receptor-targeting PET radiotracers may include 4-fluoro-11β-methoxy-16α-^{18}F-fluoroestradiol, for which early trials suggested improved tumor-to-background imaging[137] and 21-[^{18}F]fluorofuranyl-norprogesterone, which targets the progesterone receptor (PR), a downstream effector of ER.[138] HER2-targeted agents provide another opportunity for PET targeting of a specific molecule to help guide therapy selection. Multiple HER2-targeted therapies prolong survival in patients with HER2-positive tumors.[139] There is particular renewed interest in HER2-targeting imaging given the recent success of HER2-targeted therapies in newly defined "HER2-low" tumors, allowing possible HER2-targeted therapy for tumors that previously would not be considered eligible.[140–142] Multiple HER2-targeted PET radiotracers are currently in clinical trials.[7,143,144] Anti-1-amino-3-18F-fluorocyclobutane-1-carboxylic acid is an amino acid analog PET radiotracer, approved for prostate cancer imaging. Initial studies suggest it may have applications in ILC.[145,146] Cancer-associated fibroblasts found in most breast malignancies and other cancers often express fibroblast activation protein (FAP).[147,148] PET radiotracers targeting FAP are of growing interest with several recent successes in patients with breast cancer.[147,148]

TECHNOLOGIC DEVELOPMENTS

Technological developments during the past quarter century have also greatly improved the sensitivity and accuracy of PET imaging. Installation of the digital systems using silicon photomultipliers has improved performance and imaging quality.[149,150] Total-body PET/CT allows increased sensitivity and dynamic/pharmacokinetic studies of the entire body.[150,151] Both digital and total-body PET/CT enable faster acquisition or lower administered activity. PET/MRI is being evaluated for breast cancer diagnosis, staging, and treatment response.[73,152] Artificial intelligence software, semiquantification algorithms and radiomics analysis are aiming to better define radiotracer uptake as predictive and prognostic biomarkers.[112,153]

SUMMARY

The discussion of the transformative nature of PET imaging in oncology would be incomplete without a discussion of the role of PET in the care of patients with breast cancer. During the past quarter-century, PET imaging has demonstrated remarkable and growing success in the management of patients with breast cancer. Clearly, the most influential PET radiotracer to date has been ^{18}F-FDG, which has prospective trial evidence supporting its use for systemic staging of breast cancer at initial diagnosis, detecting recurrent disease, and measuring treatment response after therapy. Bone imaging with ^{18}F-NaF has increased and decreased over time, although may still be used for more sensitive detection of bone metastases than gamma bone scan agents. The more recently FDA-approved ^{18}F-FES has its own unique clinical uses, including selection of appropriate patients for endocrine-targeted therapies, assessing lesions that are difficult or dangerous to biopsy, and assessing lesions when other tests are inconclusive. Many investigational radiotracers may further the application of PET in patients with breast cancer by targeting PR, HER2, or FAP. The next quarter-century portends to be as exciting and clinically valuable as the last.

CLINICS CARE POINTS

- There are prospective data supporting the use 18F-FDG PET for systemic staging of patients with newly diagnosed large or locally advanced disease (stages IIB–IIIC), detecting sites of recurrence, and monitoring treatment response.

- ^{18}F-FDG PET is mostly recommended for the invasive ductal carcinoma histology because invasive lobular carcinoma (ILC) histology has lower FDG-avidity and less supporting data.

- ^{18}F-NaF has superior sensitivity for osseous metastases than 99mTc-MDP or CT.

- Appropriate use criteria for ^{18}F-FES PET support its use for selecting patients for use of endocrine therapies, assessing lesions that are difficult or dangerous to biopsy, and assessing lesions when other tests are inconclusive.

- There are many additional PET radiotracers under investigation for patients with breast cancer.

DISCLOSURE

G.A. Ulaner discloses grants, consulting fees, honoraria, and/or speaker fees from Curium, GE Heathcare, Lantheus, Nuclidium, POINT, RayzeBio, Briacell, and ImaginAb. S.C. Vaz has no disclosures to declare. D. Groheux has no disclosures to declare.

REFERENCES

1. Perou CM, Sorlie T, Eisen MB, et al. Molecular portraits of human breast tumours. Nature 2000; 406(6797):747–52.
2. Sorlie T, Perou CM, Tibshirani R, et al. Gene expression patterns of breast carcinomas distinguish tumor subclasses with clinical implications. Proc Natl Acad Sci U S A 2001;98(19):10869–74.
3. Houssami N, Macaskill P, von Minckwitz G, et al. Meta-analysis of the association of breast cancer subtype and pathologic complete response to neoadjuvant chemotherapy. Eur J Cancer 2012;48(18): 3342–54.
4. Groheux D, Espie M, Giacchetti S, et al. Performance of FDG PET/CT in the clinical management of breast cancer. Radiology 2013;266(2):388–405.
5. Ulaner GA. 16α-18F-fluoro-17β-Fluoroestradiol (FES): clinical applications for patients with breast cancer. Semin Nucl Med 2022;52:574–83.
6. Kurland BF, Wiggins JR, Coche A, et al. Whole-body characterization of estrogen receptor status in metastatic breast cancer with 16α-18F-Fluoro-17β-Estradiol positron emission tomography: meta-analysis and recommendations for integration into clinical applications. Oncol 2020;25(10): 835–44.
7. Ducharme M, Mansur A, Sligh L, et al. Human epidermal growth factor receptor 2/human epidermal growth factor receptor 3 PET imaging: challenges and opportunities. Pet Clin 2023;18(4): 543–55.
8. Provenzano E, Ulaner GA, Chin SF. Molecular classification of breast cancer. Pet Clin 2018;13(3): 325–38.
9. Roy M, Fowler AM, Ulaner GA, et al. Molecular classification of breast cancer. Pet Clin 2023; 18(4):441–58.
10. Ciriello G, Gatza ML, Beck AH, et al. Comprehensive molecular portraits of invasive lobular breast cancer. Cell 2015;163(2):506–19.
11. Berg WA, Gutierrez L, NessAiver MS, et al. Diagnostic accuracy of mammography, clinical examination, US, and MR imaging in preoperative assessment of breast cancer. Radiology 2004; 233(3):830–49.
12. Lopez JK, Bassett LW. Invasive lobular carcinoma of the breast: spectrum of mammographic, US, and MR imaging findings. Radiographics 2009; 29(1):165–76.
13. Avril N, Menzel M, Dose J, et al. Glucose metabolism of breast cancer assessed by 18F-FDG PET: histologic and immunohistochemical tissue analysis. J Nucl Med 2001;42(1):9–16.
14. Cecil K, Huppert L, Mukhtar R, et al. Metabolic positron emission tomography in breast cancer. Pet Clin 2023;18(4):473–85.
15. Pauwels EK, Ribeiro MJ, Stoot JH, et al. FDG accumulation and tumor biology. Nucl Med Biol 1998; 25(4):317–22.
16. Minn H, Soini I. [18F]fluorodeoxyglucose scintigraphy in diagnosis and follow up of treatment in advanced breast cancer. Eur J Nucl Med 1989; 15(2):61–6.
17. Groheux D, Groheux D. Breast cancer systemic staging (comparison of computed tomography, bone scan, and 18F-fluorodeoxyglucose PET/ computed tomography) FDG-PET/CT for primary staging and detection of recurrence of breast cancer. Pet Clin 2023;52(5):508–19.
18. Ulaner GA. PET/CT for patients with breast cancer: where is the clinical impact? AJR Am J Roentgenol 2019;213(2):254–65.
19. Groheux D. FDG-PET/CT for primary staging and detection of recurrence of breast cancer. Semin Nucl Med 2022;52(5):508–19.
20. Groheux D, Moretti JL, Baillet G, et al. Effect of (18) F-FDG PET/CT imaging in patients with clinical stage II and III breast cancer. Int J Radiat Oncol Biol Phys 2008;71(3):695–704.
21. Dayes IS, Metser U, Hodgson N, et al. Impact of (18) F-Labeled fluorodeoxyglucose positron emission tomography-computed tomography versus conventional staging in patients with locally advanced breast cancer. J Clin Oncol 2023. https://doi.org/ 10.1200/jco.23.00249. Jco2300249.
22. Groheux D, Hindie E, Delord M, et al. Prognostic impact of (18)FDG-PET-CT findings in clinical stage III and IIB breast cancer. J Natl Cancer Institute 2012;104(24):1879–87.
23. Hildebrandt MG, Gerke O, Baun C, et al. [18F]Fluorodeoxyglucose (FDG)-Positron Emission Tomography (PET)/computed tomography (CT) in suspected recurrent breast cancer: a prospective comparative study of dual-time-point FDG-PET/ CT, contrast-enhanced CT, and bone scintigraphy. J Clin Oncol 2016;34(16):1889–97.
24. Ulaner GA, Saura C, Piha-Paul SA, et al. Impact of FDG PET imaging for expanding patient eligibility and measuring treatment response in a genome-driven basket trial of the pan-HER kinase inhibitor, neratinib. Clin Cancer Res 2019;3(5):666–71.
25. Kitajima K, Higuchi T, Yamakado K, et al. Early assessment of tumor response using (18)F-FDG PET/CT after one cycle of systemic therapy in

patients with recurrent and metastatic breast cancer. Hell J Nucl Med 2022;25(2):155–62.

26. Makhlin I, Korhonen KE, Martin ML, et al. (18)F-FDG PET/CT for the evaluation of therapy response in hormone receptor-positive bone-dominant metastatic breast cancer. Radiol Imaging Cancer 2022; 4(6):e220032.

27. Vogsen M, Harbo F, Jakobsen NM, et al. Response monitoring in metastatic breast cancer: a prospective study comparing (18)F-FDG PET/CT with conventional CT. J Nucl Med 2023;64(3):355–61.

28. Vogsen M, Naghavi-Behzad M, Harbo FG, et al. 2-[(18)F]FDG-PET/CT is a better predictor of survival than conventional CT: a prospective study of response monitoring in metastatic breast cancer. Sci Rep 2023;13(1):5552.

29. Lebron-Zapata L, Jochelson MS. Overview of breast cancer screening and diagnosis. Pet Clin 2018;13(3):301–23.

30. Avril N, Rose CA, Schelling M, et al. Breast imaging with positron emission tomography and fluorine-18 fluorodeoxyglucose: use and limitations. J Clin Oncol 2000;18(20):3495–502.

31. Caldarella C, Treglia G, Giordano A. Diagnostic performance of dedicated positron emission mammography using fluorine-18-fluorodeoxyglucose in women with suspicious breast lesions: a meta-analysis. Clin Breast Cancer 2014;14(4):241–8.

32. Narayanan D, Berg WA. Dedicated breast gamma camera imaging and breast PET: current status and future directions. Pet Clin 2018;13(3):363–81.

33. Berg WA, Madsen KS, Schilling K, et al. Breast cancer: comparative effectiveness of positron emission mammography and MR imaging in presurgical planning for the ipsilateral breast. Radiology 2011;258(1):59–72.

34. Pinker K, Bogner W, Baltzer P, et al. Improved differentiation of benign and malignant breast tumors with multiparametric 18fluorodeoxyglucose positron emission tomography magnetic resonance imaging: a feasibility study. Clin Cancer Res 2014; 20(13):3540–9.

35. Moo TA, Sanford R, Dang C, et al. Overview of breast cancer therapy. Pet Clin 2018;13(3):339–54.

36. Veronesi U, Viale G, Paganelli G, et al. Sentinel lymph node biopsy in breast cancer: ten-year results of a randomized controlled study. Ann Surg 2010;251(4):595–600.

37. Wahl RL, Siegel BA, Coleman RE, et al. Prospective multicenter study of axillary nodal staging by positron emission tomography in breast cancer: a report of the staging breast cancer with PET Study Group. J Clin Oncol 2004;22(2):277–85.

38. Veronesi U, De Cicco C, Galimberti VE, et al. A comparative study on the value of FDG-PET and sentinel node biopsy to identify occult axillary metastases. Ann Oncol 2007;18(3):473–8.

39. Choi YJ, Shin YD, Kang YH, et al. The effects of preoperative (18)F-FDG PET/CT in breast cancer patients in comparison to the conventional imaging study. J Breast Cancer 2012;15(4):441–8.

40. Shien T, Akashi-Tanaka S, Yoshida M, et al. Evaluation of axillary status in patients with breast cancer using thin-section CT. Int J Clin Oncol 2008;13(4): 314–9.

41. Alberini JL, Lerebours F, Wartski M, et al. 18F-fluorodeoxyglucose positron emission tomography/computed tomography (FDG-PET/CT) imaging in the staging and prognosis of inflammatory breast cancer. Cancer 2009;115(21):5038–47.

42. Fuster D, Duch J, Paredes P, et al. Preoperative staging of large primary breast cancer with [18F] fluorodeoxyglucose positron emission tomography/computed tomography compared with conventional imaging procedures. J Clin Oncol 2008; 26(29):4746–51.

43. Groheux D, Giacchetti S, Espie M, et al. The yield of 18F-FDG PET/CT in patients with clinical stage IIA, IIB, or IIIA breast cancer: a prospective study. J Nucl Med 2011;52(10):1526–34.

44. Ulaner GA, Castillo R, Goldman DA, et al. (18)F-FDG-PET/CT for systemic staging of newly diagnosed triple-negative breast cancer. Eur J Nucl Med Mol Imaging 2016;43(11):1937–44.

45. Ulaner GA, Castillo R, Wills J, et al. 18F-FDG-PET/CT for systemic staging of patients with newly diagnosed ER-positive and HER2-positive breast cancer. Eur J Nucl Med Mol Imaging 2017;44(9): 1420–7.

46. Riedl CC, Slobod E, Jochelson M, et al. Retrospective analysis of 18F-FDG PET/CT for staging asymptomatic breast cancer patients younger than 40 years. J Nucl Med 2014;55(10):1578–83.

47. Bruckmann NM, Kirchner J, Morawitz J, et al. Prospective comparison of CT and 18F-FDG PET/MRI in N and M staging of primary breast cancer patients: initial results. PLoS One 2021;16(12): e0260804.

48. Morawitz J, Bruckmann NM, Dietzel F, et al. Comparison of nodal staging between CT, MRI, and [(18)F]-FDG PET/MRI in patients with newly diagnosed breast cancer. Eur J Nucl Med Mol Imaging 2022;49(3):992–1001.

49. Heusner TA, Kuemmel S, Umutlu L, et al. Breast cancer staging in a single session: whole-body PET/CT mammography. J Nucl Med 2008;49(8): 1215–22.

50. Segaert I, Mottaghy F, Ceyssens S, et al. Additional value of PET-CT in staging of clinical stage IIB and III breast cancer. Breast J 2010;16(6):617–24.

51. Yang WT, Le-Petross HT, Macapinlac H, et al. Inflammatory breast cancer: PET/CT, MRI, mammography, and sonography findings. Breast Cancer Res Treat 2008;109(3):417–26.

52. Cochet A, Dygai-Cochet I, Riedinger JM, et al. ^{18}F-FDG PET/CT provides powerful prognostic stratification in the primary staging of large breast cancer when compared with conventional explorations. Eur J Nucl Med Mol Imaging 2014;41(3):428–37.

53. Jacene HA, DiPiro PJ, Bellon J, et al. Discrepancy between FDG-PET/CT and contrast-enhanced CT in the staging of patients with inflammatory breast cancer: implications for treatment planning. Breast Cancer Res Treat 2020;181(2):383–90.

54. Ko H, Baghdadi Y, Love C, et al. Clinical utility of 18F-FDG PET/CT in staging localized breast cancer before initiating preoperative systemic therapy. J Natl Compr Cancer Netw 2020;18(9):1240–6.

55. Han S, Choi JY. Impact of 18F-FDG PET, PET/CT, and PET/MRI on staging and management as an initial staging modality in breast cancer: a systematic review and meta-analysis. Clin Nucl Med 2021; 46(4):271–82.

56. Catalano OA, Nicolai E, Rosen BR, et al. Comparison of CE-FDG-PET/CT with CE-FDG-PET/MR in the evaluation of osseous metastases in breast cancer patients. Br J Cancer 2015;112(9):1452–60.

57. Botsikas D, Bagetakos I, Picarra M, et al. What is the diagnostic performance of 18-FDG-PET/MR compared to PET/CT for the N- and M- staging of breast cancer? Eur Radiol 2019;29(4):1787–98.

58. Melsaether AN, Raad RA, Pujara AC, et al. Comparison of whole-body (18)F FDG PET/MR imaging and whole-body (18)F FDG PET/CT in terms of lesion detection and radiation dose in patients with breast cancer. Radiology 2016;281(1):193–202.

59. Dashevsky BZ, Goldman DA, Parsons M, et al. Appearance of untreated bone metastases from breast cancer on FDG PET/CT: importance of histologic subtype. Eur J Nucl Med Mol Imaging 2015; 42(11):1666–73.

60. Hogan MP, Goldman DA, Dashevsky B, et al. Comparison of 18F-FDG PET/CT for systemic staging of newly diagnosed invasive lobular carcinoma versus invasive ductal carcinoma. J Nucl Med 2015;56(11):1674–80.

61. Gradishar WJ, Moran MS, Abraham J, et al. NCCN Guidelines® Insights: Breast Cancer, Version 4.2023. J Natl Compr Canc Netw 2023;21(6): 594–608.

62. Gradishar WJ, Moran MS, Abraham J, et al. NCCN Guidelines® insights: breast cancer, version 4.2023. J Natl Compr Cancer Netw 2023;21(6): 594–608.

63. Cochet A, David S, Moodie K, et al. The utility of 18 F-FDG PET/CT for suspected recurrent breast cancer: impact and prognostic stratification. Cancer Imag 2014;14(1):13.

64. Vogsen M, Jensen JD, Gerke O, et al. Benefits and harms of implementing [(18)F]FDG-PET/CT for diagnosing recurrent breast cancer: a prospective clinical study. EJNMMI Res 2021;11(1):93.

65. Radan L, Ben-Haim S, Bar-Shalom R, et al. The role of FDG-PET/CT in suspected recurrence of breast cancer. Cancer 2006;107(11):2545–51.

66. Schmidt GP, Baur-Melnyk A, Haug A, et al. Comprehensive imaging of tumor recurrence in breast cancer patients using whole-body MRI at 1.5 and 3 T compared to FDG-PET-CT. Eur J Radiol 2008;65(1):47–58.

67. Evangelista L, Baretta Z, Vinante L, et al. Tumour markers and FDG PET/CT for prediction of disease relapse in patients with breast cancer. Eur J Nucl Med Mol Imaging 2011;38(2):293–301.

68. Champion L, Brain E, Giraudet AL, et al. Breast cancer recurrence diagnosis suspected on tumor marker rising: value of whole-body 18FDG-PET/CT imaging and impact on patient management. Cancer 2011;117(8):1621–9.

69. Dirisamer A, Halpern BS, Flory D, et al. Integrated contrast-enhanced diagnostic whole-body PET/CT as a first-line restaging modality in patients with suspected metastatic recurrence of breast cancer. Eur J Radiol 2010;73(2):294–9.

70. Pan L, Han Y, Sun X, et al. FDG-PET and other imaging modalities for the evaluation of breast cancer recurrence and metastases: a meta-analysis. J Cancer Res Clin Oncol 2010;136(7):1007–22.

71. Pennant M, Takwoingi Y, Pennant L, et al. A systematic review of positron emission tomography (PET) and positron emission tomography/computed tomography (PET/CT) for the diagnosis of breast cancer recurrence. Health Technol Assess 2010;14(50):1–103.

72. Xiao Y, Wang L, Jiang X, et al. Diagnostic efficacy of 18F-FDG-PET or PET/CT in breast cancer with suspected recurrence: a systematic review and meta-analysis. Nucl Med Commun 2016;37(11): 1180–8.

73. Fowler AM, Strigel RM. Clinical advances in PET–MRI for breast cancer. Lancet Oncol 2022;23(1):e32–43.

74. Kirchner J, Martin O, Umutlu L, et al. Impact of 18F-FDG PET/MR on therapeutic management in high risk primary breast cancer patients – a prospective evaluation of staging algorithms. Eur J Radiol 2020; 128:108975.

75. Schelling M, Avril N, Nahrig J, et al. Positron emission tomography using [(18)F]Fluorodeoxyglucose for monitoring primary chemotherapy in breast cancer. J Clin Oncol 2000;18(8):1689–95.

76. Schwarz-Dose J, Untch M, Tiling R, et al. Monitoring primary systemic therapy of large and locally advanced breast cancer by using sequential positron emission tomography imaging with [18F]fluorodeoxyglucose. J Clin Oncol 2009;27(4):535–41.

77. Humbert O, Berriolo-Riedinger A, Riedinger JM, et al. Changes in 18F-FDG tumor metabolism after

a first course of neoadjuvant chemotherapy in breast cancer: influence of tumor subtypes. Ann Oncol 2012;23(10):2572–7.

78. Groheux D, Hindie E, Giacchetti S, et al. Triple-negative breast cancer: early assessment with 18F-FDG PET/CT during neoadjuvant chemotherapy identifies patients who are unlikely to achieve a pathologic complete response and are at a high risk of early relapse. J Nucl Med 2012; 53(2):249–54.

79. Humbert O, Cochet A, Riedinger JM, et al. HER2-positive breast cancer: (1)(8)F-FDG PET for early prediction of response to trastuzumab plus taxane-based neoadjuvant chemotherapy. Eur J Nucl Med Mol Imaging 2014;41(8):1525–33.

80. Groheux D, Giacchetti S, Delord M, et al. Prognostic impact of 18F-FDG PET/CT staging and of pathological response to neoadjuvant chemotherapy in triple-negative breast cancer. Eur J Nucl Med Mol Imaging 2015;42(3):377–85.

81. Groheux D, Hatt M, Hindie E, et al. Estrogen receptor-positive/human epidermal growth factor receptor 2-negative breast tumors: early prediction of chemosensitivity with (18)F-fluorodeoxyglucose positron emission tomography/computed tomography during neoadjuvant chemotherapy. Cancer 2013;119(11):1960–8.

82. Groheux D. Role of fludeoxyglucose in breast cancer: treatment response. Pet Clin 2018;13(3): 395–414.

83. Connolly RM, Leal JP, Solnes L, et al. Updated results of TBCRC026: phase II trial correlating standardized uptake value with pathological complete response to pertuzumab and trastuzumab in breast cancer. J Clin Oncol 2021;39(20):2247–56.

84. Han S, Choi JY. Prognostic value of (18)F-FDG PET and PET/CT for assessment of treatment response to neoadjuvant chemotherapy in breast cancer: a systematic review and meta-analysis. Breast Cancer Res 2020;22(1):119.

85. Coudert B, Pierga JY, Mouret-Reynier MA, et al. Use of [(18)F]-FDG PET to predict response to neoadjuvant trastuzumab and docetaxel in patients with HER2-positive breast cancer, and addition of bevacizumab to neoadjuvant trastuzumab and docetaxel in [(18)F]-FDG PET-predicted non-responders (AVATAXHER): an open-label, randomised phase 2 trial. Lancet Oncol 2014;15(13): 1493–502.

86. Pérez-García JM, Gebhart G, Borrego MR, et al. Trastuzumab and pertuzumab without chemotherapy in early-stage HER2+ breast cancer: a plain language summary of the PHERGain study. Future Oncol 2022;18(33):3677–88.

87. Pérez-García JM, Gebhart G, Ruiz Borrego M, et al. Chemotherapy de-escalation using an (18)F-FDG-PET-based pathological response-adapted strategy in patients with HER2-positive early breast cancer (PHERGain): a multicentre, randomised, open-label, non-comparative, phase 2 trial. Lancet Oncol 2021;22(6):858–71.

88. Groheux D, Mankoff D, Espie M, et al. (1)(8)F-FDG PET/CT in the early prediction of pathological response in aggressive subtypes of breast cancer: review of the literature and recommendations for use in clinical trials. Eur J Nucl Med Mol Imaging 2016;43(5):983–93.

89. Johnson P, Federico M, Kirkwood A, et al. Adapted treatment guided by interim PET-CT scan in advanced Hodgkin's lymphoma. N Engl J Med 2016;374(25):2419–29.

90. Gennari A, Donati S, Salvadori B, et al. Role of 2-[18F]-fluorodeoxyglucose (FDG) positron emission tomography (PET) in the early assessment of response to chemotherapy in metastatic breast cancer patients. Clin Breast Cancer 2000;1(2): 156–61 [discussion: 162–163].

91. Dose Schwarz J, Bader M, Jenicke L, et al. Early prediction of response to chemotherapy in metastatic breast cancer using sequential 18F-FDG PET. J Nucl Med 2005;46(7):1144–50.

92. Eisenhauer EA, Therasse P, Bogaerts J, et al. New response evaluation criteria in solid tumours: revised RECIST guideline (version 1.1). European J Cancer 2009;45(2):228–47.

93. Hutchings M, Barrington SF. PET/CT for therapy response assessment in lymphoma. J Nucl Med 2009;50(Suppl 1):21S–30S.

94. Wahl RL, Jacene H, Kasamon Y, et al. From RECIST to PERCIST: evolving considerations for PET response criteria in solid tumors. J Nucl Med 2009;50(Suppl 1). 122S-150S.

95. Mayer IA, Abramson VG, Isakoff SJ, et al. Stand up to cancer phase Ib study of pan-phosphoinositide-3-kinase inhibitor buparlisib with letrozole in estrogen receptor-positive/human epidermal growth factor receptor 2-negative metastatic breast cancer. J Clin Oncol 2014;32(12):1202–9.

96. Lin NU, Guo H, Yap JT, et al. Phase II study of lapatinib in combination with trastuzumab in patients with human epidermal growth factor receptor 2-positive metastatic breast cancer: clinical outcomes and predictive value of early [18F]Fluorodeoxyglucose positron emission tomography imaging (TBCRC 003). J Clin Oncol 2015;33(24): 2623–31.

97. Du Y, Cullum I, Illidge TM, et al. Fusion of metabolic function and morphology: sequential [18F]fluorodeoxyglucose positron-emission tomography/computed tomography studies yield new insights into the natural history of bone metastases in breast cancer. J Clin Oncol 2007;25(23):3440–7.

98. Tateishi U, Gamez C, Dawood S, et al. Bone metastases in patients with metastatic breast cancer:

morphologic and metabolic monitoring of response to systemic therapy with integrated PET/CT. Radiology 2008;247(1):189–96.

99. Riedl CC, Pinker K, Ulaner GA, et al. Comparison of FDG-PET/CT and contrast-enhanced CT for monitoring therapy response in patients with metastatic breast cancer. Eur J Nucl Med Mol Imaging 2017; 44(9):1428–37.

100. Naghavi-Behzad M, Vogsen M, Vester RM, et al. Response monitoring in metastatic breast cancer: a comparison of survival times between FDG-PET/CT and CE-CT. Br J Cancer 2022;126(9): 1271–9.

101. Muzahir S, Ulaner GA, Schuster DM. Evaluation of treatment response in patients with breast cancer. Pet Clin 2023;18(4):517–30.

102. Grant FD, Fahey FH, Packard AB, et al. Skeletal PET with 18F-fluoride: applying new technology to an old tracer. J Nucl Med 2008;49(1):68–78.

103. Czernin J, Satyamurthy N, Schiepers C. Molecular mechanisms of bone 18F-NaF deposition. J Nucl Med 2010;51(12):1826–9.

104. Schirrmeister H, Guhlmann A, Kotzerke J, et al. Early detection and accurate description of extent of metastatic bone disease in breast cancer with fluoride ion and positron emission tomography. J Clin Oncol 1999;17(8):2381–9.

105. Even-Sapir E, Metser U, Flusser G, et al. Assessment of malignant skeletal disease: initial experience with 18F-fluoride PET/CT and comparison between 18F-fluoride PET and 18F-fluoride PET/CT. J Nucl Med 2004;45(2):272–8.

106. Hillner BE, Siegel BA, Hanna L, et al. Impact of (18) F-Fluoride PET on intended management of patients with cancers other than prostate cancer: results from the national oncologic PET registry. J Nucl Med 2014;55(7):1054–61.

107. Hillner BE, Siegel BA, Hanna L, et al. 18F-fluoride PET used for treatment monitoring of systemic cancer therapy: results from the National Oncologic PET Registry. J Nucl Med 2015;56(2):222–8.

108. Bridges RL, Wiley CR, Christian JC, et al. An introduction to Na(18)F bone scintigraphy: basic principles, advanced imaging concepts, and case examples. J Nucl Med Technol 2007;35(2):64–76 [quiz: 78–9].

109. Wade AA, Scott JA, Kuter I, et al. Flare response in 18F-fluoride ion PET bone scanning. AJR Am J Roentgenol 2006;186(6):1783–6.

110. Peterson LM, O'Sullivan J, Wu QV, et al. Prospective study of serial (18)F-FDG PET and (18)F-Fluoride PET to predict time to skeletal-related events, time to progression, and survival in patients with bone-dominant metastatic breast cancer. J Nucl Med 2018;59(12):1823–30.

111. Hwang KT, Kim J, Jung J, et al. Impact of breast cancer subtypes on prognosis of women with operable invasive breast cancer: a population-based study using SEER database. Clin Cancer Res 2019;25(6):1970–9.

112. Ulaner GA, Riedl CC, Dickler MN, et al. Molecular imaging of biomarkers in breast cancer. J Nucl Med 2016;57(Suppl 1). 53S-59S.

113. Harris L, Fritsche H, Mennel R, et al. American Society of Clinical Oncology 2007 update of recommendations for the use of tumor markers in breast cancer. J Clin Oncol 2007;25(33):5287–312.

114. (EBCTCG) EBCTCG. Effects of chemotherapy and hormonal therapy for early breast cancer on recurrence and 15-year survival: an overview of the randomised trials. Lancet 2005;365(9472):1687–717.

115. Davies C, Godwin J, Gray R, et al. Relevance of breast cancer hormone receptors and other factors to the efficacy of adjuvant tamoxifen: patient-level meta-analysis of randomised trials. Lancet 2011; 378(9793):771–84.

116. Katzenellenbogen JA. The quest for improving the management of breast cancer by functional imaging: the discovery and development of 16α-[(18) F]fluoroestradiol (FES), a PET radiotracer for the estrogen receptor, a historical review. Nucl Med Biol 2021;92:24–37.

117. van Geel JJL, Boers J, Elias SG, et al. Clinical validity of 16α-[(18)F]Fluoro-17β-Estradiol positron emission tomography/computed tomography to assess estrogen receptor status in newly diagnosed metastatic breast cancer. J Clin Oncol 2022;40(31):3642–52.

118. Ulaner GA, Mankoff DA, Clark AS, et al. Summary: appropriate use criteria for estrogen receptor-targeted PET Imaging with 16α-(18)F-Fluoro-17β-Fluoroestradiol. J Nucl Med 2023;64(3):351–4.

119. Ulaner GA, Fowler AM, Clark AS, et al. Estrogen receptor-targeted and progesterone receptor-targeted PET for patients with breast cancer. Pet Clin 2023. https://doi.org/10.1016/j.cpet.2023.04. 008.

120. Linden HM, Peterson LM, Fowler AM. Clinical potential of estrogen and progesterone receptor imaging. Pet Clin 2018;13(3):415–22.

121. Mortimer JE, Dehdashti F, Siegel BA, et al. Positron emission tomography with 2-[18F]Fluoro-2-deoxy-D-glucose and 16alpha-[18F]fluoro-17beta-estradiol in breast cancer: correlation with estrogen receptor status and response to systemic therapy. Clin Cancer Res 1996;2(6):933–9.

122. Dehdashti F, Flanagan FL, Mortimer JE, et al. Positron emission tomographic assessment of "metabolic flare" to predict response of metastatic breast cancer to antiestrogen therapy. Eur J Nucl Med 1999;26(1):51–6.

123. Linden HM, Stekhova SA, Link JM, et al. Quantitative fluoroestradiol positron emission tomography

imaging predicts response to endocrine treatment in breast cancer. J Clin Oncol 2006;24(18):2793–9.

124. van Kruchten M, de Vries EG, Glaudemans AW, et al. Measuring residual estrogen receptor availability during fulvestrant therapy in patients with metastatic breast cancer. Cancer Discov 2015; 5(1):72–81.

125. Boers J, Venema CM, de Vries EFJ, et al. Molecular imaging to identify patients with metastatic breast cancer who benefit from endocrine treatment combined with cyclin-dependent kinase inhibition. Eur J Cancer 2020;126:11–20.

126. Mariotto AB, Etzioni R, Hurlbert M, et al. Estimation of the number of women living with metastatic breast cancer in the United States. Cancer Epidemiol Biomarkers Prev 2017;26(6):809–15.

127. van Kruchten M, Glaudemans AW, de Vries EF, et al. PET imaging of estrogen receptors as a diagnostic tool for breast cancer patients presenting with a clinical dilemma. J Nucl Med 2012;53(2): 182–90.

128. Sun Y, Yang Z, Zhang Y, et al. The preliminary study of 16α-[18F]fluoroestradiol PET/CT in assisting the individualized treatment decisions of breast cancer patients. PLoS One 2015;10(1):e0116341.

129. Yang Z, Xie Y, Liu C, et al. The clinical value of (18) F-fluoroestradiol in assisting individualized treatment decision in dual primary malignancies. Quant Imaging Med Surg 2021;11(9):3956–65.

130. Boers J, Loudini N, Brunsch CL, et al. Value of (18) F-FES PET in solving clinical dilemmas in breast cancer patients: a retrospective study. J Nucl Med 2021;62(9):1214–20.

131. Jager A, de Vries EGE, der Houven van Oordt CWM, et al. A phase 1b study evaluating the effect of elacestrant treatment on estrogen receptor availability and estradiol binding to the estrogen receptor in metastatic breast cancer lesions using (18)F-FES PET/CT imaging. Breast Cancer Res 2020;22(1):97.

132. Wang Y, Ayres KL, Goldman DA, et al. 18F-Fluoroestradiol PET/CT measurement of estrogen receptor suppression during a phase i trial of the novel estrogen receptor-targeted therapeutic GDC-0810: using an imaging biomarker to guide drug dosage in subsequent trials. Clin Cancer Res 2017;23(12):3053–60.

133. Iqbal R, Yaqub M, Oprea-Lager DE, et al. Biodistribution of (18)F-FES in patients with metastatic ER+ breast cancer undergoing treatment with rintodestrant (G1T48), a novel selective ER degrader. J Nucl Med 2022;63(5):694–9.

134. Ulaner GA, Jhaveri K, Chandarlapaty S, et al. Head-to-head evaluation of (18)F-FES and (18)F-FDG PET/CT in metastatic invasive lobular breast cancer. J Nucl Med 2021;62(3):326–31.

135. Covington MF, Hoffman JM, Morton KA, et al. Prospective pilot study of (18)F-Fluoroestradiol PET/CT in patients with invasive lobular carcinomas. AJR Am J Roentgenol 2023;1–12. https://doi.org/10.2214/ajr.22.28809.

136. Bottoni G, Fiz F, Puntoni M, et al. Diagnostic effectiveness of [(18)F]Fluoroestradiol PET/CT in oestrogen receptor-positive breast cancer: the key role of histopathology. Evidence from an international multicentre prospective study. Eur J Nucl Med Mol Imaging 2023;50(8):2477–85.

137. Paquette M, Lavallée É, Phoenix S, et al. Improved estrogen receptor assessment by PET using the novel radiotracer (18)F-4FMFES in estrogen receptor-positive breast cancer patients: an ongoing phase II clinical trial. J Nucl Med 2018; 59(2):197–203.

138. Dehdashti F, Wu N, Ma CX, et al. Association of PET-based estradiol-challenge test for breast cancer progesterone receptors with response to endocrine therapy. Nat Commun 2021;12(1):733.

139. Graff SL, Yan F, Abdou Y, et al. Newly approved and emerging agents in HER2-positive metastatic breast cancer trastuzumab deruxtecan in previously treated HER2-low advanced breast cancer. Clin Breast Cancer 2023;387(1):9–20.

140. Modi S, Saura C, Yamashita T, et al. Trastuzumab deruxtecan in previously treated HER2-positive breast cancer. N Engl J Med 2020;382(7):610–21.

141. Modi S, Jacot W, Yamashita T, et al. Trastuzumab deruxtecan in previously treated HER2-low advanced breast cancer. N Engl J Med 2022; 387(1):9–20.

142. Tarantino P, Viale G, Press MF, et al. ESMO expert consensus statements (ECS) on the definition, diagnosis, and management of HER2-low breast cancer. Ann Oncol 2023. https://doi.org/10.1016/j.annonc.2023.05.008.

143. Dijkers EC, Oude Munnink TH, Kosterink JG, et al. Biodistribution of 89Zr-trastuzumab and PET imaging of HER2-positive lesions in patients with metastatic breast cancer. Clin Pharmacol Ther 2010; 87(5):586–92.

144. Ulaner GA, Carrasquillo JA, Riedl CC, et al. Identification of HER2-positive metastases in patients with HER2-negative primary breast cancer by using HER2-targeted (89)Zr-Pertuzumab PET/CT. Radiology 2020;296(2):370–8.

145. Ulaner GA, Goldman DA, Gonen M, et al. Initial results of a prospective clinical trial of 18F-Fluciclovine PET/CT in newly diagnosed invasive ductal and invasive lobular breast cancers. J Nucl Med 2016;57(9):1350–6.

146. Tade FI, Cohen MA, Styblo TM, et al. Anti-3-18F-FACBC (18F-Fluciclovine) PET/CT of breast cancer: an exploratory study. J Nucl Med 2016;57(9):1357–63.

147. Backhaus P, Burg MC, Roll W, et al. Simultaneous FAPI PET/MRI targeting the fibroblast-activation protein for breast cancer. Radiology 2021204677. https://doi.org/10.1148/radiol.2021204677.

148. Elboga U, Sahin E, Kus T, et al. Superiority of (68) Ga-FAPI PET/CT scan in detecting additional lesions compared to (18)FDG PET/CT scan in breast cancer (68)Ga-FAPI PET/CT: tracer uptake in 28 different kinds of cancer. Ann Nucl Med 2021; 35(12):1321–31.

149. López-Mora DA, Carrió I, Flotats A. Digital PET vs analog PET: clinical implications? Semin Nucl Med 2022;52(3):302–11.

150. Alberts I, Sachpekidis C, Prenosil G, et al. Digital PET/CT allows for shorter acquisition protocols or reduced radiopharmaceutical dose in [(18)F]-FDG PET/CT. Ann Nucl Med 2021;35(4):485–92.

151. Katal S, Eibschutz LS, Saboury B, et al. Advantages and applications of total-body PET scanning. Diagnostics 2022;(2):12. https://doi.org/10.3390/diagnostics12020426.

152. Ruan D, Sun L. Diagnostic performance of PET/MRI in breast cancer: a systematic review and Bayesian bivariate meta-analysis. Clin Breast Cancer 2023;23(2):108–24.

153. Sollini M, Cozzi L, Ninatti G, et al. PET/CT radiomics in breast cancer: mind the step. Methods 2021; 188:122–32.

Quarter-Century PET/Computed Tomography Transformation of Oncology
Hepatobiliary and Pancreatic Cancer

Asha Kandathil, MBBS, DMRD, MD[a],*, Rathan Subramaniam, MD, PhD, MPH, MBA[b,c,d]

KEYWORDS

- Hepatocellular carcinoma • Cholangiocarcinoma • Gall bladder carcinoma • Pancreatic carcinoma
- FDG PET/CT

KEY POINTS

- [18F] Fluorodeoxyglucose[18]F-FDG) PET/CT can improve the staging accuracy and clinical management of patients with hepatobiliary and pancreatic cancers, by detection of unsuspected metastases.
- ^{18}F-FDG PET/CT metabolic parameters are valuable in predicting treatment response and survival.
- Metabolic response on ^{18}F-FDG PET/CT can predict preoperative pathologic response to neoadjuvant therapy in patients with pancreatic cancer and determine prognosis.
- Several novel non-FDG tracers, such as 68-Ga prostate-specific membrane antigen and ^{68}Ga-fibroblast activation protein inhibitor PET/CT, show promise for imaging hepatobiliary and pancreatic cancers with potential for radioligand therapy.

INTRODUCTION

Multiphase CT or MR imaging is the mainstay in diagnosis, staging, and surveillance of patients with hepatobiliary and pancreatic malignancies. [18F] Fluorodeoxyglucose (FDG) PET/CT offers added value in therapeutic decision-making and in determining prognosis. Several studies have shown that non-FDG tracers such as gallium-68 (^{68}Ga)-labeled fibroblast activation protein (FAP) inhibitor (FAPI) PET/CT have potential in diagnosis, staging, and possibly radioligand therapy of hepatobiliary and pancreatic malignancies.

HEPATOCELLULAR CARCINOMA

Worldwide, hepatocellular carcinoma (HCC) is the seventh most common malignancy and second most common cause of cancer mortality. Cirrhosis, primarily caused by alcoholism or chronic infection with hepatitis B virus or hepatitis C virus, is the critical risk factor for HCC.[1] Therapeutic options, which vary based on tumor stage and resectability, patient performance status, and degree of hepatic dysfunction, include resection, liver transplantation, radiofrequency ablation, radiotherapy, chemoembolization, targeted molecular therapy such as sorafenib, vascular endothelial growth factor (VEGF) receptor inhibitors, or immunotherapy.

Liver ultrasound is recommended as the primary surveillance modality for HCC.[2] A lesion detected on surveillance ultrasound is characterized and diagnosed by triple-phase helical CT or triple-phase dynamic contrast-enhanced MR imaging.[3] The National Comprehensive Cancer Network (NCCN)

[a] Department of Radiology, University of Texas Southwestern Medical Center, Dallas, TX, USA; [b] Faculty of Medicine, Nursing, Midwifery and Health Sciences, University of Notre Dame Australia, Sydney, Australia; [c] Department of Radiology, Duke University, Durham, NC, USA; [d] Department of Medicine, University of Otago Medical School, Dunedin, New Zealand
* Corresponding author.
E-mail address: Asha.Kandathil@utsouthwestern.edu

PET Clin 19 (2024) 163–175
https://doi.org/10.1016/j.cpet.2023.12.003
1556-8598/24/Published by Elsevier Inc.

guidelines do not recommend ^{18}F-FDG PET/CT for diagnosis, staging, or surveillance of patients with HCC.[4]

[18F] FLUORODEOXYGLUCOSE PET/ COMPUTED TOMOGRAPHY

^{18}F-FDG PET/CT is not currently used in the initial workup of HCC patients. It, however, plays a role in determining prognosis, detecting extrahepatic metastases, selecting liver transplantation candidates, and assessing residual tumors after local therapy of HCC. It has the advantage of surveying the entire body and becomes more valuable than CT and MR imaging in detecting nodal and distant metastases.

HCC accumulates ^{18}F-FDG to varying degrees due to differing amounts of FDG-6-phosphatase activity and glucose transporters. Therefore ^{18}F-FDG PET CT has limited sensitivity (50%–70%) for detecting intra-hepatic HCC.[5,6] In a retrospective study by Wudel and colleagues,[7] 43 of 67 (64%) of the HCCs accumulated FDG. In a prospective study by Park and colleagues,[8] the overall sensitivity of ^{18}F-FDG PET for the detection of primary HCC was 60.9%. This was however related to tumor size, number, and degree of differentiation. Larger number and size of tumors and poor tumor differentiation were significantly associated with increased sensitivity for detection of primary HCC on ^{18}F-FDG PET/CT. Elevated serum alpha-fetoprotein levels, an advanced tumor stage, and portal vein tumor thrombosis were also significantly associated with positive FDG-PET results.

In a prospective study by Seo and colleagues in 70 patients who underwent curative resection of HCC, standardized uptake values (SUVs) were significantly higher in poorly differentiated HCC (10.1 ± 6.5) than in well-differentiated HCCs (3.4 ± 1.4) and moderately differentiated HCCs (4.5 ± 1.8). Tumor-to-non-tumor SUV ratio (TNR) was significantly higher in poorly differentiated HCCs (3.9 ± 2.9) than in well-differentiated HCCs (1.1 ± 0.4) and moderately differentiated HCCs (1.6 ± 0.7).[9]

Staging: ^{18}F-FDG PET/CT is useful in evaluating extrahepatic metastases, despite its limited sensitivity in detecting primary HCC (**Fig. 1**). In a study by Sugiyama and colleagues,[10] 18F-FDG PET detected 83% of extrahepatic metastases larger than 1 cm and 13% of metastatic lesions ≤ 1 cm. Ho and colleagues[11] showed that ^{18}F-FDG PET/CT had a patient-based sensitivity of 79% and a lesion-based sensitivity of 77% in the detection of extrahepatic metastases, including lymph node, lung, and bone metastases. In the study by Wudel and colleagues, ^{18}F-FDG had the highest sensitivity (88%) in detecting HCC metastasis when the primary HCC tumor was also ^{18}F-FDG avid.[7] FDG-PET imaging had a clinically significant impact in 26 of 91 (28%) patients with HCC including detection of unsuspected metastatic disease in high-risk patients and liver transplant candidates.

Prognosis: ^{18}F-FDG PET/CT is useful in predicting prognosis of HCC patients. Well-differentiated

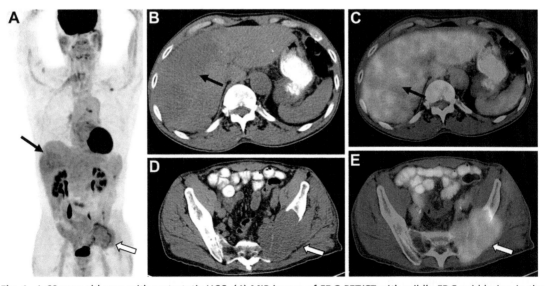

Fig. 1. A 68-year-old man with metastatic HCC. (*A*) MIP image of FDG PET/CT with mildly FDG-avid lesion in the right hepatic lobe (*narrow black arrow*) and left pelvis (*broad white arrow*). (*B, C*) CT and fused PET/CT images demonstrate FDG-avid hypodense hepatic mass with SUVmax 3 (*narrow black arrows*). (*D, E*) CT and fused PET/ CT images demonstrate large lytic lesion in the left iliac bone with FDG-avid soft tissue and SUVmax 2.5 (*broad white arrows*).

tumors tend to not accumulate ^{18}F-FDG, whereas the poorly differentiated and moderate-to-poorly differentiated tumors show increased ^{18}F-FDG uptake. In a meta-analysis of 22 studies on the prognostic role of pretreatment ^{18}F-FDG PET/CT on HCC patients, high tumor SUV and high tumor SUV/liver SUV ratio were associated with poor prognosis.[12] Kornberg and colleagues[13] showed that preoperative ^{18}F-FDG uptake was highly associated with the presence of poor tumor differentiation and microvascular invasion. In a retrospective review of 56 patients who had surgical resection of HCC, Cho and colleagues noted that SUVmax was higher ($\geq$4.9) in larger tumors and correlated with serum alpha-fetoprotein and recurrence rate.[14] As such, pretreatment ^{18}F-FDG PET has been shown to predict early recurrence after curative resection, liver transplantation, and local therapy such as radiofrequency ablation and transarterial chemoembolization (TACE).

Resection: Preoperative ^{18}F-FDG PET is helpful in predicting recurrence in HCC patients following liver resection.[15–17] Hatano and colleagues[15] showed that overall survival (OS) following resection (5-year survival rate: 63 vs 29%; median survival time: 2310 vs182 days) was significantly longer in patients with lower TNR than in those with higher SUV ratio (SUV ratio >2). In a study by Ahn and colleagues[16] in 93 patients with HCC who underwent resection, predictors of early tumor recurrence in less than a year were large tumor size ($\geq$5 cm), high TNR ($\geq$2), high SUV$_{tumor}$ ($\geq$4) **(Fig. 2)**.

Liver transplant: In liver transplantation for HCC, preoperative ^{18}F-FDG PET is a valuable tool in patient selection, helpful in predicting tumor recurrence.[13,18,19] Lee and colleagues found that the pretransplant TNR significantly predicted tumor recurrence, with a cutoff value of 1.15.[18] Kornberg and colleagues [13] found that transplant recipients

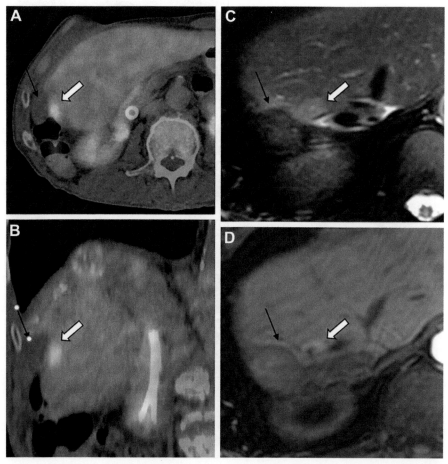

Fig. 2. 74-year-old man with local recurrence of resected HCC. (*A, B*) Axial and coronal-fused PET/CT images with FDG-avid local recurrence (*broad white arrows*) adjacent to the resection cavity (*narrow black arrow*). (*C*) T2W hyperintense lesion demonstrating peripheral arterial enhancement (*D*) adjacent to the resection cavity (*narrow black arrow*) on axial MR imaging is consistent with local tumor recurrence (*broad white arrows*).

outside the Milan criteria with no tumor FDG up-take had excellent recurrence-free survival (RFS) at 3 years comparable to recipients within the Milan criteria. In a study by Yang and colleagues[19] in 38 HCC patients who underwent liver transplantation, FDG uptake by tumor was associated with tumor recurrence even in patients who satisfied the Milan criteria. They suggest a cautious selection of PET-positive HCC patients for liver transplantation (**Fig. 3**).

Transarterial chemoembolization: Song and colleagues[20] found that ^{18}F-FDG PET predicted treatment response in patients who underwent TACE and systemic chemotherapy for HCC. The response rates in patients with a high tumor maximal SUV to the liver mean SUV ($Tsuv_{max}/Lsuv_{mean}$) ratio (≥ 1.90) were significantly better than those with a low SUV ratio (<1.90). In a study by Lee and colleagues[21] in 214 intermediate-to-advanced-stage HCC TACE or concurrent intra-arterial chemotherapy with external-beam radiotherapy (CCRT), tumor-to-normal liver ^{18}F-FDG uptake ratio (TLR) was an independent prognostic factor for survival. When the TLR was greater than 2.0, patients treated with CCRT showed significantly better progression free survival (PFS) and overall survival (OS) than those treated with TACE. They concluded that ^{18}F-FDG PET/CT may help determine the treatment modality for intermediate-to-advanced-stage HCCs (**Fig. 4**).

Sorafenib: Sorafenib, a multitargeted kinase inhibitor with antiproliferative and anti-angiogenic effects, has survival benefits over supportive care in advanced HCC. The drug targets the Raf/MAPK/ERK signaling pathway and the tyrosine kinase VEGFR-2 and -3 and PDGF receptors. In a study by Lee and colleagues[22] in 30 patients with HCC treated with sorafenib, patients with SUV less than 5 showed significantly longer OS and progression-free survival than those with SUV ≥ 5.00.

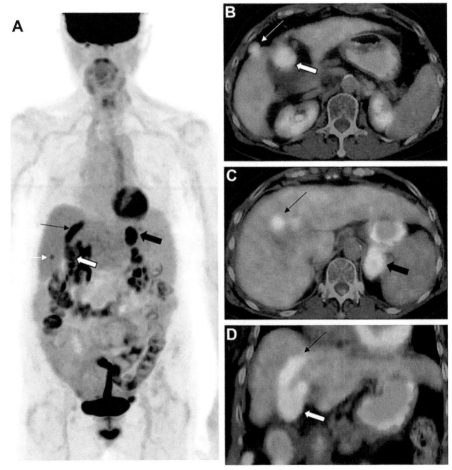

Fig. 3. A 82-year-old woman with recurrent metastatic HCC following TACE. (*A–D*) MIP and fused axial FDG PET/CT images demonstrate recurrent FDG-avid HCC (*broad white arrows*), with tumor thrombus in the hepatic vein (*narrow black arrow*), left adrenal metastasis (*broad black arrow*), and peritoneal metastasis (*narrow white arrow*).

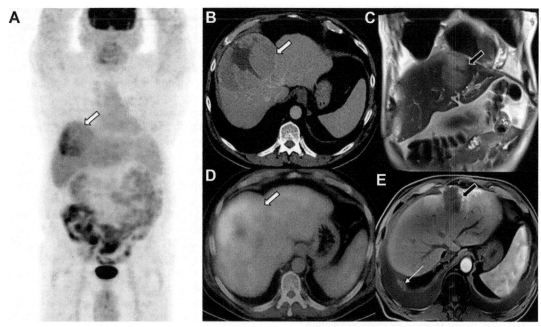

Fig. 4. A 66-year-old man with recurrent metastatic HCC following liver transplant. (*A,B,D*) Pretransplant FDG PET/CT demonstrates an 8 cm partially necrotic HCC in the right hepatic lobe with SUVmax of 4.8 (broad white arrow). (*C, E*) Posttransplant MR imaging—coronal T2W and axial post-contrast MR imaging demonstrate recurrent T2W hyperintense, peripherally enhancing tumor in the left hepatic lobe (*broad black arrows*), and bilateral small pleural effusions with enhancing right pleural metastases (*narrow white arrow*).

Atezolizumab plus bevacizumab (ATEZO/BEV), which combines an immune checkpoint inhibitor (ATEZO) with a VEGF inhibitor (BEV), was FDA-approved in May 2020 for treatment of HCC. In 20 patients treated with ATEZO/BEV, Kawamura and colleagues found that a (TLR ≥2 on pretreatment FDG PET/CT was associated with early progressive disease.[23]

Non-FDG tracers such as ^{68}Ga prostate-specific membrane antigen (PSMA) and ^{68}Ga-fibroblast activation protein inhibitor (FAPI) PET/CT are being evaluated for imaging HCCs.

Gallium-68-prostate-specific membrane antigen: PSMA is overexpressed in prostate cancer cells and neovasculature associated with other neoplasms. On retrospective pathologic analysis of PSMA expression in 148 surgically resected HCCs, Thompson and colleagues found that patients with moderate or poorly differentiated HCCs which expressed PSMA had a longer OS trend than those with lesions without PSMA expression. They also prospectively performed ^{68}Ga-PSMA PET/CT in 31 newly diagnosed patients with 39 biopsy-proven or image-based HCC lesions liver imaging reporting and data system (LI-RADS 5). Twenty-five lesions (64%) had marked PSMA uptake with median SUV_{max} 9.2 (range: 4.9–28.4). PSMA expression in HCC has the potential for PSMA radioligand therapy[24]

GALLIUM-68-FIBROBLAST ACTIVATION PROTEIN INHIBITOR PET/COMPUTED TOMOGRAPHY

Gallium-68-labeled FAPI PET/CT detects FAP, which is highly expressed in cancer-associated fibroblasts. Initial studies suggest ^{68}Ga-FAPI-04 PET/CT is more sensitive than 18F-FDG PET/CT in detecting primary and metastatic HCC lesions. Wang and colleagues compared the performance of 18F-FDG and 68Ga-FAPI-04 PET/CT in 35 intrahepatic lesions in 25 patients with HCC. Lesions had a greater target-to-background ratio (TBR) on ^{68}Ga-FAPI-04 PET/CT than ^{18}F-FDG PET/CT. ^{68}Ga-FAPI-04 PET/CT had higher sensitivity of 85.7% in the detection of HCC than ^{18}F-FDG PET/CT with a sensitivity of 57.1%, including for lesions ≤ 2 cm in diameter and well- or moderately-differentiated lesions. The SUVmax and TBR in lesions with ^{68}Ga-FAPI-04 uptake correlated with tumor size.[25]In a study by Guo and colleagues comparing the performance of [^{68}Ga]Ga-FAPI-04 PET/CT with contrast-enhanced CT, liver MR imaging, and [^{18}F]-FDG PET/CT in 34 patients with 20 HCC, 12 intrahepatic cholangiocarcinomas, and two benign hepatic nodules [[68] Ga]Ga-FAPI-04 PET/CT performed better than [^{18}F]-FDG PET/CT in detecting hepatic and extrahepatic lesions. The sensitivity of [^{68}Ga] Ga-FAPI-04 (96%) was equivalent to MR imaging (100%) and contrast-enhanced CT (96%) and superior to ^{18}F FDG PET/CT (65%) for the detection of primary liver tumors. The tumor detection rate for hepatic and extrahepatic disease was 87.4% with [^{68}Ga] Ga-FAPI-04 PET/CT and 65% for [^{18}F]-FDG PET/CT.[26]

BILIARY MALIGNANCY

Intra- and extrahepatic cholangiocarcinoma and gall bladder carcinoma are aggressive tumors characterized by early lymphatic and hematogenous metastases. Ultrasound, CT, MR imaging, magnetic resonance cholangiopancreatography (MRCP), and endoscopic retrograde cholangiopancreatography (ERCP) are the primary imaging modalities for diagnosis and staging in these patients who often present with symptoms of biliary colic or obstructive jaundice. Surgery remains the only curative modality. However, most patients are diagnosed at an advanced stage and are treated with chemotherapy or chemoradiation.

CHOLANGIOCARCINOMA

In addition to classification as intrahepatic or extrahepatic cholangiocarcinomas based on anatomic location, these tumors may be subclassified into mass forming, periductal infiltrating, or intraductal tumors based on macroscopic appearance.

[18F] FLUORODEOXYGLUCOSE PET/ COMPUTED TOMOGRAPHY

The clinical usefulness of ^{18}F-FDG PET/CT in the differential diagnosis of bile duct cancers is related to the primary disease site. Albazaz and colleagues found that the overall sensitivity of FDG PET/CT for the detection of primary cholangiocarcinoma was 77% (48/62), with a much higher sensitivity for intrahepatic than for extrahepatic cholangiocarcinoma (92%, 36/39 vs 52%, 12/23).[27] In a study comparing ^{18}F FDG PET/CT and contrast-enhanced CT scans, Petrowsky and colleagues reported that PET/CT demonstrated a sensitivity of 93% and a specificity of 80% in detecting intrahepatic cholangiocarcinoma and a sensitivity of 55% and a specificity of 33% in detecting extrahepatic cholangiocarcinoma.[28] Corvera and colleagues also found that the sensitivity of PET for detecting intrahepatic CCA was 95% but only 69% for extrahepatic CCA.[29]This is likely due to the infiltrating nature and low cellularity of extrahepatic cholangiocarcinoma (**Fig. 5**).

PET/CT is sensitive and specific for the detection of metastases and tumor recurrence.[30,31]In the study by Corvera and colleagues, PET had a sensitivity of 78% and specificity of 75% for detecting the primary biliary tumor and a sensitivity of 96% and specificity of 89% for detecting metastatic disease.[29]In a study to determine whether PET/CT is superior to conventional imaging in the diagnosis of primary cholangiocarcinoma, regional lymph node metastasis, and distant metastasis, Kim and colleagues found that PET/CT improved the accuracy of preoperative staging. The sensitivity, specificity, and accuracy of PET/CT in primary tumor detection were 84.0%, 79.3%, and 82.9%, respectively, comparable to that of CT and MR imaging/ MRCP. PET/CT had higher accuracy than CT and MR imaging in the diagnosis of regional lymph node metastases (75.9% vs 60.9%) and distant metastases (88.3% vs 78.7%)[32] (**Fig. 6**).

Seo and colleagues investigated the usefulness of ^{18}F-FDG PET/CT as a marker for lymph node metastasis and recurrence in intrahepatic cholangiocarcinoma. The reported diagnostic accuracies of FDG-PET, CT, and MR imaging for detection of lymph node metastasis were 86%, 68%, and 57%, the sensitivities were 43%, 43%, and 43%, and the specificities were 100%, 76%, and 64%, respectively. The disease-free survival rates in the high SUV group ($\geq$8.5) were significantly lower than in the low SUV group (<8.5), and a high SUV was an independent predictor of postoperative recurrence on multivariate analysis.[33] Albazaz and colleagues evaluated the impact of F-18 FDG PET/CT scans on the management pathway of patients with primary biliary malignancy. FDG PET/CT impacted patient management in 24% (21/87) of cholangiocarcinomas, finding occult sites of disease and characterizing indeterminate lesions on CT and MR imaging. FDG PET/CT upstaged 19% (12/62) and downstaged 3% (2/ 62) of the scans performed for initial staging.[27]

GALLBLADDER CARCINOMA

Several studies have demonstrated high sensitivity (75%–100%) of FDG PET/CT in detecting gall bladder cancer.[28,34,35] In a study by Petrowsky and colleagues, PET/CT had a high sensitivity of 100% (14/14) in detecting primary or recurrent gallbladder cancer.[28] Corvera and colleagues showed that PET had a sensitivity of 86% for detecting the primary tumor (gallbladders in situ) or detecting residual disease in postcholecystectomy patients and 87% sensitivity for detecting metastases.[29] Albazaz and colleagues evaluated the impact of ^{18}F-FDG PET/CT scans on the management pathway of patients with gallbladder malignancy. FDG PET/CT changed management in 39% (12/31) of cases by identifying occult sites

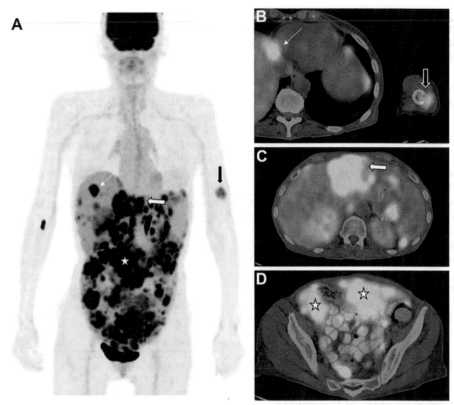

Fig. 5. A 73-year-old woman with metastatic cholangiocarcinoma. (*A–D*) Maximum intensity projection (MIP) and fused axial FDG PET/CT images demonstrate FDG-avid intrahepatic cholangiocarcinoma (*broad white arrows*), hepatic metastases (*narrow white arrow*), left humeral metastasis (*broad black arrow*), and peritoneal metastasis (*white stars*).

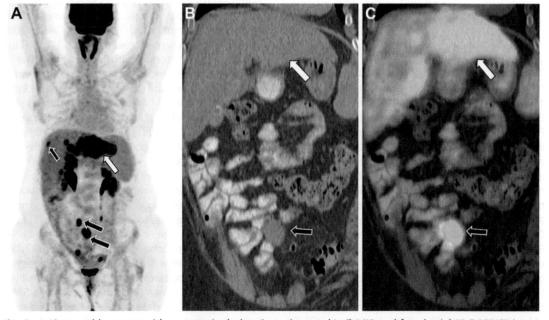

Fig. 6. A 48-year-old woman with metastatic cholangiocarcinoma. (*A–C*) MIP and fused axial FDG PET/CT images demonstrate FDG-avid intrahepatic cholangiocarcinoma (*broad white arrows*) and peritoneal metastasis (*broad black arrows*).

of disease not detected by CT/MR imaging and finding unsuspected sites of disease recurrence. It, however, may fail to identify small-volume peritoneal metastases.[27]

PANCREATIC CANCER
Introduction

Pancreatic cancer is an aggressive neoplasm with a 5-year survival rate of approximately 10%. The incidence has risen among younger women and older individuals.[36] Poor prognosis is attributed to early micro-metastasis, late diagnosis, and drug resistance. More than 90% are ductal adenocarcinomas, often associated with K-ras mutation. Dedicated pancreatic CT of the abdomen is the preferred imaging modality for diagnosing and determining the local extent of pancreatic cancer. For therapeutic purposes, pancreatic tumors are classified as resectable, borderline resectable, and locally advanced pancreatic cancer or metastatic tumors. Surgery is often the only potentially curative option. Neoadjuvant chemotherapy is offered before surgery for borderline resectable tumors. Patients with unresectable tumors or postoperative recurrence are treated with chemotherapy.[37]

[^{18}F] fluorodeoxyglucose PET/computed tomography

According to the NCCN guidelines, ^{18}F-FDG PET/CT may be performed to detect extra-pancreatic metastases in high-risk patients after formal pancreatic protocol CT. The NCCN guidelines do not recommend FDG PET/CT for posttreatment response assessment.[38]

Diagnosis

^{18}F-FDG PET/CT has reported sensitivity of 85% to 100%, specificity of 61% to 94%, and accuracy of 84% to 95% in diagnosing pancreatic cancer.[39–42] FDG uptake by pancreatic cancer correlates with increased Ki-67 and is highest in poorly differentiated tumors. Medium- or well-differentiated pancreatic cancers may not have increased FDG uptake. Inflammatory lesions such as chronic lymphoplasmacytic pancreatitis, autoimmune pancreatitis, and tuberculosis may have increased FDG uptake. On comparing the diagnostic accuracy of ^{18}F-FDG PET/CT, CA19-9, contrast-enhanced CT and contrast-enhanced MR imaging in discrimination between malignant and benign pancreatic lesions, Huang and colleagues found that SUVmax of malignant lesions (7.34 ± 4.17) was higher than SUVmax of benign lesions (1.70 ± 2.68). Combined PET/CT and CA19-9 with cutoff points of 3.75 SUVmax and 105.35 for CA19-9 level of 105.35 achieved the best diagnostic performance. In this study, for differentiating malignant from benign pancreatic lesions, PET/CT had sensitivity, specificity, and accuracy of 91.9%, 96.3%, and 94.0%, respectively, contrast-enhanced CT had sensitivity, specificity, and accuracy of 83.6%, 77.8%, 81.2%, and contrast-enhanced MR imaging had sensitivity, specificity, and accuracy of 91.2%, 75.0%, and 81.7%.[43] In a multicenter prospective study conducted in 18 UK pancreatic tertiary referral centers, Ghaneh and colleagues evaluated the performance of multidetector CT (MDCT) in 589 patients and FDG PET/CT in 550 patients with suspected pancreatic cancer. MDCT had a sensitivity of 88.5% and specificity of 70.6%; FDG PET/CT had a sensitivity of 92.7% and specificity of 75.8% for the diagnosis of pancreatic cancer. Pancreatic cancer had a higher median SUVmax of 7.5 compared with median SUVmax of 5.7 for other lesions. Adding PET/CT to standard workup improved pancreatic cancer diagnosis, staging, and management.[42]

Staging and Resection

Surgical resection is the only curative option for pancreatic cancer; however, more than 80% of patients present unresectable disease due to locally advanced disease or distant metastases. Borderline resectable pancreatic cancer (BRPC) patients who could be eligible for radical surgery following neoadjuvant chemotherapy may have local arterial or venous (superior mesenteric vein/portal vein) invasion.[44] PET has less spatial resolution and accuracy than CT in assessing locoregional involvement, which is critical in therapeutic decision-making in pancreatic cancer. CT, MR imaging, and endoscopic ultrasound are better at defining tumor's border and local spread.[45] However, PET/CT performs better than CT in identifying unsuspected metastases, reducing the frequency of futile surgeries. In a 2017 meta-analysis of 17 clinical studies in 1343 patients, PET/CT had greater ability than CT in detecting true positive distant metastases (OR = 1.52, 95% CI 1.23–1.88) with no significant difference in the detection of regional nodal metastases (OR = 0.97, 95% CI 0.63–1.47).[46] In a meta-analysis by Lee and colleagues of nine studies that evaluated the diagnostic performance of FDG PET/CT and one which evaluated the diagnostic performance of PET/MR imaging in staging pancreatic adenocarcinoma, the pooled sensitivity for detection of lymph node metastasis was 55%, specificity 94%, and pooled sensitivity for detection of distant metastasis was 80%, specificity 100% leading to management change in 19% of patients[47] (**Fig. 7**).

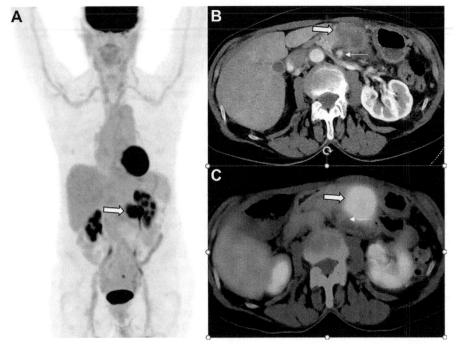

Fig. 7. A 81-year-old woman with locally advanced pancreatic cancer. (*A*) MIP image of FDG PET/CT demonstrates FDG-avid pancreatic mass with no sites of metastases and (*B, C*) contrast-enhanced CT and fused axial FDG PET/CT images demonstrate 4 cm FDG-avid pancreatic mass with central necrosis and surrounding fat stranding (*broad white arrows*) abutting the superior mesenteric vein (SMV) (*narrow white arrow*).

Neoadjuvant Therapy

Neoadjuvant therapy (NAT) with induction chemotherapy followed by consolidative chemoradiation enables some patients with locally advanced pancreatic cancer (LAPC) or BRPC to access margin-negative resection and may treat occult metastases. Cross-sectional imaging is unreliable in predicting posttreatment response due to the inability to distinguish tumor from fibrosis.

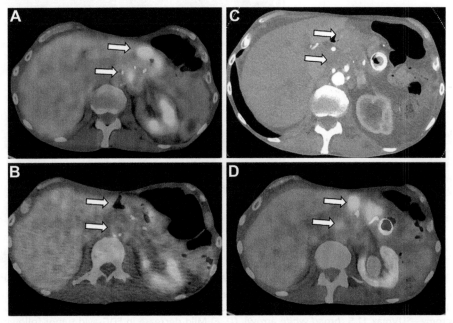

Fig. 8. A 74-year-old man with postsurgical and post-RT recurrence of pancreatic cancer. (*A*) Fused axial FDG PET/CT demonstrates FDG-avid recurrent pancreatic carcinoma, following distal pancreatectomy (*broad white arrow*). (*B*) Significant decrease in FDG-avid tumor following radiation therapy (*broad white arrow*). (*C, D*) Local tumor recurrence on CECT and fused axial PET/CT (*broad white arrows*).

Normalization of Ca 19-9 is often used to determine biochemical response.[48] Recent studies demonstrate the usefulness of FDG PET/CT in predicting preoperative pathologic response to NAT and survival.

In a study of the utility of ^{18}F-FDG PET/CT in assessing treatment response in 20 patients with LAPC treated with neoadjuvant chemo-RT, Choi and colleagues observed that mean survival was longer (23.2 months) in patients with $\geq$ 50% decrease in SUV between pre-study PET scan and PET scan after the first cycle of chemotherapy, as compared with 11.3 months in patients with less than 50% decrease in SUV[49] (**Fig. 8**).

In a retrospective study on 202 patients with BRPC/LAPC who underwent surgical resection following NAT, Abdelrehman and colleagues found that metabolic response on post-NAT PET/CT performed within 60 days of resection as defined by FDG uptake below hepatic FDG uptake and similar to adjacent pancreatic parenchyma was associated with both RFS and OS. They noted that major

pathologic response was more likely in patients with significant CA 19-9 response and major metabolic response on PET/CT al.[50]

In a cohort study of 115 consecutive patients treated for pancreatic cancer, Itchins and colleagues performed PET/CT at baseline and following NAT. Improvement in SUVmax to less than 5 following NAT was associated with improved OS. PET/CT upstaged the tumor in 12% of patients following NAT, avoiding futile surgery.[51]

In 86 patients who had preoperative 18F-FDG PET/CT after completion of neoadjuvant treatment, Ikenaga and colleagues found that elevated posttreatment SUVmax ($\geq$4.5) was an independent predictor of early recurrence within 6 months after surgery and decreased OS. Dynamic changes in maximum standardized uptake during NAT were associated with pathologic response to NAT but not with radiological response or change in CA19-9 level[52] (**Fig. 9**).

Prognosis: In a 2017 meta-analysis of 16 studies by Zhu and colleagues, high SUVmax on

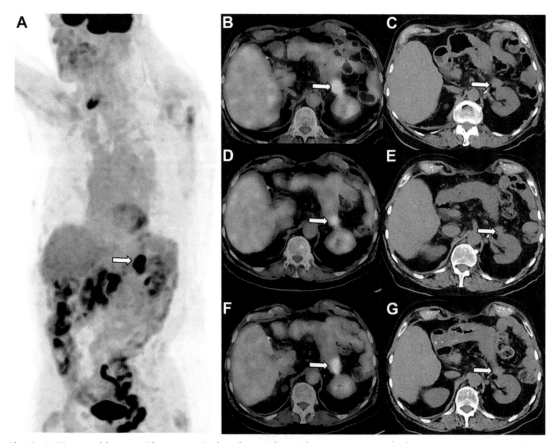

Fig. 9. A 70-year-old man with postsurgical and post-chemotherapy recurrence of pancreatic cancer. (*A–C*) MIP, fused axial FDG PET/CT, and CT images demonstrate FDG-avid recurrent pancreatic carcinoma, following distal pancreatectomy—SUVmax 11.5 (*broad white arrow*). (*D, E*) Mild decrease in FDG-avid tumor following chemotherapy—SUVmax 5.3 (*broad white arrow*). (*F, G*) Subsequent disease progression with increased FDG avidity of the tumor—SUVmax 6.9 (*broad white arrows*).

pretreatment ^{18}F-FDG PET/CT was associated with poor prognosis, including event-free survival and OS. High volumetric parameter values, such as metabolic tumor volume (MTV) and total lesion glycolysis (TLG), were also significantly correlated with prognosis.[53] In a retrospective review, Hwang found that SUVmax of the tumor on pretreatment ^{18}F-FDG PET/CT was related to survival at each stage. Patients with a low SUV (≤4.1), lower serum level of CA19-9, and lower stage survived longer.[54-55] Sperti and colleagues evaluated the prognostic significance of SUVmax on preoperative PET/CT scan in 144 patients with resectable pancreatic cancer; 62 patients with low SUVmax (≤3.65) had significantly better survival than 82 patients with high SUVmax greater than 3.65. Disease-free survival and OS rates were also significantly influenced by tumor stage, lymph node involvement, pathologic grade, and resection margins.[55] Mohamed and colleagues performed a retrospective data analysis on 89 patients with pancreatic cancer who underwent FDP PET/CT. Patients were stratified into low-risk groups based on median values of 7.8 for SUVmax, 5.15 for SUV mean, 10 mm^3 for MTV, and 55 for TLG. On univariate analysis SUVmax, SUVmax, MTV, TLG, tumor size, tumor differentiation, and presence of distant metastasis were prognostic factors for OS. On multivariable analysis, TLG and presence of distant metastasis were independent prognostic factors with TLG (median value 55) remaining as the only significant PET metric after adjusting for the presence of distant metastasis on subgroup analysis.[56]Ren and colleagues also found that TLG (median value 49.3) was an independent prognostic factor of OS and progression-free survival in 73 patients with LAPC treated with stereotactic body radiation therapy.[57]

Gallium-68-Fibroblast Activation Protein Inhibitor PET/Computed Tomography

In early studies ^{68}Ga-labeled FAPI PET/CT is found to be useful for detection of tumors with a strong desmoplastic reaction, such as pancreatic cancer. There is potential for theragnostics by radiolabeling FAPI with therapeutic nuclides such as 177Lu, 90Y, and 225Ac. In 19 patients with pancreatic cancer (7 primary and 12 progressive/recurrent), ^{68}Ga-FAPI PET/CT led to restaging in half of the patients with primary pancreatic cancer and most patients with recurrent disease compared with contrast-enhanced CT.[58]

SUMMARY

^{18}F-FDG PET/CT can improve staging, therapeutic response assessment, and prognostication in patients with hepatobiliary and pancreatic malignancies. Non-FDG tracers, such as ^{68}Ga-PSMA and ^{68}Ga-FAPI PET/CT, seem to have good sensitivity for staging hepatobiliary and pancreatic cancers with potential for radioligand therapy with therapeutic nuclides such as 177Lu, 90Y, and 225Ac.

CLINICS CARE POINTS

- 18F FDG-PET/CT can improve clinical staging and therapeutic response assessment of patients with hepatobiliary and pancreatic cancer, optimizing management strategies.
- In early studies non-FDG tracers, such as 68Ga-PSMA and 68Ga-FAPI PET/CT, have good sensitivity for staging hepatobiliary and pancreatic cancers with potential for radioligand therapy.

REFERENCES

1. McGlynn KA, Petrick JL, El-Serag HB. Epidemiology of hepatocellular carcinoma. Hepatology 2021; 73(Suppl 1):4–13.
2. Singal A, Volk ML, Waljee A, et al. Meta-analysis: surveillance with ultrasound for early-stage hepatocellular carcinoma in patients with cirrhosis. Aliment Pharmacol Ther 2009;30(1):37–47.
3. Lee YJ, Lee JM, Lee JS, et al. Hepatocellular carcinoma: diagnostic performance of multidetector CT and MR imaging-a systematic review and meta-analysis. Radiology 2015;275(1):97–109.
4. Benson AB, D'Angelica MI, Abbott DE, et al. Hepatobiliary Cancers, Version 2.2021, NCCN Clinical Practice Guidelines in Oncology. J Natl Compr Canc Netw 2021;19(5):541–65.
5. Enomoto K, Fukunaga T, Okazumi S, et al. [Can fluorodeoxyglucose-positron emission tomography evaluate the functional differentiation of hepatocellular carcinoma]. Kaku Igaku 1991;28(11):1353–6.
6. Khan MA, Combs CS, Brunt EM, et al. Positron emission tomography scanning in the evaluation of hepatocellular carcinoma. J Hepatol 2000;32(5):792–7.
7. Wudel LJ Jr, Delbeke D, Morris D, et al. The role of [18F]fluorodeoxyglucose positron emission tomography imaging in the evaluation of hepatocellular carcinoma. Am Surg 2003;69(2):117–24 [discussion: 124–6].
8. Park JW, Kim JH, Kim SK, et al. A prospective evaluation of 18F-FDG and 11C-acetate PET/CT for detection of primary and metastatic hepatocellular carcinoma. J Nucl Med 2008;49(12):1912–21.
9. Seo S, Hatano E, Higashi T, et al. Fluorine-18 fluorodeoxyglucose positron emission tomography predicts

tumor differentiation, P-glycoprotein expression, and outcome after resection in hepatocellular carcinoma. Clin Cancer Res 2007;13(2 Pt 1):427–33.

10. Sugiyama M, Sakahara H, Torizuka T, et al. 18F-FDG PET in the detection of extrahepatic metastases from hepatocellular carcinoma. J Gastroenterol 2004;39(10):961–8.

11. Ho CL, Chen S, Yeung DW, et al. Dual-tracer PET/CT imaging in evaluation of metastatic hepatocellular carcinoma. J Nucl Med 2007;48(6):902–9.

12. Sun DW, An L, Wei F, et al. Prognostic significance of parameters from pretreatment (18)F-FDG PET in hepatocellular carcinoma: a meta-analysis. Abdom Radiol (NY) 2016;41(1):33–41.

13. Kornberg A, Küpper B, Thrum K, et al. Increased 18F-FDG uptake of hepatocellular carcinoma on positron emission tomography independently predicts tumor recurrence in liver transplant patients. Transplant Proc 2009;41(6):2561–3.

14. Cho KJ, Choi NK, Shin MH, et al. Clinical usefulness of FDG-PET in patients with hepatocellular carcinoma undergoing surgical resection. Ann Hepatobiliary Pancreat Surg 2017;21(4):194–8.

15. Hatano E, Ikai I, Higashi T, et al. Preoperative positron emission tomography with fluorine-18-fluorodeoxyglucose is predictive of prognosis in patients with hepatocellular carcinoma after resection. World J Surg 2006;30(9):1736–41.

16. Ahn SG, Kim SH, Jeon TJ, et al. The role of preoperative [18F]fluorodeoxyglucose positron emission tomography in predicting early recurrence after curative resection of hepatocellular carcinomas. J Gastrointest Surg 2011;15(11):2044–52.

17. Kitamura K, Hatano E, Higashi T, et al. Preoperative FDG-PET predicts recurrence patterns in hepatocellular carcinoma. Ann Surg Oncol 2012;19(1):156–62.

18. Lee JW, Paeng JC, Kang KW, et al. Prediction of tumor recurrence by 18F-FDG PET in liver transplantation for hepatocellular carcinoma. J Nucl Med 2009;50(5):682–7.

19. Yang SH, Suh KS, Lee HW, et al. The role of (18)F-FDG-PET imaging for the selection of liver transplantation candidates among hepatocellular carcinoma patients. Liver Transpl 2006;12(11):1655–60.

20. Song MJ, Bae SH, Yoo IeR, et al. Predictive value of 1F-fluorodeoxyglucose PET/CT for transarterial chemolipiodolization of hepatocellular carcinoma. World J Gastroenterol 2012;18(25):3215–22.

21. Lee JD, Yun M. Prognostic Significance of 1F-FDG Uptake in Hepatocellular Carcinoma Treated with Transarterial Chemoembolization or Concurrent Chemoradiotherapy: A Multicenter Retrospective Cohort Study. J Nucl Med 2016;57(4):509–16.

22. Lee JH, Park JY, Kim DY, et al. Prognostic value of 18F-FDG PET for hepatocellular carcinoma patients treated with sorafenib. Liver Int 2011;31(8):1144–9.

23. Kawamura Y, Kobayashi M, Shindoh J, et al. Pretreatment Positron Emission Tomography with 18F-Fluorodeoxyglucose May Be a Useful New Predictor of Early Progressive Disease following Atezolizumab plus Bevacizumab in Patients with Unresectable Hepatocellular Carcinoma. Oncology 2022;100(6):320–30.

24. Thompson SM, Suman G, Torbenson MS, et al. PSMA as a Theranostic Target in Hepatocellular Carcinoma: Immunohistochemistry and 68 Ga-PSMA-11 PET Using Cyclotron-Produced 68 Ga. Hepatol Commun 2022;6(5):1172–85.

25. Wang H, Zhu W, Ren S, et al. 68Ga-FAPI-04 Versus 18F-FDG PET/CT in the Detection of Hepatocellular Carcinoma. Front Oncol 2021;11:693640.

26. Guo W, Pang Y, Yao L, et al. Imaging fibroblast activation protein in liver cancer: a single-center post hoc retrospective analysis to compare [68Ga]Ga-FAPI-04 PET/CT versus MRI and [18F]-FDG PET/CT. Eur J Nucl Med Mol Imaging 2021;48(5):1604–17.

27. Albazaz R, Patel CN, Chowdhury FU, et al. Clinical impact of FDG PET-CT on management decisions for patients with primary biliary tumours. Insights Imaging 2013;4(5):691–700.

28. Petrowsky H, Wildbrett P, Husarik DB, et al. Impact of integrated positron emission tomography and computed tomography on staging and management of gallbladder cancer and cholangiocarcinoma. J Hepatol 2006;45(1):43–50.

29. Corvera CU, Blumgart LH, Akhurst T, et al. 18F-fluorodeoxyglucose positron emission tomography influences management decisions in patients with biliary cancer. J Am Coll Surg 2008;206(1):57–65.

30. Moon CM, Bang S, Chung JB, et al. Usefulness of 18F-fluorodeoxyglucose positron emission tomography in differential diagnosis and staging of cholangiocarcinomas. J Gastroenterol Hepatol 2008;23(5):759–65.

31. Li J, Kuehl H, Grabellus F, et al. Preoperative assessment of hilar cholangiocarcinoma by dual-modality PET/CT. J Surg Oncol 2008;98(6):438–43.

32. Kim JY, Kim MH, Lee TY, et al. Clinical role of 18F-FDG PET-CT in suspected and potentially operable cholangiocarcinoma: a prospective study compared with conventional imaging. Am J Gastroenterol 2008;103(5):1145–51.

33. Seo S, Hatano E, Higashi T, et al. Fluorine-18 fluorodeoxyglucose positron emission tomography predicts lymph node metastasis, P-glycoprotein expression, and recurrence after resection in mass-forming intrahepatic cholangiocarcinoma. Surgery 2008;143(6):769–77.

34. Rodríguez-Fernández A, Gómez-Río M, Llamas-Elvira JM, et al. Positron-emission tomography with fluorine-18-fluoro-2-deoxy-D-glucose for gallbladder cancer diagnosis. Am J Surg 2004;188(2):171–5.

35. Koh T, Taniguchi H, Yamaguchi A, et al. Differential diagnosis of gallbladder cancer using positron

emission tomography with fluorine-18-labeled fluoro-deoxyglucose (FDG-PET). J Surg Oncol 2003;84(2): 74–81.

36. Gaddam S, Abboud Y, Oh J, et al. Incidence of Pancreatic Cancer by Age and Sex in the US, 2000-2018. JAMA 2021;326(20):2075–7.

37. Jiang S, Fagman JB, Ma Y, et al. A comprehensive review of pancreatic cancer and its therapeutic challenges. Aging (Albany NY) 2022;14(18):7635–49.

38. Tempero MA, Malafa MP, Al-Hawary M, et al. Pancreatic adenocarcinoma, version 2.2021, NCCN clinical Practice guidelines in Oncology. J Natl Compr Canc Netw 2021;19(4):439–57.

39. Buchs NC, Bühler L, Bucher P, et al. Value of contrast-enhanced 18F-fluorodeoxyglucose positron emission tomography/computed tomography in detection and presurgical assessment of pancreatic cancer: a prospective study. J Gastroenterol Hepatol 2011;26(4):657–62.

40. Kauhanen SP, Komar G, Seppänen MP, et al. A prospective diagnostic accuracy study of 18F-fluoro-deoxyglucose positron emission tomography/computed tomography, multidetector row computed tomography, and magnetic resonance imaging in primary diagnosis and staging of pancreatic cancer. Ann Surg 2009;250(6):957–63.

41. Ergul N, Gundogan C, Tozlu M, et al. Role of (18)F-fluorodeoxyglucose positron emission tomography/computed tomography in diagnosis and management of pancreatic cancer; comparison with multidetector row computed tomography, magnetic resonance imaging and endoscopic ultrasonography. Rev Esp Med Nucl Imagen Mol 2014;33(3): 159–64.

42. Ghaneh P, Hanson R, Titman A, et al. PET-PANC: multicentre prospective diagnostic accuracy and health economic analysis study of the impact of combined modality 18fluorine-2-fluoro-2-deoxy-d-glucose positron emission tomography with computed tomography scanning in the diagnosis and management of pancreatic cancer. Health Technol Assess 2018;22(7):1–114.

43. Huang S, Chong H, Sun X, et al. The value of (18)F-FDG PET/CT in diagnosing pancreatic lesions: comparison with CA19-9, enhanced CT or enhanced MR. Front Med 2021;8:668697.

44. Lopez NE, Prendergast C, Lowy AM. Borderline resectable pancreatic cancer: definitions and management. World J Gastroenterol 2014;20(31):10740–51.

45. Izuishi K, Yamamoto Y, Sano T, et al. Impact of 18-fluorodeoxyglucose positron emission tomography on the management of pancreatic cancer. J Gastrointest Surg 2010;14(7):1151–8.

46. Wang L, Dong P, Wang WG, et al. Positron emission tomography modalities prevent futile radical resection of pancreatic cancer: A meta-analysis. Int J Surg 2017;46:119–25.

47. Lee JW, O JH, Choi M, et al. Impact of F-18 Fluoro-deoxyglucose PET/CT and PET/MRI on Initial Staging and Changes in Management of Pancreatic Ductal Adenocarcinoma: A Systemic Review and Meta-Analysis. Diagnostics (Basel) 2020;10(11): 952.

48. Gugenheim J, Crovetto A, Petrucciani N. Neoadjuvant therapy for pancreatic cancer. Updates Surg 2022;74(1):35–42.

49. Choi M, Heilbrun LK, Venkatramanamoorthy R, et al. Using 18F-fluorodeoxyglucose positron emission tomography to monitor clinical outcomes in patients treated with neoadjuvant chemo-radiotherapy for locally advanced pancreatic cancer. Am J Clin Oncol 2010;33(3):257–61.

50. Abdelrahman AM, Goenka AH, Alva-Ruiz R, et al. FDG-PET Predicts Neoadjuvant Therapy Response and Survival in Borderline Resectable/Locally Advanced Pancreatic Adenocarcinoma. J Natl Compr Canc Netw 2022;20(9):1023–32.e3.

51. Itchins M, Chua TC, Arena J, et al. Evaluation of Fluorodeoxyglucose Positron Emission Tomography Scanning in the Neoadjuvant Therapy Paradigm in Pancreatic Ductal Adenocarcinoma. Pancreas 2020;49(2):224–9.

52. Ikenaga N, Nakata K, Hayashi M, et al. Clinical Implications of FDG-PET in Pancreatic Ductal Adenocarcinoma Patients Treated with Neoadjuvant Therapy. J Gastrointest Surg 2023;27(2):337–46.

53. Zhu D, Wang L, Zhang H, et al. Prognostic value of 18F-FDG-PET/CT parameters in patients with pancreatic carcinoma: A systematic review and meta-analysis. Medicine (Baltimore) 2017;96(33): e7813.

54. Hwang JP, Lim I, Chang KJ, et al. Prognostic value of SUVmax measured by Fluorine-18 Fluorodeoxyglucose Positron Emission Tomography with Computed Tomography in Patients with Pancreatic Cancer. Nucl Med Mol Imaging 2012;46(3):207–14.

55. Sperti C, Friziero A, Serafini S, et al. Prognostic Implications of 18-FDG Positron Emission Tomography/Computed Tomography in Resectable Pancreatic Cancer. J Clin Med 2020;9(7):2169.

56. Mohamed E, Needham A, Psarelli E, et al. Prognostic value of 18FDG PET/CT volumetric parameters in the survival prediction of patients with pancreatic cancer. Eur J Surg Oncol 2020;46(8):1532–8.

57. Ren S, Zhu X, Zhang A, et al. Prognostic value of 18F-FDG PET /CT metabolic parameters in patients with locally advanced pancreatic Cancer treated with stereotactic body radiation therapy. Cancer Imaging 2020;20:22.

58. Röhrich M, Naumann P, Giesel FL, et al. Impact of 68Ga-FAPI PET/CT Imaging on the Therapeutic Management of Primary and Recurrent Pancreatic Ductal Adenocarcinomas. J Nucl Med 2021;62(6): 779–86.

Role of PET/Computed Tomography in Gastric and Colorectal Malignancies

Yogita Khandelwal, MD[a], Ashwin Singh Parihar, MBBS, MD[b],
Golmehr Sistani, MD[c], Marigdalia K. Ramirez-Fort, MD[d],
Katherine Zukotynski, MD, PhD[e,*],
Rathan M. Subramaniam, MD, PhD, MPH, MBA[f]

KEYWORDS

- Gastric cancer • Colorectal cancer • PET/CT • FDG

KEY POINTS

- 18F-FDG PET plays an important role in the evaluation of patients with cancer of the gastrointestinal tract both at the time of initial staging and at the time of subsequent treatment strategy
- Somatostatin-targeting radiopharmaceuticals have become key in the evaluation of patients with NETs
- Newer radiopharmaceuticals are being developed that may provide additional insights

INTRODUCTION

The glucose analog 2-deoxy-2-^{18}F-D-glucose (FDG) is the most widely used radiopharmaceutical for imaging of cancers using PET. ^{18}F-FDG is transported into tissues by glucose transporters (GLUTs) and is intracellularly phosphorylated into ^{18}F-FDG-6-phosphate. The greater glucose demand required to sustain anaerobic metabolism in tumor cells results in upregulation of non-insulin-dependent transporters, GLUT-1 and GLUT-3. Since most neoplasms have low concentrations of glucose 6-phosphatase, ^{18}F-FDG-6-phosphate accumulates in tumor cells, which results in enhanced tumor-to-background activity.

Gastric cancer (GC) is a prevalent gastrointestinal malignancy and is the fourth leading cause of cancer-related deaths worldwide.[1] Although less deadly, colorectal cancer (CRC) is the most common malignancy of the gastrointestinal tract and is the third most common malignancy worldwide. GC and CRC comprise several histologic types/subtypes, such as adenocarcinomas, neuroendocrine tumors (NETs), gastrointestinal stromal tumors (GISTs), lymphomas, mesenchymal tumors, and mixed tumor types. Histologic characterization is important to guide imaging and to determine if ^{18}F-FDG PET/CT is useful. For example, signet ring cell mucinous adenocarcinomas tend to have low ^{18}F-FDG avidity due to limited tumor cellularity. Intestinal adenocarcinomas and lymphomas of the gastrointestinal tissue are typically highly ^{18}F-FDG avid.[2]

Gastric and colorectal malignancies often spread first by local extension to adjacent organs, with subsequent peritoneal involvement and distant metastases (lymphatic or hematogenous).[3,4] Hematogenous spread is also common, typically to the liver, lungs, and bones.

^{a} Department of Nuclear Medicine, AIIMS Campus, Ansari Nagar East, New Delhi, Delhi 110016, India; ^{b} Mallinckodt Institute of Radiology, Washington University School of Medicine, 510 South Kingshighway Boulevard, St. Louis, MO 63110, USA; ^{c} Medical Imaging Department, Royal Victoria Regional Health Centre, 201 Georgian Drive, Barrie, ON L4M 6M2, Canada; ^{d} BioFort, 1 Fort Estate, PR-1 Km 20.6 Bo. Rios, Sector, La Muda, Guaynabo 00970, Puerto Rico; ^{e} Department of Medical Imaging, McMaster University, 1280 Main Street West, Hamilton, ON L8S 4L8, Canada; ^{f} Faculty of Medicine, Nursing, Midwifery & Health Sciences, 160 Oxford Street, Darlinghurst, NSW 2010, Australia
* Corresponding author.
E-mail address: katherine.zukotynski@utoronto.ca

PET Clin 19 (2024) 177–186
https://doi.org/10.1016/j.cpet.2023.12.004
1556-8598/24/© 2023 Elsevier Inc. All rights reserved.

The goal of oncological imaging is detection and characterization of malignant disease, determining disease extent, staging, assessment of therapeutic response, recurrence, and prognosis.[5,6] Ultrasound, computed tomography (CT), and MRI are the most commonly used modalities for staging; if a biopsy is required, endoscopy or colonoscopy is typically needed. However, anatomic imaging is limited in differentiating benign from malignant nodal disease, post-therapy change from tumor recurrence, and even non-opacified bowel loops from metastasis. PET/CT with ^{18}F-FDG is a functional imaging modality that includes anatomic information (provided by CT). This is a powerful tool for the evaluation of gastric and colorectal carcinoma. This article focuses on the role of PET/CT in evaluating and managing GC and CRC. The authors start with describing the common aspects of imaging with ^{18}F-FDG, followed by tumor-specific discussions of gastric and colorectal malignancies. Finally, the authors provide a brief overview of non-FDG tracers including their potential clinical applications, and describe future directions in imaging these malignancies.

^{18}F-FDG PET TECHNIQUE

Several technical considerations are important for performing ^{18}F-FDG PET/CT in GC/CRC.[7,8]

Patient Preparation

Patients should fast for 4 to 6 hours before the scan to ensure optimal uptake of ^{18}F-FDG. Patients should also avoid strenuous physical activity before the scan. To improve imaging of the stomach, gastric distension is helpful and may be achieved by asking the patient to drink approximately 500 mL of water before scanning. The intravenous injection of 20 mg hyoscine butylbromide (antispasmodic) prior to imaging may be helpful.[9,10] When the scan is being performed for radiation therapy planning, a small amount of oral contrast may be used instead of the 500 mL of water. The use of negative oral contrast can help delineate the bowel and surrounding structures. Additionally, bowel preparation using an iso-osmotic solution given a day before the scan (cleansing) may decrease physiologic bowel uptake.

Image Acquisition

Images are usually acquired approximately 60 minutes after the intravenous injection of ^{18}F-FDG ($\sim$0.15 mCi/kg) with the patient lying supine. Additional static and delayed images maybe acquired to differentiate physiologic ^{18}F-FDG uptake in the bowel from that due to malignancy.[11] Intravenous diuretic administration for faster emptying of the urinary bladder may be considered in select cases with rectal carcinoma to increase the signal-to-noise ratio in the pelvis. Obtaining additional delayed images at 100 to 150 min post injection can be helpful in select patients to improved differentiate between inflammatory versus neoplastic etiologies.[12,13]

Image Quantification and Interpretation

For semiquantitative analysis, regions of interest (ROI) can be drawn to obtain standardized uptake values (SUVs). The maximum SUV is the most commonly used metric, although others such as the SUVpeak, SUVmean, and the lean body mass–adjusted SUV have shown to be of benefit.[14] Additional derived parameters such as metabolic tumor volume (MTV) and total lesion glycolysis (TLG), although not routinely calculated, may have prognostic significance.[15] Image interpretation is typically qualitative and takes into account both the metabolic features on PET and the morphologic features on CT or MRI. As with other oncologic indications, it is important to be aware of infective and inflammatory conditions that can mimic a malignancy on ^{18}F-FDG PET/CT.[2,16] The major limitations of evaluation of GC and CRC with ^{18}F-FDG PET/CT include:

- Variable physiologic uptake in the gastrointestinal tract. Additionally, metformin can lead to an intense ^{18}F-FDG uptake in the small intestine and the colon.
- Infective/inflammatory conditions—Bacterial and fungal infections, enterocolitis, inflammatory bowel disease, diverticulitis, and post-surgery or post-radiation therapy inflammation.
- Small liver lesions may be missed due to physiologic FDG uptake in the liver, unless the lesional avidity leads to a significantly high tumor to background activity.
- Mucinous-type malignancies, well-differentiated NETs.

^{18}F-FDG PET/CT findings should be interpreted in conjunction with other imaging modalities and clinical information to ensure accurate staging and treatment response evaluation. Timing in relation to treatment received is important along with reviewing previous studies and correlation with other imaging and tumor markers.

GASTRIC CANCER

Epithelial tumors are the most common histologic type, accounting for over 80% of gastric tumors, with the predominant subtype being adenocarcinoma.[17] Gastric adenocarcinoma is further classified into intestinal and non-intestinal (diffuse and indeterminate) subtypes based on the Lauren classification.[18] Using a different classification scheme, the World Health Organization (WHO) classification of gastric adenocarcinoma includes papillary, tubular, and mucinous subtypes (equivalent to the Lauren intestinal subtype), signet-ring cell and other poorly cohesive carcinomas (equivalent to diffuse subtype), and rare subtypes (eg, mixed, squamous, adenosquamous) equivalent to the Lauren indeterminate subtype.[19] Mesenchymal and NETs account for the second and third most common types of gastric malignancies, respectively, followed by gastric lymphoma.[18] (**Fig. 1**).

CLINICAL INDICATIONS OF PET/COMPUTED TOMOGRAPHY IMAGING
Diagnosis

Histopathologic evaluation of gastric tissue, following endoscopic biopsy is the gold standard for the diagnosis of GC. ^{18}F-FDG PET/CT has variable and often limited sensitivity in detecting primary GC due to interference from physiologic FDG uptake in the stomach and ^{18}F-FDG-avid non-neoplastic and benign pathology such as gastritis and leiomyoma.[20,21] Correlation with multimodal imaging, endoscopy, and clinical features is recommended in patients with diffuse or focal increased ^{18}F-FDG uptake in the stomach. There is variability of ^{18}F-FDG uptake among the various histo-types, with the intestinal subtypes having a higher ^{18}F-FDG avidity and mucincous subtypes having low ^{18}F-FDG avidity due to their pauci-cellular nature.

Initial Staging

The role of ^{18}F-FDG PET/CT is limited for T- and N-staging gastro-esophageal junction tumors and GC. The primary role is detecting distant metastases, that is, M-staging per the tumor, node, and metastasis (TNM) staging system.[21–23] The National Comprehensive Cancer Network (NCCN) guidelines for esophageal and gastro-esophageal junction tumors recommend endoscopic ultrasound (EUS) and CT for T and N staging, and ^{18}F-FDG PET/CT for staging occult distant metastases on CT.[24] ^{18}F-FDG-PET/CT does not have a major role in early-stage tumors (T1) due to the low likelihood of distant metastases and the false-positive PET/CT findings resulting in additional investigations that are often low yield and potentially delay treatment.[25] Similar to gastro-esophageal junction tumors, the NCCN guideline recommends EUS and CT for initial staging of gastric cancer. The NCCN guidelines permit use of ^{18}F-FDG PET/CT in GC with the following indications: staging if there is no evidence of M1 disease (may not be appropriate for T1 disease) and if clinically indicated; for the evaluation of response to neoadjuvant and adjuvant chemotherapy or chemoradiation, and for surveillance following neoadjuvant or adjuvant therapy in stage I-III disease.[26]

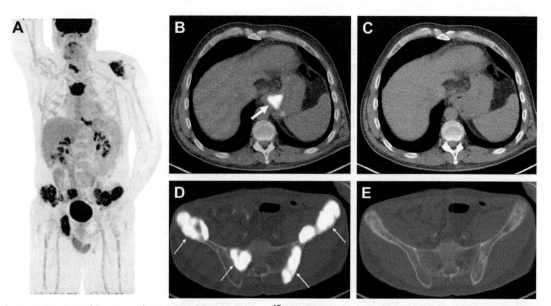

Fig. 1. A 52-year-old-man with gastric adenocarcinoma. ^{18}F-FDG PET/CT maximum intensity projection image (*A*) shows extensive hypermetabolic metastatic disease. The trans-axial fused PET/computed tomography (CT) and CT images show the hypermetabolic primary lesion involving the gastric cardia and the distal esophagus (*thick arrow; B, C*) with multifocal osseous metastases, including both the iliac bones and the sacrum (*thin arrows; D, E*).

Radiation Treatment Planning

Analogous to the incorporation of CT-based radiation treatment planning in the 1990s, the current incorporation CT through FDG PET/CT can improve target delineation and reduce acute (eg, diarrhea, constipation, bleeding, mucositis, etc.) and late (eg, small-nerve neuropathy, accelerated atherosclerosis, strictures, fistulas, etc.) radiation toxicities, thereby decreasing overall patient morbidity and mortality. Traditionally radiotherapy delivery was done using an anteroposterior conformal technique; currently, with increasing accessibility to newer technology, multi field techniques are more commonly used. Multi field techniques (eg, 3D-Conformal Radiation Therapy, Intensity Modulated Radiation Therapy) allow increased flexibility in determining which regions including normal tissue are likely to be incidentally irradiated. The Quantitative Analysis of Normal Tissue Effects in the Clinic (QUANTEC) criteria establishe dose-volume constraints for organs at risk (OAR) when irradiating cancer. The OARs during radiotherapy planning for GC are the heart, kidneys, esophagus, liver, and spinal cord. The gross tumor volume (GTV) is defined as the region containing known disease (ie, stomach, colon, rectum) as seen in the planning CT (ie, CT simulation). Clinical target volume (CTV) is the GTV plus an extension contour that includes anatomic regions likely involved with microscopic disease. A third extension is then made to the CTV to create the planning target volume (PTV) margins; these expansion margins are based on set-up uncertainty and internal organ motion so as to ensure the CTV receives the full prescription dose during each fraction.[27] Dose-volume constraints are then used in routine inverse dose planning to optimize the therapeutic ratio of the radiotherapy prescribed to the PTV.[28] As PET-avid regions help define the GTV, fusing or co-registering an FDG PET/CT with a CT simulation helps to improve GTV delineation for gastric and colorectal cancers, optimizes the therapeutic ratio between the OARs and PTV, and allows for dose variation in different areas of the tumor [5]. The value of FDG PET/CT may also be seen in GTV delineation of oligometastatic disease for stereotactic body radiotherapy, where tighter dose constraints are required. Further, the NCCN increasingly recognizes the usefulness of FDG PET/CT in radiation treatment planning [27].

Assessment of Treatment Response

Apart from initial staging, the NCCN guidelines recommend ^{18}F-FDG PET/CT for assessment of treatment response in esophageal and GE junction tumors following neoadjuvant or definitive chemoradiation.[29] The curative treatment of gastric cancer includes surgical resection of tumor and lymph node dissection. Studies show that perioperative chemotherapy or radiochemotherapy can improve relapse-free and overall survival in patients with gastric cancer.[30,31] So, the evaluation of the therapy response is important in management. There is evidence that ^{18}F-FDG PET/CT can be effective in response evaluation in gastric cancer.[32–34] In a study performed on 40 gastric cancer patients, the tumoral FDG uptake reduction 2 weeks post chemotherapy was significantly different between responding and non-responding tumors with 35% FDG uptake reduction as optimal cutoff of differentiation.[34] Another study evaluating response to neoadjuvant chemotherapy found FDG PET superior to response evaluation criteria in solid tumors (RECIST) evaluation by CT in predicting the median time to disease progression and overall survival.[32]

Re-staging and Surveillance

Distant lymphatic and peritoneal metastatic disease can be detected in up to 40% of patients approximately 2 to 3 years after definitive treatment of locally advanced GC.[20,35,36] Both the NCCN and the European Society for Medical Oncology guidelines support the use of FDG PET/CT to detect disease dissemination.[37]

Colorectal Cancer

Colorectal cancers (CRC) can be found from the cecum to the rectum, with the rectosigmoid being the most common location for colorectal adenocarcinoma.[38] In less than 10% of patients, CRC is associated with familial syndromes including familial adenomatous polyposis, hereditary nonpolyposis colon cancer syndrome, and Peutz–Jeghers syndrome. The most common histologic subtype comprising more than 90% of colorectal cancer is adenocarcinoma, originating from epithelial cells of colorectal mucosa.[39] Other subtypes include mucinous carcinoma of the colon, neuroendocrine, squamous cell, adenosquamous, spindle cell, lymphoma, and undifferentiated carcinomas. As discussed previously, the mucinous subtypes commonly show poor uptake on FDG due to low cellularity and high mucin content of the tumor mass. These tumors frequently produce cystic or calcified hepatic metastases and have widespread intraperitoneal metastases.[40] Among large bowel lymphomas, diffuse large B-cell lymphoma is the most common.[41] In comparison with adenocarcinoma, colonic lymphoma often presents with circumferential wall thickening, and, can affect longer as well as multiple colonic segments.[42] Another major histologic category of colorectal malignancies are the family of neuroendocrine neoplasms (NENs) of the large bowel, with a predilection for the rectum.[43] These include indolent well differentiated NETs to poorly differentiated carcinomas which are highly aggressive. The majority of NETs express somatostatin receptors that can be targeted in diagnostic imaging and therapy (theranostics).[44–46]

CLINICAL INDICATIONS OF PET/COMPUTED TOMOGRAPHY IMAGING
Diagnosis

Colonoscopy is the modality of choice for initial diagnosis as it allows evaluation of the entire large intestine and the capability to take biopsies/resection of polyps in a single session.[47] Focal ^{18}F-FDG uptake in the bowel on PET/CT, especially when correlating with a mass on CT, suggests a malignant lesion and requires further evaluation with colonoscopy. PET/CT can also identify incidental synchronous/metachronous primary tumors, affecting management. However, ^{18}F-FDG PET/CT has low specificity as premalignant lesions such as adenomas, and focal infection/inflammation also show increased ^{18}F-FDG uptake and can be found incidentally in PET. Thus, a single time point PET/CT alone cannot reliably differentiate between benign and malignant disease.[48] (Fig. 2).

Initial Staging

The NCCN guidelines recommend CT and MRI for the initial staging of colorectal carcinoma. ^{18}F-FDG PET/CT is useful for detecting lymph node involvement and distant metastases. There is limited added value of ^{18}F-FDG PET/CT in the local staging of CRC, and it is thus not routinely performed for pre-operative staging.[49,50] Around 30% of patients with CRC have distant metastases at initial presentation, including involvement of the liver, lungs, and bones.[51] In patients with suspected metastatic disease, ^{18}F-FDG PET/CT is useful for determining overall stage and prognosis as the management and long-term outcomes are heavily influenced by the initial stage of the disease. Surgical resection of limited metastatic disease with curative intent has demonstrated favorable long-term outcomes.[12–15]

Radiation Therapy Planning

NCCN guidelines recognize the usefulness of ^{18}F-FDG PET/CT in radiation therapy planning.[52] ^{18}F-FDG PET/CT helps improve tumor delineation, minimizing exposure to non-tumor areas, allowing for radiation dose adjustment to different areas of the tumor.

Assessment of Treatment Response

Anatomic changes lag behind metabolic changes when assessing response to therapy.[6] ^{18}F-FDG uptake is proportional to the number of viable cells; hence, reduction in FDG uptake usually denotes treatment response which precedes changes in tumor size.[14] ^{18}F-FDG PET/CT can assess treatment response in the early course of therapy, which can help guide treatment decisions and predict prognosis.[53] Treatment response is frequently assessed using both qualitative (visual analysis) and quantitative methods including parameters such as standardized uptake value (SUV).[54] Other volumetric PET parameters like metabolic tumor volume (MTV) and total lesion glycolysis (TLG) can also be used.

^{18}F-FDG PET/CT has been utilized for response assessment in a variety of treatment settings, including neoadjuvant and adjuvant chemotherapy, radiation therapy, and metastasis-directed therapies, including selective internal radiation therapy (SIRT), radiofrequency ablation, and transcatheter arterial chemoembolization, predominantly in locally advanced disease, oligometastatic disease, or potentially resectable metastatic disease.[55,56] It also helps in the optimal selection of patients for surgical resection and early identification of non-responders.

Multiple studies have been performed using different treatment regimens, imaging timepoints, and assessment criteria for analyzing the role of ^{18}F-FDG PET/CT after neoadjuvant chemotherapy.[57,58] Assessment of response using ^{18}F-FDG PET utilizing parameters like SUVmax, MTV, and TLG are predictors for long-term outcomes, but there is a lack of uniform, ideal timing of PET during and after neoadjuvant chemotherapy for CRC.[59] PET response criteria in solid tumors (PERCIST) has been established as the metabolic response criteria for the assessment of treatment response in solid tumors, predominantly in a clinical trial setting.[14]

Immunotherapy is an emerging treatment modality for advanced CRC. Assessing treatment response after immunotherapy is challenging as the post-treatment changes in the tumor microenvironment can mimic progression of disease, a phenomenon also known as "pseudoprogression."[60] A few immunotherapy-specific response assessment criteria have been described based on FDG PET/CT; however, most lack validation in large cohorts.[61–64]

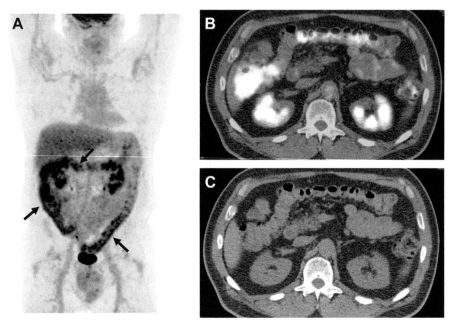

Fig. 2. A 58-year-old-man with adenocarcinoma of the sigmoid colon diagnosed on a colonoscopy biopsy. The maximum intensity projection (A) and the transaxial images (B, C) show diffusely increased FDG uptake throughout the colon (*arrows*) that limits the detection of the primary site. The patient had type 2 diabetes mellitus and was taking metformin at the time of the ^{18}F-FDG PET/CT study.

Re-staging and Surveillance

Disease recurrence is seen in up to 30% of patients within 2 years of initial resection, with the liver being the most common site for metastatic disease.[65,66] Guidelines recommend intensive follow-up during the first 3 to 5 years. Patients with rising serum carcino-embryonic antigen (CEA) levels without detectable disease on anatomic imaging pose a clinical challenge. Various studies have suggested the positive value of performing ^{18}F-FDG PET/CT in the evaluation of disease recurrence.[67–69] A few studies have evaluated the role of ^{18}F-FDG PET/CT for recurrent CRC with normal CEA levels, suggesting satisfactory sensitivities and specificities for detecting recurrence regardless of level of biomarkers.[70,71]

The major concern in detecting recurrence is differentiating recurrence from post-treatment scarring and radiation fibrosis. ^{18}F-FDG PET/CT has proven to be efficient and superior to both CT and MRI in this regard.[72] PET/CT can localize disease recurrence earlier than conventional imaging modalities with more accurate restaging, allowing for earlier intervention and potentially better outcomes. Accurate detection of loco-regional recurrence may be hindered by substantial distortion of anatomy post surgery.[73] The altered anatomy may limit the utility of structural imaging, but ^{18}F-FDG avidity can facilitate detection of disease sites.

To increase the specificity of lesion characterization, dual time imaging can be done with ^{18}F-FDG by performing scans at 2 different time periods usually 1 to 3 hours apart. Increase of ^{18}F-FDG uptake with time favors a malignant etiology (**Fig. 3**).

OTHER RADIOPHARMACEUTICALS AND FUTURE DIRECTIONS

Fibroblast activation protein (FAP) is a type II transmembrane protease with dipeptidyl peptidase and endopeptidase activities that mainly exists in fibroblasts activated by cancer, chronic inflammation, and fibrosis.[74] A recently published meta-analysis of 148 patients with gastric cancer showed that ^{68}Ga-FAPI-04 PET/MRI or PET/CT was superior to ^{18}F-FDG PET/MRI or PET/CT in detection of the primary tumor, lymph node, and peritoneal metastases. There is low hepatic background with ^{68}Ga-FAPI-04 which may be advantageous for the detection of liver metastasis. Further studies are required to evaluate the sensitivity and specificity of ^{68}Ga-FAPI-04 PET in different pathologic types of gastric and colorectal malignancies.

Prostate-specific membrane antigen (PSMA) is a type II transmembrane receptor used primarily for imaging and therapy of prostate cancer.[75–79] In addition to the prostate cancer cells, PSMA is expressed in the tumor neovasculature of several non-prostate

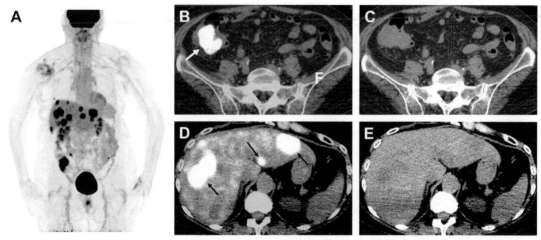

Fig. 3. A 78-year-old-woman with adenocarcinoma of the cecum. ^{18}F-FDG PET/CT maximum intensity projection image (*A*) and trans-axial fused PET/CT and CT images show (*B* and *C*) the hypermetabolic primary soft tissue mass at the cecum (*white arrow*) and (*D* and *E*) multiple hypermetabolic hypoattenuating lesions in the liver (*black arrows*) that were biopsy proven as metastases from the colorectal primary.

malignancies that can facilitate their diagnosis and potentially, therapy. These include several gastric and colorectal malignancies.[80–83] A prospective clinical trial has comparatively evaluated PSMA PET/CT to ^{18}F-FDG PET/CT of primary gastric and colorectal cancer; this study concluded with the feasibility of PSMA PET/CT for these aforementioned malignancies; however, ^{18}F-FDG PET/CT outperformed PSMA PET/CT due to the poor tumor-to-background ratio of latter, in the primary locations of these tumors.[84] Therefore, PSMA PET/CT may be better suited toward increasing the diagnostic certainty of imaging in the setting of metastatic disease.[85,86]

Somatostatin-targeting radiopharmaceuticals are excellent for the evaluation of NETs. Other radiotracers including ^{64}Cu-ATSM, ^{68}Ga-Pentixafor, ^{18}F-FLT, and ImmunoPET have been investigated as an alternative to ^{18}F-FDG PET. ^{18}F-FLT serves as a proliferative marker by reporting on the activity of thymidine salvage pathway.[87] A few pilot studies using ^{18}F-FLT have been performed for various indications in CRC, but has not gained much traction.[88] ^{64}Cu-ATSM is a promising theranostic agent with high tissue permeability and targeting of over-reduced state under hypoxia within tumors.[89]

SUMMARY

^{18}F-FDG PET plays an important role in the evaluation of patients with cancer of the gastrointestinal tract both at the time of initial staging and at the time of subsequent treatment strategy. While, to date, ^{18}F-FDG continues to be the most ubiquitous radiopharmaceutical used, somatostatin-targeting radiopharmaceuticals have become key in the evaluation of patients with NETs and it is likely that newer radiopharmaceuticals will become available in the near future, although their exact clinical indications remain to be determined.

CLINICS CARE POINTS

- 18F-FDG PET is useful in staging and subsequent treatment strategy of patients with gastrointestical and colorectal malignancies
- Somatostatin-targeting radiopharmaceuticals have become key in the evaluation of patients with NETs

DISCLOSURE

M.K. Ramirez-Fort is CEO of BioFort Corp. The other authors report no conflicts of interest related to gastric and colorectal cancer.

REFERENCES

1. Machlowska J, Baj J, Sitarz M, et al. Gastric cancer: epidemiology, risk factors, classification, genomic characteristics and treatment strategies. Int J Mol Sci 2020;21.
2. Jayaprakasam VS, Paroder V, Schoder H. Variants and pitfalls in PET/CT imaging of gastrointestinal cancers. Semin Nucl Med 2021;51:485–501.

3. Young JJ, Pahwa A, Patel M, et al. Ligaments and lymphatic pathways in gastric adenocarcinoma. Radiographics 2019;39:668–89.

4. Riihimaki M, Hemminki A, Sundquist J, et al. Patterns of metastasis in colon and rectal cancer. Sci Rep 2016;6:29765.

5. Howard BA, Wong TZ. ^{18}F-FDG-PET/CT imaging for gastrointestinal malignancies. Radiol Clin 2021;59: 737–53.

6. Parihar AS, Dehdashti F, Wahl RL. FDG PET/CT-based response assessment in malignancies. Radiographics 2023;43:e220122.

7. Boellaard R, Delgado-Bolton R, Oyen WJ, et al. Fdg pet/CT: EANM procedure guidelines for tumour imaging: version 2.0. Eur J Nucl Med Mol Imag 2015; 42:328–54.

8. Delbeke D, Coleman RE, Guiberteau MJ, et al. Procedure guideline for tumor imaging with 18F-FDG PET/CT 1.0. J Nucl Med 2006;47:885–95.

9. Le Roux PY, Duong CP, Cabalag CS, et al. Incremental diagnostic utility of gastric distension FDG PET/CT. Eur J Nucl Med Mol Imag 2016;43:644–53.

10. Dyde R, Chapman AH, Gale R, et al. Precautions to be taken by radiologists and radiographers when prescribing hyoscine-N-butylbromide. Clin Radiol 2008;63:739–43.

11. Kuker RA, Mesoloras G, Gulec SA. Optimization of FDG-PET/CT imaging protocol for evaluation of patients with primary and metastatic liver disease. Int Semin Surg Oncol 2007;4:17.

12. Perry C, Herishanu Y, Metzer U, et al. Diagnostic accuracy of PET/CT in patients with extranodal marginal zone MALT lymphoma. Eur J Haematol 2007;79:205–9.

13. Saleh Farghaly HR, Mohamed Sayed MH, Nasr HA, et al. Dual time point fluorodeoxyglucose positron emission tomography/computed tomography in differentiation between malignant and benign lesions in cancer patients. Does it always work? Indian J Nucl Med 2015;30:314–9.

14. Wahl RL, Jacene H, Kasamon Y, et al. From RECIST to PERCIST: evolving Considerations for PET response criteria in solid tumors. J Nucl Med 2009; 50(Suppl 1):122S–50S.

15. Kido H, Kato S, Funahashi K, et al. The metabolic parameters based on volume in PET/CT are associated with clinicopathological N stage of colorectal cancer and can predict prognosis. EJNMMI Res 2021;11:87.

16. Vadi SK, Kumar R, Mittal BR, et al. 18F-FDG PET/CT in an atypical case of relapsed IgG4-related disease presenting as inflammatory pseudotumor in gall bladder fossa with extensive disease involvement. Clin Nucl Med 2018;43:e357–9.

17. Hu B, El Hajj N, Sittler S, et al. Gastric cancer: classification, histology and application of molecular pathology. J Gastrointest Oncol 2012;3:251–61.

18. Lauren P. The two histological main types of gastric carcinoma: diffuse and so-called intestinal-type carcinoma. An attempt at a histo-clinical classification. Acta Pathol Microbiol Scand 1965;64:31–49.

19. Flejou JF. [WHO Classification of digestive tumors: the fourth edition]. Ann Pathol 2011;31:S27–31.

20. Wu CX, Zhu ZH. Diagnosis and evaluation of gastric cancer by positron emission tomography. World J Gastroenterol 2014;20:4574–85.

21. Bosch KD, Chicklore S, Cook GJ, et al. Staging FDG PET-CT changes management in patients with gastric adenocarcinoma who are eligible for radical treatment. Eur J Nucl Med Mol Imag 2020;47:759–67.

22. Amin MB, Greene FL, Edge SB, et al. The Eighth Edition AJCC Cancer Staging Manual: continuing to build a bridge from a population-based to a more "personalized" approach to cancer staging. CA Cancer J Clin 2017;67:93–9.

23. Tirumani H, Rosenthal MH, Tirumani SH, et al. Esophageal carcinoma: current concepts in the role of imaging in staging and management. Can Assoc Radiol J 2015;66:130–9.

24. Ajani JA, D'Amico TA, Bentrem DJ, et al. Esophageal and esophagogastric junction cancers, version 2.2023, NCCN clinical practice guidelines in Oncology. J Natl Compr Cancer Netw 2023;21:393–422.

25. Cuellar SL, Carter BW, Macapinlac HA, et al. Clinical staging of patients with early esophageal adenocarcinoma: does FDG-PET/CT have a role? J Thorac Oncol 2014;9:1202–6.

26. Koppula BR, Fine GC, Salem AE, et al. PET-CT in clinical adult Oncology: III. Gastrointestinal malignancies. Cancers 2022;14.

27. Ramirez-Fort MK, Rogers MJ, Santiago R, et al. Prostatic irradiation-induced sexual dysfunction: a review and multidisciplinary guide to management in the radical radiotherapy era (Part I defining the organ at risk for sexual toxicities). Rep Practical Oncol Radiother 2020;25:367–75.

28. Bentzen SM, Constine LS, Deasy JO, et al. Quantitative analyses of normal tissue Effects in the clinic (QUANTEC): an introduction to the scientific issues. Int J Radiat Oncol Biol Phys 2010;76:S3–9.

29. Ajani JA, D'Amico TA, Bentrem DJ, et al. Esophageal and esophagogastric junction cancers, version 2.2019, NCCN clinical practice guidelines in Oncology. J Natl Compr Cancer Netw 2019;17:855–83.

30. Wildiers H, Neven P, Christiaens MR, et al. Neoadjuvant capecitabine and docetaxel (plus trastuzumab): an effective non-anthracycline-based chemotherapy regimen for patients with locally advanced breast cancer. Ann Oncol 2011;22:588–94.

31. Biffi R, Fazio N, Luca F, et al. Surgical outcome after docetaxel-based neoadjuvant chemotherapy in locally-advanced gastric cancer. World J Gastroenterol 2010;16:868–74.

32. Di Fabio F, Pinto C, Rojas Llimpe FL, et al. The predictive value of 18F-FDG-PET early evaluation in patients with metastatic gastric adenocarcinoma treated with

chemotherapy plus cetuximab. Gastric Cancer 2007; 10:221–7.

33. Ott K, Herrmann K, Lordick F, et al. Early metabolic response evaluation by fluorine-18 fluorodeoxyglucose positron emission tomography allows in vivo testing of chemosensitivity in gastric cancer: long-term results of a prospective study. Clin Cancer Res 2008;14:2012–8.

34. Weber WA, Ott K, Becker K, et al. Prediction of response to preoperative chemotherapy in adenocarcinomas of the esophagogastric junction by metabolic imaging. J Clin Oncol 2001;19:3058–65.

35. Yoo CH, Noh SH, Shin DW, et al. Recurrence following curative resection for gastric carcinoma. Br J Surg 2000;87:236–42.

36. Smyth EC, Shah MA. Role of (1)(8)F 2-fluoro-2-deoxyglucose positron emission tomography in upper gastrointestinal malignancies. World J Gastroenterol 2011;17:5059–74.

37. Smyth EC, Verheij M, Allum W, et al. Gastric cancer: ESMO Clinical Practice Guidelines for diagnosis, treatment and follow-up. Ann Oncol 2016;27(Supp 5):v38–49.

38. Horton KM, Abrams RA, Fishman EK. Spiral CT of colon cancer: imaging features and role in management. Radiographics 2000;20:419–30.

39. Fleming M, Ravula S, Tatishchev SF, et al. Colorectal carcinoma: pathologic aspects. J Gastrointest Oncol 2012;3:153–73.

40. Okuno M, Ikehara T, Nagayama M, et al. Mucinous colorectal carcinoma: clinical pathology and prognosis. Am Surg 1988;54:681–5.

41. Quayle FJ, Lowney JK. Colorectal lymphoma. Clin Colon Rectal Surg 2006;19:49–53.

42. Lee WK, Lau EW, Duddalwar VA, et al. Abdominal manifestations of extranodal lymphoma: spectrum of imaging findings. AJR Am J Roentgenol 2008;191:198–206.

43. Yao JC, Hassan M, Phan A, et al. One hundred years after "carcinoid": epidemiology of and prognostic factors for neuroendocrine tumors in 35,825 cases in the United States. J Clin Oncol 2008;26:3063–72.

44. Ashwathanarayana AG, Biswal CK, Sood A, et al. Imaging-guided use of combined (177)Lu-dotatate and capecitabine therapy in metastatic mediastinal paraganglioma. J Nucl Med Technol 2017;45:314–6.

45. Iravani A, Parihar AS, Akhurst T, et al. Molecular imaging phenotyping for selecting and monitoring radioligand therapy of neuroendocrine neoplasms. Cancer Imag 2022;22:25.

46. Park S, Parihar AS, Bodei L, et al. Somatostatin receptor imaging and theranostics: current practice and future prospects. J Nucl Med 2021;62:1323–9.

47. Rodriguez-Fraile M, Cozar-Santiago MP, Sabate-Llobera A, et al. FDG PET/CT in colorectal cancer. Rev Española Med Nucl Imagen Mol 2020;39:57–66.

48. Yasuda S, Fujii H, Nakahara T, et al. 18F-FDG PET detection of colonic adenomas. J Nucl Med 2001; 42:989–92.

49. Veit-Haibach P, Kuehle CA, Beyer T, et al. Diagnostic accuracy of colorectal cancer staging with whole-body PET/CT colonography. JAMA 2006;296: 2590–600.

50. Kinner S, Antoch G, Bockisch A, et al. Whole-body PET/CT-colonography: a possible new concept for colorectal cancer staging. Abdom Imag 2007;32: 606–12.

51. Briggs RH, Chowdhury FU, Lodge JP, et al. Clinical impact of FDG PET-CT in patients with potentially operable metastatic colorectal cancer. Clin Radiol 2011;66:1167–74.

52. Frankel TL, Gian RK, Jarnagin WR. Preoperative imaging for hepatic resection of colorectal cancer metastasis. J Gastrointest Oncol 2012;3:11–8.

53. Joo Hyun O, Lodge MA, Wahl RL. Practical percist: a simplified guide to PET response criteria in solid tumors 1.0. Radiology 2016;280:576–84.

54. Maffione AM, Marzola MC, Capirci C, et al. Value of (18)F-FDG PET for predicting response to neoadjuvant therapy in rectal cancer: systematic review and meta-analysis. AJR Am J Roentgenol 2015; 204:1261–8.

55. Maffione AM, Chondrogiannis S, Capirci C, et al. Early prediction of response by (1)(8)F-FDG PET/CT during preoperative therapy in locally advanced rectal cancer: a systematic review. Eur J Surg Oncol 2014;40:1186–94.

56. Fendler WP, Philippe Tiega DB, Ilhan H, et al. Validation of several SUV-based parameters derived from 18F-FDG PET for prediction of survival after SIRT of hepatic metastases from colorectal cancer. J Nucl Med 2013;54:1202–8.

57. Nishioka Y, Yoshioka R, Gonoi W, et al. Fluorine-18-fluorodeoxyglucose positron emission tomography as an objective substitute for CT morphologic response criteria in patients undergoing chemotherapy for colorectal liver metastases. Abdom Radiol (NY) 2018;43:1152–8.

58. Lastoria S, Piccirillo MC, Caraco C, et al. Early PET/CT scan is more effective than RECIST in predicting outcome of patients with liver metastases from colorectal cancer treated with preoperative chemotherapy plus bevacizumab. J Nucl Med 2013;54: 2062–9.

59. Bampo C, Alessi A, Fantini S, et al. Is the standardized uptake value of FDG-PET/CT predictive of pathological complete response in locally advanced rectal cancer treated with capecitabine-based neoadjuvant chemoradiation? Oncology 2013;84:191–9.

60. Borcoman E, Kanjanapan Y, Champiat S, et al. Novel patterns of response under immunotherapy. Ann Oncol 2019;30:385–96.

61. Unterrainer M, Ruzicka M, Fabritius MP, et al. PET/CT imaging for tumour response assessment to immunotherapy: current status and future directions. European radiology experimental 2020;4.

62. Costa LB, Queiroz MA, Barbosa FG, et al. Reassessing patterns of response to immunotherapy with pet: from morphology to metabolism. Radiographics 2021;41:120–43.

63. Iravani A, Hicks RJ. Imaging the cancer immune environment and its response to pharmacologic intervention, Part 1: the role of 18F-FDG PET/CT. J Nucl Med 2020;61:943–50.

64. Lopci E, Hicks RJ, Dercle L, et al. FDG PET/CT imaging during immunomodulatory treatments in patients with solid tumors European Association of. Nuclear Medicine, Eur J Nucl Med Mol Imag 2022; 49:2323–41.

65. Valk PE, Abella-Columna E, Haseman MK, et al. Whole-body PET imaging with [18F]fluorodeoxyglucose in management of recurrent colorectal cancer. Arch Surg 1999;134:503–11 [discussion: 511-503].

66. Scheele J, Stang R, Altendorf-Hofmann A, et al. Resection of colorectal liver metastases. World J Surg 1995;19:59–71.

67. Liu FY, Chen JS, Changchien CR, et al. Utility of 2-fluoro-2-deoxy-D-glucose positron emission tomography in managing patients of colorectal cancer with unexplained carcinoembryonic antigen elevation at different levels. Dis Colon Rectum 2005;48: 1900–12.

68. Flamen P, Hoekstra OS, Homans F, et al. Unexplained rising carcinoembryonic antigen (CEA) in the postoperative surveillance of colorectal cancer: the utility of positron emission tomography (PET). Eur J Cancer 2001;37:862–9.

69. Milardovic R, Beslic N, Sadija A, et al. Role of 18F-FDG PET/CT in the follow-up of colorectal cancer. Acta Inf Med 2020;28:119–23.

70. Sanli Y, Kuyumcu S, Ozkan ZG, et al. The utility of FDG-PET/CT as an effective tool for detecting recurrent colorectal cancer regardless of serum CEA levels. Ann Nucl Med 2012;26:551–8.

71. Chiaravalloti A, Fiorentini A, Palombo E, et al. Evaluation of recurrent disease in the re-staging of colorectal cancer by (18)F-FDG PET/CT: use of CEA and CA 19-9 in patient selection. Oncol Lett 2016; 12:4209–13.

72. Buchmann I, Ganten TM, Haberkorn U. [[18F]-FDG-PET in the diagnostics of gastrointestinal tumors]. Z Gastroenterol 2008;46:367–75.

73. de Geus-Oei LF, Ruers TJ, Punt CJ, et al. FDG-PET in colorectal cancer. Cancer Imag 2006;6:S71–81.

74. Zhao L, Chen J, Pang Y, et al. Fibroblast activation protein-based theranostics in cancer research: a state-of-the-art review. Theranostics 2022;12: 1557–69.

75. Afshar-Oromieh A, Babich JW, Kratochwil C, et al. The rise of PSMA ligands for diagnosis and therapy of prostate cancer. J Nucl Med 2016;57:79S–89S.

76. Chatalic KLS, Heskamp S, Konijnenberg M, et al. Towards personalized treatment of prostate cancer: PSMA I&T, a promising prostate-specific membrane antigen-targeted theranostic agent. Theranostics 2016;6:849–61.

77. Afshar-Oromieh A, Malcher A, Eder M, et al. Pet imaging with a [68ga]gallium-labelled psma ligand for the diagnosis of prostate cancer: biodistribution in humans and first evaluation of tumour lesions. Eur J Nucl Med Mol Imag 2013;40:486–95.

78. Afshar-Oromieh A, Haberkorn U, Zechmann C, et al. Repeated PSMA-targeting radioligand therapy of metastatic prostate cancer with 131I-MIP-1095. Eur J Nucl Med Mol Imag 2017;44:950–9.

79. Parihar AS, Hofman MS, Iravani A. (177)Lu-Prostate-specific membrane antigen radioligand therapy in patients with metastatic castration-resistant prostate cancer. Radiology 2023;306:e220859.

80. Laurens ST, Witjes F, Janssen M, et al. 68Ga-Prostate-Specific membrane antigen uptake in gastrointestinal stromal tumor. Clin Nucl Med 2018;43:60–1.

81. Malik D, Kumar R, Mittal BR, et al. 68)Ga-labelled PSMA (prostate specific membrane antigen) expression in signet-ring cell gastric carcinoma. Eur J Nucl Med Mol Imag 2018;45:1276–7.

82. Han XD, Liu C, Liu F, et al. 64)Cu-PSMA-617: a novel PSMA-targeted radio-tracer for PET imaging in gastric adenocarcinoma xenografted mice model. Oncotarget 2017;8:74159–69.

83. Sasikumar A, Joy A, Pillai M, et al. 68Ga-PSMA uptake in an incidentally detected gastrointestinal stromal tumor in a case of suspected carcinoma prostate. Clin Nucl Med 2017;42:e447–8.

84. Vuijk FA, Kleiburg F, Noortman WA, et al. Prostate-specific membrane antigen targeted pet/CT imaging in patients with colon, gastric and pancreatic cancer. Cancers 2022;14.

85. Ozcan PP, Serdengecti M, Koc ZP, et al. Cancers and benign processes on (68) Ga PSMA PET-CT imaging other than prostate cancer. World J Nucl Med 2022;21:106–11.

86. Kesim S, Oksuzoglu K. 68Ga-PSMA uptake in brain metastasis of gastric carcinoma. Clin Nucl Med 2022;47:e585–6.

87. Schelhaas S, Wachsmuth L, Hermann S, et al. Thymidine metabolism as a confounding factor for 3'-deoxy-3'-(18)F-fluorothymidine uptake after therapy in a colorectal cancer model. J Nucl Med 2018;59:1063–9.

88. Dehdashti F, Grigsby PW, Myerson RJ, et al. Positron emission tomography with [(18)F]-3'-deoxy-3'fluorothymidine (FLT) as a predictor of outcome in patients with locally advanced resectable rectal cancer: a pilot study. Mol Imag Biol 2013;15:106–13.

89. Yoshii Y, Yoshimoto M, Matsumoto H, et al. 64)Cu-ATSM internal radiotherapy to treat tumors with bevacizumab-induced vascular decrease and hypoxia in human colon carcinoma xenografts. Oncotarget 2017;8:88815–26.

Quarter Century PET/ Computed Tomography Transformation of Oncology
Neuroendocrine Tumors

Charles Marcus, MD[a],*, Saima Muzahir, MD, FCPS, FRCPE[a], Rathan M. Subramaniam, MD, PhD, MPH, MBA[b,c,d]

KEYWORDS

- PET/CT • Neuroendocrine • DOTATATE • Gastroenteropancreatic • Theranostics • Somatostatin
- Octreoscan

KEY POINTS

- PET imaging of neuroendocrine tumors (NETs) outperforms anatomic (computed tomography [CT]/ MRI), nuclear medicine planar, and single-photon emission computed tomography imaging.
- Somatostatin receptor–targeted PET/CT provides accurate staging, treatment response assessment, and restaging of NET patients.
- Somatostatin receptor–targeted PET/CT can have a significant impact on management decisions in these patients.
- Radionuclide therapy has become an important therapeutic option in patients with metastatic disease with disease progression while on somatostatin analogues.

INTRODUCTION

Neuroendocrine tumors (NETs) encompass a wide group of tumors arising from the secretory cells of the neuroendocrine cells and can secrete peptides making them "functional" or "non-functional" without secreting active peptides. These tumors can arise from a wide variety of structures within the human body, with the most common origin being the gastroenteropancreatic (GEP) system.[1] These tumors exhibit varying biological properties with indolent tumors being the most encountered tumors. However, some of these tumors (10%–20%) can behave aggressively.[2] There has been a steady increase in the incidence of NETs in the last few decades. In the United States, the prevalence of NETs is approximately 170, 000, with 22,744 GEP NETs recorded between 1975 and 2012, with the highest incidence in patients older than 70 years of age. The most common location of the primary disease is the bowel, followed by the pancreas, stomach, and appendix. Metastatic disease is detected at diagnosis in a large proportion of these patients (40%–76%), especially in patients with pancreatic NETs. Gastroenteric tumors demonstrate a higher overall survival rate (55%–89%), compared to pancreatic tumors (38%).[3]

Significant advances have been made in the last few decades in the diagnosis, imaging evaluation, and management of NETs. Detailed discussion of the evaluation and management of NETs is beyond the scope of this article and will focus on the molecular imaging and theranostics in the management of NETs. Anatomic imaging (computed

[a] Division of Nuclear Medicine, Department of Radiology and Imaging Sciences, Emory University School of Medicine, 1364 Clifton Road Northeast, E163, Atlanta, GA 30322, USA; [b] Faculty of Medicine, Nursing, Midwifery and Health Sciences, The University of Notre Dame Australia, 160 Oxford Street, Darlinghurst, New South Wales 2010, Australia; [c] Department of Radiology, Duke University, Durham, NC, USA; [d] Department of Medicine, Otago Medical School, The University of Otago, New Zealand
* Corresponding author.
E-mail address: cvmarcu@emory.edu

PET Clin 19 (2024) 187–196
https://doi.org/10.1016/j.cpet.2023.12.005
1556-8598/24/© 2023 Elsevier Inc. All rights reserved.

tomography [CT]/MRI) is performed to image the primary tumor site, and depending on the suspicion of distant disease, additional imaging of other sites can be considered. Multiphasic contrast-enhanced imaging is preferred for the imaging of the liver, a common site of hypervascular NET metastases. Somatostatin receptor (SSTR)-targeted imaging is useful in the evaluation of metastatic disease and determining SSTR expression for treatment planning. Octreotide planar or single-photon emission computed tomography (SPECT)/CT imaging has fallen out of favor over the years and is reserved in cases when SSTR-targeted PET imaging either with CT or MRI is not available. Surveillance imaging is usually recommended for 10 years after initial curative treatment.[4]

This review will aim to provide a summary of PET/CT imaging in NETs, with special focus on the evolution of molecular imaging in the evaluation of NETs. A brief overview of the role of theranostics in the management of metastatic NETs will also be discussed.

MANAGEMENT OF NEUROENDOCRINE TUMORS

Many NET patients present with advanced disease at the time of initial diagnosis.[5] Multiple therapeutic options are available for NET based on current guidelines,[6] including cytoreductive operations, catheter-based liver-directed treatment and needle ablation, somatostatin analogs (SSAs), mammalian target of rapamycin (mTOR) inhibitors, tyrosine kinase inhibitors, systemic chemotherapy, and peptide receptor radionuclide therapy (PRRT).

Locoregional disease: Surgical resection is considered as the only curative treatment based on current National Comprehensive Cancer Network (NCCN) guidelines.[4] Patients with early-stage disease (stage I to III) should be evaluated for possible curative resection.[7] Small intraluminal lung or gastrointestinal neuroendocrine neoplasm (T1-T2) without nodal metastases can undergo curative endoscopic resection.[8] The size and intraluminal growth on CT are predictors of treatment. Reuling and colleagues showed that lesions below 2.0 cm were successfully resected in 72% of patients.[9]

Liver-directed therapies: The liver is the most common site of distant NET metastases and is considered the major prognosticator of survival irrespective of the primary site.[10] Approximately 80% to 90% of small bowel and 60% to 70% of pancreatic NET metastasize to the liver.[11] The management and eligibility is considerably different for patients with metastatic NETs than from those with other types of cancer. In liver- dominant

disease, cytoreductive surgery is an option if more than 90% of the imaged liver volume can be safely removed with an operative mortality of less than 10%.[12] If the patient is not a surgical candidate, multiple liver-directed therapies are available.[13] The choice of liver- directed therapy depends upon hepatic tumor burden, growth rate, liver function, and the presence of extrahepatic metastases.[14] Liver-directed embolization options include trans arterial bland embolization causing tumor ischemia, trans arterial chemoembolization, and trans arterial radioembolization using Y-90.[15]

Somatostatin analogues (SSAs): Well-differentiated NETs overexpress SSTR. The use of non-radioactive SSAs in the management of NETs was based on overexpression of the SSTR in these tumors. Before 2009, SSAs were used to treat symptoms of patients with functionally active NETs. The PROMID trial showed that octreotide long-acting repeatable (LAR) significantly lengthens time to progression in patients with functionally active and inactive metastatic midgut NETs. In 2014, the study of lanreotide autogel in non-functioning enteropancreatic NETs (CLATINET) showed that lanreotide can serve as a therapeutic modality to improve progression-free survival (PFS) in advanced NETs.[16,17]

Targeted Therapy: The primary focus of targeted therapy in GEP-NET treatment involves inhibition of mTOR pathway and tyrosine kinase pathway.[18] Oral mTOR inhibitor (everolimus) demonstrated significant antiproliferative effect. The most common reported serious adverse events include thrombocytopenia, diarrhea, and interstitial lung disease. The other agent is multi-targeted tyrosine kinase inhibitor sunitinib malate (Sutent, Pfizer). Sunitinib prolonged PFS in patients with metastatic pancreatic neuroendocrine tumors (panNETs) in a large phase III trial.[19]

Chemotherapy: Well-differentiated NETs are slow-growing tumors and there is no documented role of chemotherapy especially in small bowel NETs.[20,21] For intermediate to high-grade rapidly progressing or bulky pancreatic tumors there are data demonstrating promising results, with response rates ranging from 30% to 70%.[22]

PET IMAGING OF NEUROENDOCRINE TUMORS

There has been a significant increase in the interest and literature in somatostatin receptor–targeted PET imaging over time with most of the literature published in the early 2020s. In the United States, the Food and Drug Administration (FDA) approved Ga[68]-DOTATATE for clinical use in June 2016 for evaluation of both adult and pediatric patients with NETs.[23] In January 2018, the US FDA approved

Lu[177]-DOTATATE for clinical use in the management of metastatic GEP-NETs.[24] In September 2020, Cu[64]-DOTATATE, a second diagnostic PET radiotracer was approved.[25] *From planar and SPECT/CT scintigraphy to PET Imaging.*

Approved for clinical use in 1994, In[111]-DTPA Pentetreotide or Octreoscan was widely used for localizing NETs in patients, detecting disease especially in patients where the disease was not detected in conventional imaging.[26] With the introduction of somatostatin receptor–targeted PET imaging agents, there was increased interest in comparing the diagnostic performance of these agents to the then clinically used octreoscan. Studies clearly demonstrated the superior detection rate and diagnostic accuracy of the PET agents in comparison to planar or SPECT agents.[27] In a systemic review and metanalysis comparing Ga[68]-DOTATATE, In[111]-DTPA-Octreotide, and conventional imaging, the authors showed the sensitivity and specificity of PET/CT were 91% and 91%, respectively, significantly higher than octreotide or conventional imaging in pancreatic and GEP NETs. On a lesion level, Ga[68]-DOTATATE PET/CT was positive in approximately 75% lesions, significantly greater than octreoscan (P<.001), resulting in a significant impact on management in 70% patients.[28] Similar observations were made in other studies with positive rates around 60% for octreoscan compared to around 80% for somatostatin receptor–targeted PET imaging.[27] In pheochromocytoma and paraganglioma, SSTR PET imaging had superior lesion detection compared to other imaging modalities such as ^{18}F-DOPA, ^{18}F-FDG, [123/131]I-MIBG imaging, with certain exceptions such as polycthemia/paraganglioma syndrome.[29] Overall, in most clinical scenarios for the evaluation of NETs, somatostatin receptor PET imaging outperforms conventional and octreotide imaging and is preferred over these imaging techniques, when available (**Fig. 1**).

PET RADIOTRACERS FOR THE EVALUATION OF NEUROENDOCRINE TUMORS

One of the first evaluated PET radiotracer agents are Ga[68]-DOTATOC which demonstrated significantly higher affinity to SSTR2 and SSTR 5, in comparison to In[111]-Octreotate with superior resolution to planar and SPECT imaging.[30] This technique showed a statistically significant difference in the detection of neuroendocrine tumors in comparison to SPECT and diagnostic CT imaging.[31,32] Then came Ga[68]-DOTANOC, which exhibited all the advantages of the previous radiotracer and in addition showed affinity for SSTR 3.[33] The third

most evaluated PET radiotracer was Ga[68]-DOTATATE, which then became more widely used in research and clinical applications with the highest affinity for SSTR 2.[34] The latest introduction of Cu[64]-DOTATATE has raised much interest, given the added practical advantage of a longer half-life in comparison to Ga68 (12.7 h vs 68 minutes), a shorter positron range (0.7 mm vs 3.5 mm) providing superior spatial resolution, longer shelf life (>24 hours), despite the lower positron decay (17.9% vs 89%).[35] Following the introduction of these radiotracers, there was special interest in studies comparing the performance of these different agents. Ga[68]-DOTATATE and Ga[68]-DOTANOC have been shown to have comparable diagnostic accuracy with a few studies showing higher lesion level uptake of DOTATATE. Qualitatively higher radiotracer uptake was shown in about one-third of the lesions. This was reflected in the SUV measurements (SUVmax; 29.9 ± 26.4 vs 24.5 ± 20.3; $P<.01$).[36] Ga[68]-DOTATOC on the other hand has been shown to have higher uptake in NETs, detecting more lesions in comparison to Ga[68]-DOTATATE. However, significant variation in the uptake was demonstrated between patients and lesions within the same patient, failing to demonstrate a clear advantage of one radiotracer over the other.[37] A comparative study evaluating Cu[64]-DOTATATE and Ga[68]-DOTATOC showed more lesions were detected by Cu[64]-DOTATATE, although the patient-level sensitivity was comparable.[38] The more widely used oncologic PET agent, ^{18}F-FDG, is useful in select patients with known neuroendocrine cancer with suspected poorly differentiated disease and aggressive tumors that may not be highly SSTR PET radiotracer avid. These findings are also predictive of disease progression and patient outcomes[39–42] (**Fig. 2**). ^{18}F-FDG PET can play a complementary role to SSTR-PET imaging in identifying patients who may not respond to SSTR-targeted therapy. Metabolically active high-grade tumors with high proliferation index may demonstrate loss of SSTR expression that may not respond to standard treatment and may need alternative treatment options.[43]

SOMATOSTATIN RECEPTOR PET/COMPUTED TOMOGRAPHY IMAGING IN THE STAGING OF NEUROENDOCRINE TUMORS

Accurate initial staging after the diagnosis of NETs is crucial. Additional metastatic lesions have been shown to be detected in up to half of the patients. Occult primary tumors can be detected in almost one-third of patients. In patients with unknown metastatic disease, distant metastases can be

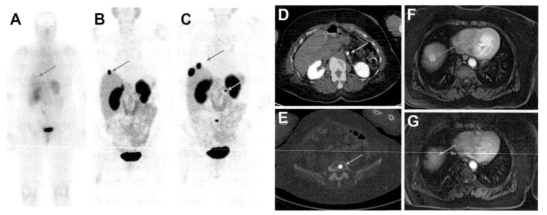

Fig. 1. Anterior planar In^{111}-octreotide scan (*A*), Ga^{68}-DOTATATE Coronal PET maximum intensity projection (MIP) (*B*) performed 2 months apart in a 75-year-old woman with pancreatic well-differentiated neuroendocrine tumor (NET) status post primary surgical management demonstrates intensely radiotracer- avid hepatic lesions on the PET scan (*blue arrows*) which demonstrated only minimal radiotracer uptake on the octreoscan. Ga^{68}-DOTATATE coronal PET (*C*), axial fused PET (*D, E*) after lanreotide therapy demonstrated progressive disease with additional metastatic lesions involving the liver (*blue arrow*), retroperitoneal lymph node (*yellow arrows*), and sacrum (*green arrows*). She subsequently underwent Lu^{177}-DOTATATE therapy. Axial postcontrast T1 pretreatment MR (*F*) and axial postcontrast T1 post-treatment MR (*G*) demonstrate significant reduction in the size and enhancement of the index liver lesion (blue *arrows*), compatible with a favorable treatment response.MR, magnetic resonance imaging.

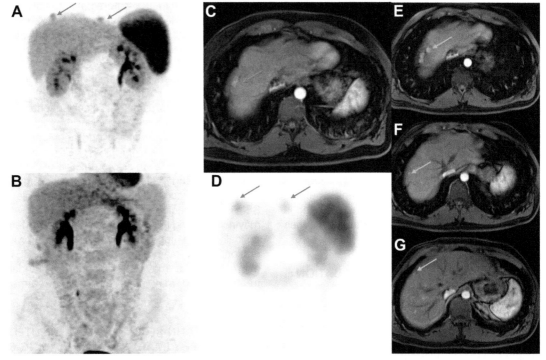

Fig. 2. Ga^{68}-DOTATATE Coronal MIP (*A*), ^{18}F-FDG Coronal MIP (*B*), Axial postcontrast T1 MR (*C*) of a 30-year-old man with well-differentiated intermediate-grade pancreatic NET, status post primary surgical management, followed by lanreotide, capecitabine, temozolomide, and everolimus for metastatic disease with subsequent imaging shown above demonstrating enhancing right subcapsular liver lesions with mild Ga^{68}-DOTATATE activity similar to thr librt and no significant ^{18}F-FDG activity (*blue arrows*). Subsequently patient underwent ^{177}Lu-DOTATATE therapy. ^{177}Lu-DOTATATE Coronal planar post- treatment image (*D*) showed radiotracer uptake within these lesions. However, subsequent axial postcontrast T1 MR images (*E–G*) demonstrated increase in the extent of the index lesions with new enhancing lesions in the liver (*yellow arrows*).

detected in up to 20% of patients. All these findings can result in a significant change in management in more than one-third of patients. Unnecessary invasive tissue sampling can be avoided in about 10% of patients. Surgical treatment plan can be changed in up to half of the patients who are scheduled to undergo primary surgical management.[24,44–47] In comparison to conventional imaging methods, SSTR PET imaging can change the stage in more than half the patients.[48] The overall sensitivity and specificity of SSTR PET imaging in the staging and diagnosis of neuroendocrine tumors are high. A meta-analysis including 1143 patients reported a pooled sensitivity of 80% and specificity of 95% in the evaluation of the primary tumor with a detection rate of 81%.[45] Another meta-analysis reported a pooled sensitivity and specificity of 91% and 94%, respectively.[49] SSTR PET imaging can detect bone metastasis with a higher diagnostic accuracy than CT.[50]

ROLE OF SOMATOSTATIN RECEPTOR PET/COMPUTED TOMOGRAPHY IN TREATMENT RESPONSE ASSESSMENT AND RESTAGING OF NEUROENDOCRINE TUMORS

Treatment response assessment can provide valuable information in management planning and prognosis prediction. In NET patients undergoing systemic therapy either with somatostatin analogues, chemotherapy, or PRRT, SSTR PET imaging can have an impact on the treatment plan in more than half the patients.[51] The level of radiotracer uptake can predict response to somatostatin analogues, with lesion demonstrating a low lesion SUVmax (<18.4) in well-differentiated grade 1 to 2 tumors, predicting progression-free survival with high specificity.[52] A higher radiotracer uptake within NET lesions can predict response to PRRT. A higher lesion SUVmean can be an indicator of response (18.0 vs 33.6; P<.05). SUVmax (>16.4) of the lesion can predict treatment response with a sensitivity and specificity of 95% and 60%, respectively. Although direct changes in the tumor uptake may not be a direct predictor of patient survival and outcomes, the changes in tumor uptake in relation to background physiologic uptake in certain organs such as the liver or the spleen can predict patient outcome[53,54] (see Fig. 1; Fig. 3). For example, change in total lesion radiotracer activity in relation to the spleen can predict overall survival after PRRT (P = .044). Three-year survival has shown to be 100% in patients who respond to PRRT compared to 50% in patients who did not respond, as predicted by the changes in tumor SUVmax in relation to the splenic uptake.[55]

Accurate detection of recurrent disease plays a crucial role in the follow-up of these patients. Studies have shown a high sensitivity (91%) and specificity (100%) in the restaging of these patients.[56] In patients with suspected recurrence, SSTR PET imaging can detect metastatic disease especially involving the peritoneum (P<.001) and bone (P = .041), resulting in a significant impact on management decisions in more than 40% of patients in comparison to conventional imaging.[57] Detection of recurrent disease can be improved with relevant clinical, other imaging, and biochemical findings.[58]

SOMATOSTATIN RECEPTOR PET/MRI IN THE EVALUATION OF NEUROENDOCRINE TUMORS

With rapid advances in PET technology, PET/MRI has come into the array of imaging options available for evaluating patients with neuroendocrine tumors. Few studies compare the role of SSTR PET/MRI to PET/CT in the evaluation of these patients. The diagnostic accuracy of SSTR PET/MR has been shown to be comparable to PET/CT.[59] A study reported a statistically significant difference in the identification of NET lesions with PET/MRI correctly identified more NET lesions than PET/CT (91% vs 87%; P = .031). The conspicuity of NET lesions was statistically higher with SSTR PET/MR Imaging (P<.01).[60]

THERANOSTICS IN THE MANAGEMENT OF NEUROENDOCRINE TUMORS

Patient screening and eligibility: This involves a multidisciplinary team, including a medical oncologist, oncologic surgeon, and nuclear medicine physician. The ideal candidates for PRRT include patients with well-differentiated and moderately differentiated neuroendocrine carcinomas defined as NET grade 1 or 2 according to the recent WHO 2019 classification.[61,62] Patients being considered for PRRT undergo diagnostic somatostatin receptor imaging to demonstrate adequate SSTR expression.[63]

Post-therapy emission scan: It is usually performed 5 to 7 days after LU[177] PRRT as ^{177}Lu emits a small percentage of gamma photons that can be imaged using a SPECT camera and absorbed dose in organs and lesions can be calculated using quantitative techniques to do dosimetry which would help in improving patient outcomes by tailoring administered therapy activities based on patient's tumor burden and tumor uptake.[64,65]

Recommended dosage: The recommended dose of ^{177}Lu-DOTATATE is 7.4 GBq (200 mCi) $\pm$ 10% every 8 weeks for a total of 4 doses (package insert,

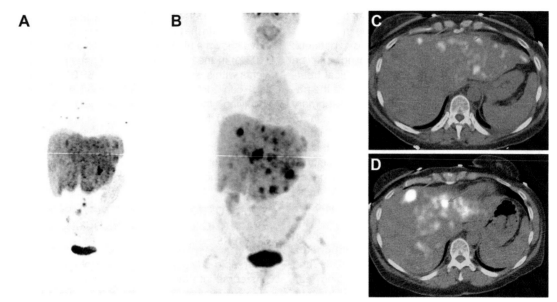

Fig. 3. Ga^{68}-DOTATATE Coronal PET MIP (*A*) and axial fused PET/CT (*C*), ^{18}F-FDG Coronal PET MIP (*B*) and axial fused PET/CT (*D*) of a 57-year-old woman with metastatic NET demonstrated metastatic disease involving the liver, bones, and lymph nodes. Some of the lesions (blue arrows) demonstrated increased ^{18}F-FDG uptake in comparison to the Ga^{68}-DOTATATE uptake suggestive of poorly differentiated disease.

Advanced Accelerator Applications). The interval between 2 treatments can be extended up to 16 weeks to allow recovery from hematologic toxicity.[66]

Evidence-based treatment algorithm and clinical practice guidelines for GEP-NETs have been proposed by a number of international oncologic societies. These guidelines have similar recommendations except for timing of PRRT in the treatment algorithm. NCCN guidelines recommend PRRT as a potential therapy for small bowel neuroendocrine tumors (SB-NETs), pancreatic neuroendocrine tumors (Pan-NETs), bronchial NETs, and paraganglioma/pheochromocytoma.[4] **Table 1** summarizes the different recommendations. There are ongoing studies assessing the efficacy of PRRT compared with other treatment options and how to optimize treatment through different dosing

Table 1
International Society recommendations for advanced GEP-NET treatment algorithm

Organization	SBNET	PNET
NCCN	PRRT as a potential therapy for SB-NETs, Pan-NETs, bronchial NETs, and paraganglioma/pheochromocytomas[4]	
SNMMI	PRRT before everolimus as a second-line therapy[72]	PRRT and chemotherapy, both as second-line options
NANETS	PRRT before everolimus as a second-line therapy[72]	PRRT and chemotherapy, both as second-line options
ESMO	PRRT before everolimus if Ki-67 < 10%, if Ki-67 > 10 then everolimus before PRRT[73]	Place PRRT after chemotherapy (capecitabine/temozolomide)
ENETS	PRRT and everolimus as second-line options[11]	Place PRRT after chemotherapy (capecitabine/temozolomide)

Abbreviations: ENETS, European Neuroendocrine Tumor Society; ESMO, European Society for Medical Oncology; NANETS, North American Neuroendocrine Tumor Society; NCCN, National Comprehensive Cancer Network; PNET, pancreatic neuroendocrine tumor; SBNET, small bowel neuroendocrine tumor; SNMMI, Society of Nuclear Medicine and Molecular Imaging.

models, using combination therapy, or use of different radionuclides and radioligands.[67]

Other somatostatin receptor–expressing tumors: In advanced neural crest tumors such as pheochromocytoma/paraganglioma, neuroblastoma, and medullary thyroid carcinoma, PRRT therapy with LU[177]-DOTATATE may be considered if tumors show adequate SSTR expression on imaging.[68,69]

PRRT Beyond beta emitters: Patients who fail ^{177}Lu-DOTATATE (PRRT) therapy have limited options. There has been a growing interest in alpha-based therapy which has emerged as an alternative treatment option. Alpha emitters have the advantage of a shorter range (<0.1 mm), sparing the surrounding healthy tissue with high linear energy transfer resulting in double-strand DNA breaks leading to cell death.[70] Actinium-225 ([225]Ac) labeled radiopharmaceuticals have been developed and following the first clinical study of [225]Ac-PRRT in NET treatment in 2011, several trials are underway for patients resistant to β-irradiation treatment.[71]

SUMMARY

PET imaging targeting somatostatin receptors has become the forefront of imaging evaluation of NET patients, and is preferred over planar or SPECT imaging, when available. It provides accurate staging, treatment response assessment, and restaging with significant impact on patient management. Somatostatin receptor–targeted radionuclide therapy has become an important treatment option for patients with metastatic disease without many treatment options with a significant impact on patient outcome and symptom management.

CLINICS CARE POINTS

- Somatostatin receptor–targeted PET imaging outperforms conventional, planar, and SPECT imaging in NET patients and should be used for evaluation when available.
- SSTR PET imaging provides accurate staging and treatment response assessment with a significant impact on patient management.
- Peptide receptor radionuclide therapy is useful in patients with metastatic disease without many treatment options and can improve patient outcome.

DISCLOSURE

C. Marcus: No relevant disclosures. S. Muzahir: No relevant disclosures.

REFERENCES

1. Yao JC, Hassan M, Phan A, et al. One hundred years after "carcinoid": epidemiology of and prognostic factors for neuroendocrine tumors in 35,825 cases in the United States. J Clin Oncol 2008;26(18):3063–72.
2. Sorbye H, Strosberg J, Baudin E, et al. Gastroenteropancreatic high-grade neuroendocrine carcinoma. Cancer 2014;120(18):2814–23.
3. Das S, Dasari A. Epidemiology, incidence, and prevalence of neuroendocrine neoplasms: are there Global differences? Curr Oncol Rep 2021;23(4):43.
4. NCCN) NCCN. NCCN Guidelines Version 2.2022 Neuroendocrine and Adrenal Tumors. Available at: https://www.nccn.org/professionals/physician_gls/pdf/neuroendocrine.pdf. Published 2022. Accessed July 25, 2023, 2023.
5. Riihimaki M, Hemminki A, Sundquist K, et al. The epidemiology of metastases in neuroendocrine tumors. Int J Cancer 2016;139(12):2679–86.
6. Shah MH, Goldner WS, Benson AB, et al. Neuroendocrine and Adrenal tumors, version 2.2021, NCCN clinical practice guidelines in oncology. J Natl Compr Canc Netw 2021;19(7):839–68.
7. Dasari A, Shen C, Halperin D, et al. Trends in the incidence, prevalence, and survival outcomes in patients with neuroendocrine tumors in the United States. JAMA Oncol 2017;3(10):1335–42.
8. Hofland J, Kaltsas G, de Herder WW. Advances in the diagnosis and management of well-differentiated neuroendocrine neoplasms. Endocr Rev 2020;41(2):371–403.
9. Reuling E, Dickhoff C, Plaisier PW, et al. Endobronchial treatment for bronchial carcinoid: patient selection and predictors of outcome. Respiration 2018;95(4):220–7.
10. Rindi G, D'Adda T, Froio E, et al. Prognostic factors in gastrointestinal endocrine tumors. Endocr Pathol 2007;18(3):145–9.
11. Pavel M, Baudin E, Couvelard A, et al. ENETS Consensus Guidelines for the management of patients with liver and other distant metastases from neuroendocrine neoplasms of foregut, midgut, hindgut, and unknown primary. Neuroendocrinology 2012;95(2):157–76.
12. Howe JR, Cardona K, Fraker DL, et al. The surgical management of small bowel neuroendocrine tumors: Consensus guidelines of the North American neuroendocrine tumor Society. Pancreas 2017;46(6):715–31.
13. Vogl TJ, Naguib NN, Zangos S, et al. Liver metastases of neuroendocrine carcinomas: interventional treatment via transarterial embolization, chemoembolization and thermal ablation. Eur J Radiol 2009;72(3):517–28.
14. Chen H, Hardacre JM, Uzar A, et al. Isolated liver metastases from neuroendocrine tumors: does resection

prolong survival? J Am Coll Surg 1998;187(1):88–92 [discussion: 92–3].

15. Lehrman ED, Fidelman N. Liver-directed therapy for neuroendocrine tumor liver metastases in the Era of peptide receptor radionuclide therapy. Semin Intervent Radiol 2020;37(5):499–507.

16. Caplin ME, Pavel M, Cwikla JB, et al. Anti-tumour effects of lanreotide for pancreatic and intestinal neuroendocrine tumours: the CLARINET open-label extension study. Endocr Relat Cancer 2016;23(3): 191–9.

17. Rinke A, Muller HH, Schade-Brittinger C, et al. Placebo-controlled, double-blind, prospective, randomized study on the effect of octreotide LAR in the control of tumor growth in patients with metastatic neuroendocrine midgut tumors: a report from the PROMID Study Group. J Clin Oncol 2009;27(28): 4656–63.

18. Puliani G, Chiefari A, Mormando M, et al. New Insights in PRRT: Lessons from 2021. Front Endocrinol 2022;13:861434.

19. Raymond E, Dahan L, Raoul JL, et al. Sunitinib malate for the treatment of pancreatic neuroendocrine tumors. N Engl J Med 2011;364(6):501–13.

20. Heetfeld M, Chougnet CN, Olsen IH, et al. Characteristics and treatment of patients with G3 gastroenteropancreatic neuroendocrine neoplasms. Endocr Relat Cancer 2015;22(4):657–64.

21. Wong MH, Chan DL, Lee A, et al. Systematic review and meta-analysis on the role of chemotherapy in advanced and metastatic neuroendocrine tumor (NET). PLoS One 2016;11(6):e0158140.

22. Strosberg J, Goldman J, Costa F, et al. The role of chemotherapy in well-differentiated gastroenteropancreatic neuroendocrine tumors. Front Horm Res 2015;44:239–47.

23. Administration FaD. FDA approves new diagnostic imaging agent to detect rare neuroendocrine tumors. In:2016.

24. (FDA) FaDA. FDA approves lutetium Lu 177 dotatate for treatment of GEP-NETS. In:2018.

25. (FDA) FaDA. Drug Trials Snapshots: DETECTNET. In:2020.

26. Olsen JO, Pozderac RV, Hinkle G, et al. Somatostatin receptor imaging of neuroendocrine tumors with indium-111 pentetreotide (Octreoscan). Semin Nucl Med 1995;25(3):251–61.

27. Poletto G, Cecchin D, Sperti S, et al. Head-to-Head comparison between peptide-based radiopharmaceutical for PET and SPECT in the evaluation of neuroendocrine tumors: a systematic review. Curr Issues Mol Biol 2022;44(11):5516–30.

28. Deppen SA, Blume J, Bobbey AJ, et al. 68Ga-DOTATATE compared with 111In-DTPA-octreotide and conventional imaging for pulmonary and gastroenteropancreatic neuroendocrine tumors: a systematic review and meta-analysis. J Nucl Med 2016;57(6):872–8.

29. Han S, Suh CH, Woo S, et al. Performance of (68)Ga-DOTA-Conjugated somatostatin receptor-targeting peptide PET in detection of pheochromocytoma and paraganglioma: a systematic review and Metaanalysis. J Nucl Med 2019;60(3):369–76.

30. Wild D, Macke HR, Waser B, et al. 68Ga-DOTANOC: a first compound for PET imaging with high affinity for somatostatin receptor subtypes 2 and 5. Eur J Nucl Med Mol Imaging 2005;32(6):724.

31. Buchmann I, Henze M, Engelbrecht S, et al. Comparison of 68Ga-DOTATOC PET and 111In-DTPAOC (Octreoscan) SPECT in patients with neuroendocrine tumours. Eur J Nucl Med Mol Imaging 2007; 34(10):1617–26.

32. Gabriel M, Decristoforo C, Kendler D, et al. 68Ga-DOTA-Tyr3-octreotide PET in neuroendocrine tumors: comparison with somatostatin receptor scintigraphy and CT. J Nucl Med 2007;48(4):508–18.

33. Pettinato C, Sarnelli A, Di Donna M, et al. 68Ga-DOTANOC: biodistribution and dosimetry in patients affected by neuroendocrine tumors. Eur J Nucl Med Mol Imaging 2008;35(1):72–9.

34. Kayani I, Bomanji JB, Groves A, et al. Functional imaging of neuroendocrine tumors with combined PET/CT using 68Ga-DOTATATE (DOTA-DPhe1,Tyr3-octreotate) and 18F-FDG. Cancer 2008;112(11): 2447–55.

35. Holland JP, Ferdani R, Anderson CJ, et al. Copper-64 radiopharmaceuticals for oncologic imaging. Pet Clin 2009;4(1):49–67.

36. Kabasakal L, Demirci E, Ocak M, et al. Comparison of (6)(8)Ga-DOTATATE and (6)(8)Ga-DOTANOC PET/CT imaging in the same patient group with neuroendocrine tumours. Eur J Nucl Med Mol Imaging 2012;39(8):1271–7.

37. Poeppel TD, Binse I, Petersenn S, et al. Differential uptake of (68)Ga-DOTATOC and (68)Ga-DOTATATE in PET/CT of gastroenteropancreatic neuroendocrine tumors. Recent Results Cancer Res 2013;194: 353–71.

38. Johnbeck CB, Knigge U, Loft A, et al. Head-to-Head comparison of (64)Cu-DOTATATE and (68)Ga-DOTATOC PET/CT: a prospective study of 59 patients with neuroendocrine tumors. J Nucl Med 2017; 58(3):451–7.

39. Binderup T, Knigge U, Loft A, et al. 18F-fluorodeoxyglucose positron emission tomography predicts survival of patients with neuroendocrine tumors. Clin Cancer Res 2010;16(3):978–85.

40. Garin E, Le Jeune F, Devillers A, et al. Predictive value of 18F-FDG PET and somatostatin receptor scintigraphy in patients with metastatic endocrine tumors. J Nucl Med 2009;50(6):858–64.

41. Kayani I, Conry BG, Groves AM, et al. A comparison of 68Ga-DOTATATE and 18F-FDG PET/CT in pulmonary neuroendocrine tumors. J Nucl Med 2009; 50(12):1927–32.

42. Zalom ML, Waxman AD, Yu R, et al. Metabolic and receptor imaging in patients with neuroendocrine tumors: comparison of fludeoxyglucose-positron emission tomography and computed tomography with indium in 111 pentetreotide. Endocr Pract 2009;15(6):521–7.

43. Burkett BJ, Dundar A, Young JR, et al. How We do it: a multidisciplinary Approach to (177)Lu DOTATATE peptide receptor radionuclide therapy. Radiology 2021;298(2):261–74.

44. Crown A, Rocha FG, Raghu P, et al. Impact of initial imaging with gallium-68 dotatate PET/CT on diagnosis and management of patients with neuroendocrine tumors. J Surg Oncol 2020;121(3):480–5.

45. Cuthbertson DJ, Barriuso J, Lamarca A, et al. The impact of (68)Gallium DOTA PET/CT in managing patients with Sporadic and Familial pancreatic neuroendocrine tumours. Front Endocrinol 2021;12: 654975.

46. Lee ONY, Tan KV, Tripathi V, et al. The role of 68 Ga-DOTA-SSA PET/CT in the management and prediction of peptide receptor radionuclide therapy response for patients with neuroendocrine tumors : a systematic review and meta-analysis. Clin Nucl Med 2022;47(9):781–93.

47. Tierney JF, Kosche C, Schadde E, et al. 68)Gallium-DOTATATE positron emission tomography-computed tomography (PET CT) changes management in a majority of patients with neuroendocrine tumors. Surgery 2019;165(1):178–85.

48. Singh D, Arya A, Agarwal A, et al. Role of Ga-68 DOTANOC positron emission tomography/computed tomography scan in clinical management of patients with neuroendocrine tumors and its Correlation with conventional imaging- experience in a Tertiary Care Center in India. Indian J Nucl Med 2022;37(1):29–36.

49. Singh S, Poon R, Wong R, et al. 68Ga PET imaging in patients with neuroendocrine tumors: a systematic review and meta-analysis. Clin Nucl Med 2018; 43(11):802–10.

50. Ambrosini V, Nanni C, Zompatori M, et al. (68)Ga-DOTA-NOC PET/CT in comparison with CT for the detection of bone metastasis in patients with neuroendocrine tumours. Eur J Nucl Med Mol Imaging 2010;37(4):722–7.

51. Tan TH, Boey CY, Lee BN. Impact of (68)Ga-DOTA-Peptide PET/CT on the management of gastrointestinal neuroendocrine tumour (GI-NET): Malaysian National Referral Centre experience. Nucl Med Mol Imaging 2018;52(2):119–24.

52. Lee H, Eads JR, Pryma DA. (68) Ga-DOTATATE positron emission tomography-computed tomography Quantification predicts response to somatostatin analog therapy in gastroenteropancreatic neuroendocrine tumors. Oncol 2021;26(1):21–9.

53. Kratochwil C, Stefanova M, Mavriopoulou E, et al. SUV of [68Ga]DOTATOC-PET/CT predicts response Probability of PRRT in neuroendocrine tumors. Mol Imaging Biol 2015;17(3):313–8.

54. Opalinska M, Morawiec-Slawek K, Kania-Kuc A, et al. Potential value of pre- and post-therapy [68Ga]Ga-DOTA-TATE PET/CT in the prognosis of response to PRRT in disseminated neuroendocrine tumors. Front Endocrinol 2022;13:929391.

55. Kepenek F, Komek H, Can C, et al. The prognostic role of whole-body volumetric 68 GA-DOTATATE PET/computed tomography parameters in patients with gastroenteropancreatic neuroendocrine tumor treated with 177 LU-DOTATATE. Nucl Med Commun 2023;44(6):509–17.

56. Haidar M, Shamseddine A, Panagiotidis E, et al. The role of 68Ga-DOTA-NOC PET/CT in evaluating neuroendocrine tumors: real-world experience from two large neuroendocrine tumor centers. Nucl Med Commun 2017;38(2):170–7.

57. Lugat A, Frampas E, Touchefeu Y, et al. Prospective Multicentric assessment of (68)Ga-DOTANOC PET/CT in Grade 1-2 GEP-NET. Cancers 2023;15(2).

58. Haug AR, Cindea-Drimus R, Auernhammer CJ, et al. Neuroendocrine tumor recurrence: diagnosis with 68Ga-DOTATATE PET/CT. Radiology 2014;270(2): 517–25.

59. Berzaczy D, Giraudo C, Haug AR, et al. Whole-body 68Ga-DOTANOC PET/MRI versus 68Ga-DOTANOC PET/CT in patients with neuroendocrine tumors: a prospective study in 28 patients. Clin Nucl Med 2017;42(9):669–74.

60. Sawicki LM, Deuschl C, Beiderwellen K, et al. Evaluation of (68)Ga-DOTATOC PET/MRI for whole-body staging of neuroendocrine tumours in comparison with (68)Ga-DOTATOC PET/CT. Eur Radiol 2017;27(10):4091–9.

61. Nagtegaal ID, Odze RD, Klimstra D, et al. The 2019 WHO classification of tumours of the digestive system. Histopathology 2020;76(2):182–8.

62. Popa O, Taban SM, Pantea S, et al. The new WHO classification of gastrointestinal neuroendocrine tumors and immunohistochemical expression of somatostatin receptor 2 and 5. Exp Ther Med 2021; 22(4):1179.

63. Kwekkeboom DJ, Kam BL, van Essen M, et al. Somatostatin-receptor-based imaging and therapy of gastroenteropancreatic neuroendocrine tumors. Endocr Relat Cancer 2010;17(1):R53–73.

64. Devasia TP, Dewaraja YK, Frey KA, et al. A novel time-activity information-sharing approach using nonlinear mixed models for patient-specific dosimetry with reduced imaging time points: application in SPECT/CT after (177)Lu-DOTATATE. J Nucl Med 2021;62(8):1118–25.

65. Lawhn-Heath C, Hope TA, Martinez J, et al. Dosimetry in radionuclide therapy: the clinical role of measuring radiation dose. Lancet Oncol 2022; 23(2):e75–87.

66. Kolasinska-Cwikla A, Lowczak A, Maciejkiewicz KM, et al. Peptide receptor radionuclide therapy for advanced gastroenteropancreatic neuroendocrine tumors - from oncology perspective. Nucl Med Rev Cent East Eur 2018;21(2). https://doi.org/10.5603/NMR.2018.0019.

67. Hope TA, Pavel M, Bergsland EK. Neuroendocrine tumors and peptide receptor radionuclide therapy: when is the right time? J Clin Oncol 2022;40(24):2818–29.

68. Kong G, Grozinsky-Glasberg S, Hofman MS, et al. Efficacy of peptide receptor radionuclide therapy for functional metastatic paraganglioma and pheochromocytoma. J Clin Endocrinol Metab 2017;102(9):3278–87.

69. Satapathy S, Mittal BR, Bhansali A. Peptide receptor radionuclide therapy in the management of advanced pheochromocytoma and paraganglioma: a systematic review and meta-analysis. Clin Endocrinol 2019;91(6):718–27.

70. Lassmann M, Eberlein U. Targeted alpha-particle therapy: imaging, dosimetry, and radiation protection. Ann ICRP 2018;47(3–4):187–95.

71. Kunikowska J, Krolicki L. Targeted alpha-Emitter therapy of neuroendocrine tumors. Semin Nucl Med 2020;50(2):171–6.

72. Hope TA, Bodei L, Chan JA, et al. NANETS/SNMMI Consensus Statement on patient selection and Appropriate Use of (177)Lu-DOTATATE peptide receptor radionuclide therapy. J Nucl Med 2020;61(2):222–7.

73. Pavel M, Oberg K, Falconi M, et al. Gastroentero-pancreatic neuroendocrine neoplasms: ESMO Clinical Practice Guidelines for diagnosis, treatment and follow-up. Ann Oncol 2020;31(7):844–60.

PET/Computed Tomography Transformation of Oncology
Kidney and Urinary Tract Cancers

Jorge D. Oldan, MD[a], Jennifer A. Schroeder, MD[a],
Jean Hoffman-Censits, MD[b], W. Kimryn Rathmell, MD, PhD[c],
Matthew I. Milowsky, MD, FASCO[d], Lilja B. Solnes, MD[e],
Sridhar Nimmagadda, PhD[e], Michael A. Gorin, MD[f], Amir H. Khandani, MD[a],
Steven P. Rowe, MD, PhD[a,*]

KEYWORDS

- Renal cell carcinoma • Urothelial carcinoma • Carbonic anhydrase IX

KEY POINTS

- Although guidelines do not postulate any utility for 18F-FDG PET in renal cell carcinoma, there may be applications in the identification of occult metastases and response to therapy.
- Despite urinary excretion of the radiotracer, 18F-FDG PET demonstrates good detection efficiency for metastatic disease from urothelial carcinoma and may have roles in tumor characterization and response assessment.
- New PET radiotracers targeting epithelial cell-surface proteins and the tumor microenvironment will allow improved non-invasive characterization of renal masses and urothelial carcinomas and may aid therapy selection and prognostication.

INTRODUCTION

Renal cell carcinoma (RCC) and urothelial carcinoma (UC) represent the third and second most common genitourinary malignancies, trailing prostate cancer.[1] Both types of tumors can be intrinsically aggressive and hypermetabolic on 2-deoxy-2-[18F]fluoro-D-glucose (18F-FDG), the most commonly used PET radiotracer in routine clinical practice. However, there are significant limitations to the use of 18F-FDG PET for imaging those tumors, which include, but are not limited to, the excretion of 18F-FDG through the kidneys, the accumulation of 18F-FDG within excreted urine along the urinary tract, and variable uptake of 18F-FDG within indeterminate renal masses. However, there may also be important biological and prognostic information in 18F-FDG PET uptake in primary tumors.[2–4] In addition, recent evaluation of 18F-FDG uptake by discrete cellular compartments of the tumor microenvironment has raised the awareness of inflammatory cells contributing substantially to the overall tumor signal.[5] In clinical practice, the difficulties in deconvoluting the

[a] Molecular Imaging and Therapeutics, Department of Radiology, University of North Carolina, Chapel Hill, NC, USA; [b] Department of Medical Oncology and Urology, Sidney Kimmel Comprehensive Cancer Center, Johns Hopkins University School of Medicine, Baltimore, MD, USA; [c] Department of Medicine, Vanderbilt University Medical Center, Nashville, TN, USA; [d] Lineberger Comprehensive Cancer Center, University of North Carolina, Chapel Hill, NC, USA; [e] The Russell H. Morgan Department of Radiology and Radiological Science, Johns Hopkins University School of Medicine, Baltimore, MD, USA; [f] Milton and Carroll Petrie Department of Urology, Icahn School of Medicine at Mount Sinai, New York, NY, USA
* Corresponding author. Molecular Imaging and Therapeutics, Department of Radiology, University of North Carolina, 101 Manning Drive, Chapel Hill, NC 27514.
E-mail address: Steven_Rowe@med.unc.edu

PET Clin 19 (2024) 197–206
https://doi.org/10.1016/j.cpet.2023.12.006

contributions of different cell types to overall tumor uptake have spurred different approaches to the molecular imaging of RCC and UC.

The focus in RCC has been 2-fold; first, the improved characterization of benign versus malignant indeterminate renal masses and differentiation between aggressive clear cell RCC (ccRCC) and more indolent/benign tumors such as oncocytomas, and second, optimizing the ability to detect metastatic disease. For decades, the high sensitivity of conventional cross-sectional imaging for the detection of small renal masses has led to the increasing incidence of such lesions,[6] but, generally, has also provided relatively limited characterization of tumor biology and metastatic potential.[7,8] Though ^{18}F-FDG is an important tool to detect metastatic RCC,[9] sensitivity likely lags compared to arterial-phase, contrast-enhanced anatomic imaging.[10]

It is perhaps best to think of the current and future applications of PET imaging agents in UC as detecting and characterizing metastatic disease. The undeniable limitation for PET imaging of UC within the luminal urinary tract is the difficulty in designing radiotracers that are not renally excreted. At times, such radiotracers require large, hydrophobic groups included in the molecular structure, which can lead to off-target, false-positive binding.[11]

In this review, the authors will discuss the role of ^{18}F-FDG PET in evaluating patients with RCC and UC. The authors will also describe emerging classes of radiotracers that may address some of the clinical shortcomings associated with ^{18}F-FDG and/or may open new avenues of investigation into the tumor microenvironment and imaging biomarker discovery.

ROLE OF 2-DEOXY-2-[^{18}F] FLUORO-D-GLUCOSE PET IN RENAL CELL CARCINOMA

RCC has historically been one of the few tumors (along with hepatocellular carcinoma, prostate cancer, invasive lobular carcinoma of the breast, and most neuroendocrine and mucinous tumors) said to be cold, or poorly visualized, on ^{18}F-FDG PET. There is also the added complication that ^{18}F-FDG is renally excreted, producing a high background that interferes with lesion detection and/or characterization by decreasing regional contrast and thus limiting sensitivity. The current National Comprehensive Cancer Network (NCCN) guidelines[12] do not postulate any use for ^{18}F-FDG PET in RCC, citing an article that showed no role in postoperative surveillance.[13]

The situation may be somewhat more complicated than it appears, and many older studies focus on PET rather than PET combined with computed tomography (CT), which is the predominant modality in the present day. The earliest meta-analysis in English[9] showed a relatively poor sensitivity and specificity of 62% and 88% for ^{18}F-FDG PET in primary renal tumors and 79% and 90% for extrarenal disease. However, the combined modality, that is, ^{18}F-FDG PET/CT, was somewhat better for extrarenal disease at 91% and 88% (**Figs. 1** and **2**). A later meta-analysis[14] reported sensitivity of 80% and specificity of 85% for ^{18}F-FDG PET/CT for detection of primary RCC, comparable to MRI (76% and 88%, respectively), whereas for overall detection sensitivity was 89% and specificity 88% for ^{18}F-FDG PET/CT, versus 90% and 80%, respectively, for MRI. Despite its weakness for detecting primary disease, ^{18}F-FDG PET/CT may be useful for kidney tumors that have metastasized outside the kidney.

Another more-recent meta-analysis[15] focused on recurrent and metastatic disease reporting both sensitivity and specificity of 88% for ^{18}F-FDG PET/CT (sensitivity was lower, at 81%, for PET without CT). Another, 2021 systematic review gave a range of 82% to 100% and 84% to 100% for recurrent and metastatic disease specifically, roughly consistent with the aforementioned.[16]

In total, in the setting of primary tumors, ^{18}F-FDG PET/CT as compared to PET alone may have value derived from the CT component. The value of ^{18}F-FDG PET/CT is well established for recurrent and metastatic disease,[16] particularly in the bone and adrenal glands.[16] ^{18}F-FDG PET/CT is more sensitive than bone scan for bone metastases,[17] given the generally lytic nature of those lesions. Further, ^{18}F-FDG PET/CT may have prognostic value, as higher maximum standardized uptake value (SUVmax) in the primary tumor is related to frequency of metastasis and decreased survival.[16] A higher SUVmax also correlates with a Fuhrman grade and sarcomatoid features, which are also poor prognostic indicators.[18] ^{18}F-FDG PET/CT can be useful in surveillance, with sensitivity 80% to 100% and specificity 70% to 100%, as well as an outstanding positive predictive value of 95% to 100%, changing management in 43% of cases.[16]

^{18}F-FDG PET/CT is currently being evaluated for the use of monitoring response to therapy. Targeted therapies used in metastatic RCC tend to be cytostatic rather than cytotoxic, and therefore cause the tumor to stabilize rather than shrink, so assessing metabolic activity may be particularly useful and more informative than anatomic imaging alone.[16] To at least some degree, uptake of ^{18}F-FDG uptake may be driven by immune cells within the tumor microenvironment as opposed to tumor epithelial cells.[5] In particular, correlation with survival has been shown with tyrosine kinase inhibitors

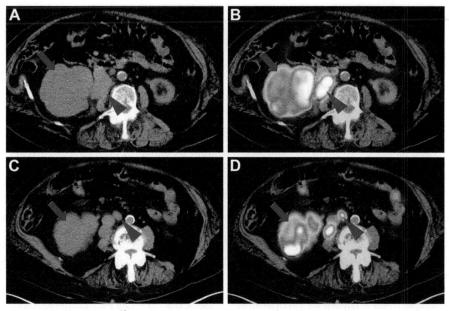

Fig. 1. (*A, C*) CT and (*B, D*) fused ^{18}F-FDG PET/CT images of right kidney unclassified RCC (*arrows*) with locoregional nodal metastases (*arrowheads*). CT, computed tomography; ^{18}F-FDG, 2-deoxy-2-[^{18}F]fluoro-D-glucose; RCC, renal cell carcinoma.

such as sunitinib or sorafenib,[4] and there is some early evidence ^{18}F-FDG PET/CT may be useful for response to immunotherapies such as nivolumab.[16,19] However, therapy with the mammalian target of rapamycin inhibitor everolimus lead to changes in ^{18}F-FDG uptake that were only modestly correlated with anatomic changes in tumor size as assessed by Response Evaluation Criteria in Solid Tumors measurements, suggesting that ^{18}F-FDG PET biomarkers may be challenging to apply in clinic.[20]

Another application is in the investigation of hereditary RCC syndromes. Tumors in some syndromes such as hereditary leiomyomatosis RCC, which is accompanied by a mutation in fumarate

hydratase, a Krebs cycle enzyme, or succinate dehydrogenase RCC, may be ^{18}F-FDG-avid due to disruptions in oxidative phosphorylation.[19,21] Defining the utility of ^{18}F-FDG PET/CT in these syndromes is difficult given their rarity.

ROLE OF 2-DEOXY-2-[^{18}F] FLUORO-D-GLUCOSE PET IN UROTHELIAL CARCINOMA

While once again acknowledging the limitation of any urinary excreted agent to adequately image intraluminal UC, ^{18}F-FDG is a valuable tool for evaluating for possible disease involvement beyond the urinary tract (**Figs. 3–5**).

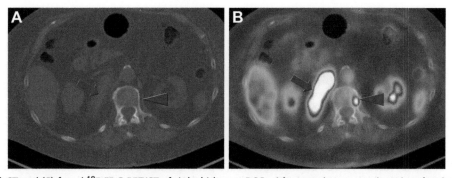

Fig. 2. (*A*) CT and (*B*) fused ^{18}F-FDG PET/CT of right kidney ccRCC with extensive venous invasion that involves the inferior vena cava (*arrows*) and a bone metastasis (*arrowheads*). ccRCC, clear cell renal cell carcinoma; CT, computed tomography; ^{18}F-FDG, 2-deoxy-2-[^{18}F]fluoro-D-glucose.

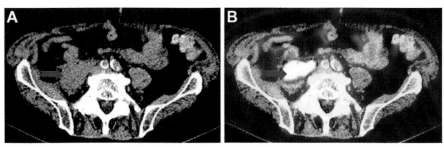

Fig. 3. (A) CT and (B) fused ^{18}F-FDG PET/CT images of recurrent UC along the right common iliac vessels demonstrating an infiltrative growth pattern (*arrows*). CT, computed tomography; ^{18}F-FDG, 2-deoxy-2-[^{18}F]fluoro-D-glucose; UC, urothelial carcinoma.

UC is divided anatomically roughly into carcinoma of the bladder (most common) and upper tract (collecting system and ureter; rare). Carcinoma of the bladder has been better studied, and in general, specificity is better than sensitivity for the PET detection of pelvic nodal involvement. There are multiple meta-analyses for preoperative nodal staging of bladder cancer,[22–24] which have generally shown similar results of 56% to 57% sensitivity and 92% to 95% specificity. For distant metastases, no (recent) meta-analysis is available, but a systematic review by Salem and colleagues[25] gives sensitivity specifically for distant metastases in muscle-invasive bladder cancer of 54% to 87%, which is better than CT (41%), though both ^{18}F-FDG PET (90%–97%) and CT (98%) show high specificity. There is at least 1 meta-analysis that has assessed the ability of ^{18}F-FDG PET to identify recurrent or residual disease for primary lesions in the bladder reporting a sensitivity of 94% and specificity of 92%, but many of the component studies used furosemide to clear the bladder of radioactive urine.[26]

In a recent meta-analysis, ^{18}F-FDG PET has also been studied to evaluate response to therapy in primary tumors,[27] which determined that this modality is more effective for assessing clinical response (94% sensitivity, 77% specificity) than pathologic complete response (68% sensitivity, 77% specificity).[27]

In regards to upper tract UC and ^{18}F-FDG PET detection of nodal involvement, management can change in 40% of cases versus 74% for the bladder.[25] There is less study of distant metastasis, but ^{18}F-FDG PET outperforms CT on detection of individual lesions although both modalities are similar in patient-level sensitivity.[25] While the NCCN does not recommend using ^{18}F-FDG PET to identify whether upper tract disease is present, it can identify abnormalities related to the tumor in 83% of patients with upper tract disease.[25] Overall, metastasis of UC in the retroperitoneum and pelvis can follow a rather diffuse and infiltrative pattern, the metabolic abnormalities of which can be apparent on ^{18}F-FDG PET[25] (see **Fig. 3**).

The inherent biological differences of UC of the bladder and upper-tract UC[28] may underlie some of the differences in sensitivity between the 2 patient populations. However, lack of sensitivity of ^{18}F-FDG for pelvic lymph nodes from UC of the bladder parallels a pattern that has been seen with other radiotracers for pelvic malignancies, namely the prostate-specific membrane antigen (PSMA)–targeted family of urea-based small molecules that are used for initial staging of men with prostate cancer.[29,30] In general, surgery will remain

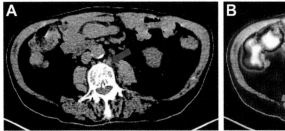
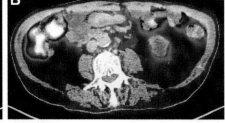

Fig. 4. (A) CT and (B) fused ^{18}F-FDG PET/CT images from a patient with UC who had evidence of retroperitoneal nodal involvement. The high contrast of PET can allow the detection of small lymph nodes that may not be anatomically abnormal. CT, computed tomography; ^{18}F-FDG, 2-deoxy-2-[^{18}F]fluoro-D-glucose; UC, urothelial carcinoma.

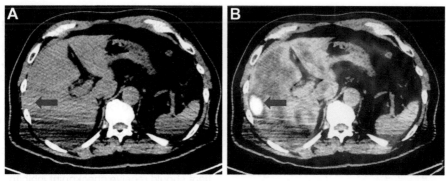

Fig. 5. (*A*) CT and (*B*) fused ^{18}F-FDG PET/CT images from a patient with UC that developed a metastasis to the liver that is not clearly visible on the noncontrast CT. CT, computed tomography; ^{18}F-FDG, 2-deoxy-2-[^{18}F]fluoro-D-glucose; UC, urothelial carcinoma.

the gold standard in pelvic nodal staging, given that low-volume disease in pelvic lymph nodes may fall below the detection limit of any radiotracer.

IMAGING OF CANCER EPITHELIAL TARGETS IN RENAL CELL AND UROTHELIAL CARCINOMAS
Carbonic Anhydrase IX

Carbonic anhydrase IX (CAIX) is a cell-surface enzyme that is constitutively overexpressed in the vast majority of ccRCC[31] and is also variably expressed in other malignancies based on their degree of hypoxia.[32] Given the potential for CAIX to serve as a noninvasive imaging biomarker for the presence of ccRCC in an otherwise indeterminate renal mass, a number of small-molecule[33–35] and monoclonal antibody[31]-based agents have been investigated in either preclinical or clinical trial settings. To date, the pivotal trials have taken place with radiolabeled versions of the g250 monoclonal antibody (girentuximab) to CAIX.

The first such trial was called REDECT and utilized ^{124}I-girentuximab and found a sensitivity of 86.2% (95% confidence interval (95% confidence interval [CI]), 75.3% to 97.1%) for ^{124}I-girentuximab PET/CT and 75.5% (95% CI, 62.6% to 88.4%) for contrast-enhanced CT.[31] In the same study, the specificity was 85.9% (95% CI, 69.4% to 99.9%) for ^{124}I-girentuximab PET/CT and 46.8% (95% CI, 18.8% to 74.7%) for contrast-enhanced CT. Intuitively, one would assume nearly 100% sensitivity for contrast-enhanced CT (all patients had an identifiable mass on anatomic imaging) and a lower specificity than was reported; although, clearly the performance characteristics of ^{124}I-girentuximab PET/CT were superior to contrast-enhanced CT. The REDECT trial established the potential for a CAIX-targeted PET agent to play a role in the noninvasive characterization of renal masses.

More recently, a confirmatory phase III trial for the girentuximab antibody has been undertaken, but utilizing the zirconium-89 radionuclide as opposed to iodine-124 (the ZIRCON trial, NCT03849118). In an open-label, multicenter design, 300 patients with clinical T1 indeterminate renal masses were dosed with ^{89}Zr-girentuximab, of whom 284 were evaluable for the primary analysis. Patients were injected on day 0 and then imaged on approximately day 5 before proceeding to resection by day 90. At the time of this writing, the final results of ZIRCON have not been published but have been announced and appear to be very promising, with the agent meeting both of its co-primary endpoints for sensitivity and specificity (86% [95% CI, 80%–90%] and 87% [95% CI, 79%–92%], respectively).[36] For masses less than 4 cm in diameter (clinical T1a), the performance of the agent remains excellent, with sensitivity of 85% (95% CI, 77%–91%] and specificity of 90% (95% CI, 79%–95%). Those findings, again, suggest that CAIX imaging can be a noninvasive means by which to characterize renal masses. It is expected that ^{89}Zr-girentuximab will be regulatory approved within a matter of months and may be available for clinical use by the time this article is published.

The most difficult hurdles for the widespread clinical use of ^{89}Zr-girentuximab are the likely high cost of the agent and how its performance characteristics compare against the very inexpensive single-photon emission CT agent ^{99m}Tc-sestamibi, as well as the need to wait 3 days between injection and imaging, which is a very different workflow than is typical in a PET center. ^{99m}Tc-sestamibi is a lipophilic cation that has high uptake in mitochondrial-rich tumors such as oncocytomas,[37] and can allow for the reliable differentiation of oncocytic neoplasm from more aggressive tumors.[38,39] In an ideal world, patients would be dual-imaged with CAIX-based radiotracers and ^{99m}Tc-sestamibi imaging to provide a comprehensive, noninvasive risk-stratification profile for their renal tumors. In reality, the vagaries of insurance coverage may make that difficult. The authors would, nonetheless, look forward to comparative trials and further, nuanced investigation into the optimized role of molecular imaging risk stratification in patients with indeterminate renal masses.[40]

Nectin-4

Antibody-drug conjugates (ADCs) have emerged as a powerful clinical tool in the treatment of advanced urothelial cancer, with 2 ADCs approved to date and multiple in development. Enfortumab vedotin is comprised of a monomethyl auristatin E chemotherapy payload linked to a nectin-4 antibody, while sacituzumab govitecan harbors an SN-38 payload, the active metabolite of irinotecan, linked to a trop-2 antibody.[41] Both agents appear to have significant clinical activity for those with visceral metastases, historically associated with the worst prognosis in advanced UC.[42] Enfortumab vedotin was Food and Drug Administration approved in late 2019 based on impressive overall response rate of 44% in platinum and checkpoint refractory UC, with a manageable safety profile.[43,44] Since that time, approval has expanded for patients who are ineligible for cisplatin in the second-line setting after checkpoint,[45] and in the frontline setting combined with pembrolizumab in cisplatin ineligible patients.[46] Ongoing trials of enfortumab alone and in combination are investigating utility in the perioperative, frontline, and even intravesical settings. Initial studies of enfortumab required tissue nectin-4 biomarker positivity for enrollment, but since nectin-4 was noted to be widely expressed in UC samples, the requirement was changed and the use of enfortumab in clinical practice is not predicated on biomarker assessment.[47]

An exciting recent advance has been the development of a small, peptide-based radiotracer targeted against nectin-4 and known as ^{68}Ga-N188.[48] In preclinical studies, ^{68}Ga-N188 demonstrated high affinity for nectin-4 and was able to localize to nectin-4–expressing xenografts.[48] In a first-in-human analysis, the agent bound to sites of suspected metastatic UC and quantified nectin-4 expression levels in various tissues.[48] Given the possible toxicities associated with enfortumab therapy, and the variable responses that can be seen, there may be a wealth of imaging biomarkers on ^{68}Ga-N188 PET scans through either baseline imaging to determine eligibility, imaging during therapy to quantify target engagement, or the use of advanced imaging methods such as radiomics and artificial intelligence (AI).

IMAGING OF THE TUMOR MICROENVIRONMENT IN RENAL CELL AND UROTHELIAL CARCINOMAS
Programmed Death Ligand-1

To date, the programmed death-1 and programmed death ligand-1 (PD-L1) axis has been the most frequently utilized for checkpoint inhibitor therapy.[49] The PD-(L)1 axis can be important in the therapy of both RCC and UC. Although it remains unclear if there is a role for noninvasive imaging of either of those cell-surface receptors in determining if a patient should receive checkpoint inhibitor therapy,[50] there are reasons to believe that whole-body target assessment may be of value.[51] Both monoclonal-antibody-[52,53] and peptide-based[54] radiotracers have been investigated.

Based on preclinical data, PET radiotracers targeted against PD-L1 are able to accurately determine target engagement.[55] More importantly, in human subjects, there are multiple studies that show that PD-L1–targeted imaging is feasible[56] and may reveal important pharmacokinetic findings such as changes in PD-L1 availability on the cell surface over time.[57] As clinical development proceeds, we should expect the emphasis for PD-L1 radiotracers to be on imaging biomarker development, as opposed to simply disease detection, as PD-L1 is expressed in normal lymph nodes,[58] which could degrade specificity. Nonetheless, the potential to optimize the eligibility of patients for anti-PD-(L)1 therapy, examine target engagement over time, dynamically track target expression, and develop prognostic imaging biomarkers provides an impetus to continue to clinically develop PD-L1 PET imaging agents.

Prostate-Specific Membrane Antigen

Despite the name, PSMA is widely expressed in normal tissues and in the tumor neovasculature of nonprostate solid tumors.[59,60] Given the highly neovascularized state of both primary[61] and metastatic tumors from ccRCC, it should not be surprising that PSMA-targeted radiotracers have high sensitivity for sites of disease involvement.[62,63] Indeed, the sensitivity for metastatic disease may be superior to ^{18}F-FDG.[64,65] In addition, uptake of PSMA-targeted diagnostic agents opens opportunities to potentially leverage theranostics for the treatment of metastatic ccRCC.[66] Nonclear cell histologies are not well imaged by PSMA radiotracers.[67] Ultimately, larger, prospective studies of the role of PSMA-targeted PET in patients with RCC are warranted in order to best understand the relative roles of ^{18}F-FDG and PSMA agents.

COMMENT AND FUTURE PERSPECTIVES

The use of ^{18}F-FDG PET across numerous malignancies is testament to its unique place as a well-studied, near-pan-cancer imaging agent.[68] Indeed, despite scant guideline recommendations regarding the use of ^{18}F-FDG PET in RCC or UC, likely partly based on the excretion of [8]F-FDG through the kidneys, it is nonetheless effective at the detection of locoregional and distant metastases in those diseases and should be more extensively utilized in patients at risk of metastatic disease. We should remain cognizant of the potential role of ^{18}F-FDG as a metabolic radiotracer that may uncover otherwise occult metastases from RCC or UC and can, potentially, provide imaging biomarkers for therapy selection or response assessment.

Recent years have seen a renaissance in nuclear medicine with the introduction of multiple new diagnostic and therapeutic agents for receptor-specific imaging and targeted therapy of multiple different cancer types,[68] most widely led by the introduction of PSMA for prostate cancer.[69] That renaissance has had direct implications on PET imaging in RCC and UC, where there are a number of targets that may have implications for therapeutic selection and/or may aid in the characterization of the tumor microenvironment.

We should be entering an era where interrogation of specific tumor biology and the tumor microenvironment are increasingly possible and desirable. Our ability to discover imaging biomarkers for prognostication, therapy selection, and response assessment should be greatly accelerated by multi-radiotracer, multi-timepoint imaging. Beyond the new radiotracers that are coming into clinical use, there is a potential synergistic effect with the rise of AI.[70] The potential for a positive feedback loop between new PET radiotracers and AI, where an advance in either domain could accelerate advances made in the other, may be the nexus for the next 25 years of the PET/CT transformation of oncology.

CLINICS CARE POINTS

- The judicious use of 18F-FDG PET in patients with renal cell carcinoma may uncover occult metastatic disease or allow therapy response monitoring.
- The high detection efficiency of 18F-FDG PET for sites of metastatic urothelial carcinoma suggests liberal use of this modality in staging and re-staging of patients may be appropriate.

- New PET agents targeting CAIX, Nectin-4, PD-L1, and PSMA may enter clinical use and provide new impetus for tumor characterization and the development of novel imaging biomarkers.

DISCLOSURE

LBS has received research funding from Precision Molecular, Inc. SN has received research funding and is a consultant for Precision Molecular, Inc. SPR owns equity in, has received research funding from, and is a consultant for Precision Molecular, Inc.

REFERENCES

1. Siegel RL, Miller KD, Wagle NS, et al. Cancer statistics, 2023. CA Cancer J Clin 2023;73(1):17–48.
2. Brooks SA, Khandani AH, Fielding JR, et al. Alternate metabolic Programs define regional Variation of Relevant biological features in renal cell carcinoma Progression. Clin Cancer Res 2016;22(12):2950–9.
3. Yin Q, Hung SC, Wang L, et al. Associations between tumor Vascularity, Vascular Endothelial growth Factor expression and PET/MRI radiomic Signatures in primary clear-cell-renal-cell-carcinoma: Proof-of-Concept study. Sci Rep 2017;7:43356.
4. Cowey CL, Fielding JR, Rathmell WK. The loss of radiographic enhancement in primary renal cell carcinoma tumors following multitargeted receptor tyrosine kinase therapy is an additional indicator of response. Urology 2010;75(5):1108–11013.e1.
5. Reinfeld BI, Madden MZ, Wolf MM, et al. Cell-programmed nutrient partitioning in the tumour microenvironment. Nature 2021;593(7858):282–8.
6. Hollingsworth JM, Miller DC, Daignault S, et al. Rising incidence of small renal masses: a need to reassess treatment effect. J Natl Cancer Inst 2006;98(18):1331–4.
7. Pierorazio PM, Hyams ES, Tsai S, et al. Multiphasic enhancement patterns of small renal masses (</=4 cm) on preoperative computed tomography: utility for distinguishing subtypes of renal cell carcinoma, angiomyolipoma, and oncocytoma. Urology 2013;81(6):1265–71.
8. Pedrosa I, Sun MR, Spencer M, et al. MR imaging of renal masses: correlation with findings at surgery and pathologic analysis. Radiographics 2008;28(4):985–1003.
9. Wang HY, Ding HJ, Chen JH, et al. Meta-analysis of the diagnostic performance of [18F]FDG-PET and PET/CT in renal cell carcinoma. Cancer Imag 2012;12(3):464–74.
10. Coquia SF, Johnson PT, Ahmed S, et al. MDCT imaging following nephrectomy for renal cell carcinoma:

protocol optimization and patterns of tumor recurrence. World J Radiol 2013;5(11):436–45.

11. Seifert R, Telli T, Opitz M, et al. Unspecific (18)F-PSMA-1007 bone uptake evaluated through PSMA-11 PET, bone Scanning, and MRI Triple Validation in patients with Biochemical recurrence of prostate cancer. J Nucl Med 2023;64(5):738–43.

12. Motzer RJ, Jonasch E, Agarwal N, et al. Kidney cancer, version 3.2022, NCCN clinical practice guidelines in oncology. J Natl Compr Canc Netw 2022; 20(1):71–90.

13. Park JW, Jo MK, Lee HM. Significance of 18F-fluorodeoxyglucose positron-emission tomography/computed tomography for the postoperative surveillance of advanced renal cell carcinoma. BJU Int 2009;103(5):615–9.

14. Yin Q, Xu H, Zhong Y, et al. Diagnostic performance of MRI, SPECT, and PET in detecting renal cell carcinoma: a systematic review and meta-analysis. BMC Cancer 2022;22(1):163.

15. Ma H, Shen G, Liu B, et al. Diagnostic performance of 18F-FDG PET or PET/CT in restaging renal cell carcinoma: a systematic review and meta-analysis. Nucl Med Commun 2017;38(2):156–63.

16. Jena R, Narain TA, Singh UP, et al. Role of positron emission tomography/computed tomography in the evaluation of renal cell carcinoma. Indian J Urol 2021;37(2):125–32.

17. Lindenberg L, Mena E, Choyke PL, et al. PET imaging in renal cancer. Curr Opin Oncol 2019;31(3): 216–21.

18. Posada Calderon L, Eismann L, Reese SW, et al. Advances in imaging-based biomarkers in renal cell carcinoma: a Critical analysis of the current Literature. Cancers 2023;15(2).

19. Karivedu V, Jain AL, Eluvathingal TJ, et al. Role of positron emission tomography imaging in Metabolically active renal cell carcinoma. Curr Urol Rep 2019; 20(10):56.

20. Chen JL, Appelbaum DE, Kocherginsky M, et al. FDG-PET as a predictive biomarker for therapy with everolimus in metastatic renal cell cancer. Cancer Med 2013;2(4):545–52.

21. Yamasaki T, Tran TA, Oz OK, et al. Exploring a glycolytic inhibitor for the treatment of an FH-deficient type-2 papillary RCC. Nat Rev Urol 2011;8(3): 165–71.

22. Crozier J, Papa N, Perera M, et al. Comparative sensitivity and specificity of imaging modalities in staging bladder cancer prior to radical cystectomy: a systematic review and meta-analysis. World J Urol 2019;37(4):667–90.

23. Ha HK, Koo PJ, Kim SJ. Diagnostic accuracy of F-18 FDG PET/CT for preoperative lymph node staging in newly diagnosed bladder cancer patients: a systematic review and meta-analysis. Oncology 2018; 95(1):31–8.

24. Soubra A, Hayward D, Dahm P, et al. The diagnostic accuracy of 18F-fluorodeoxyglucose positron emission tomography and computed tomography in staging bladder cancer: a single-institution study and a systematic review with meta-analysis. World J Urol 2016;34(9):1229–37.

25. Salem AE, Fine GC, Covington MF, et al. PET-CT in clinical Adult oncology-IV. Gynecologic and genitourinary malignancies. Cancers 2022;14(12):3000.

26. Xue M, Liu L, Du G, et al. Diagnostic evaluation of 18F-FDG PET/CT imaging in recurrent or residual urinary bladder cancer: a meta-analysis. Urol J 2020;17(6):562–7.

27. Ko WS, Kim SJ. Predictive value of 18 F-FDG PET/CT for assessment of tumor response to Neoadjuvant chemotherapy in bladder cancer. Clin Nucl Med 2023;48(7):574–80.

28. Green DA, Rink M, Xylinas E, et al. Urothelial carcinoma of the bladder and the upper tract: disparate twins. J Urol 2013;189(4):1214–21.

29. Pienta KJ, Gorin MA, Rowe SP, et al. A phase 2/3 prospective Multicenter study of the diagnostic accuracy of prostate specific membrane antigen PET/CT with (18)F-DCFPyL in prostate cancer patients (OSPREY). J Urol 2021;206(1):52–61.

30. Hope TA, Eiber M, Armstrong WR, et al. Diagnostic accuracy of 68Ga-PSMA-11 PET for pelvic nodal metastasis detection prior to radical Prostatectomy and pelvic lymph node Dissection: a Multicenter prospective phase 3 imaging trial. JAMA Oncol 2021;7(11):1635–42.

31. Divgi CR, Uzzo RG, Gatsonis C, et al. Positron emission tomography/computed tomography identification of clear cell renal cell carcinoma: results from the REDECT trial. J Clin Oncol 2013;31(2): 187–94.

32. Mondal UK, Doroba K, Shabana AM, et al. PEG linker Length Strongly Affects tumor cell Killing by PEGylated carbonic anhydrase inhibitors in hypoxic carcinomas expressing carbonic anhydrase IX. Int J Mol Sci 2021;22(3):1120.

33. Yang X, Minn I, Rowe SP, et al. Imaging of carbonic anhydrase IX with an 111In-labeled dual-motif inhibitor. Oncotarget 2015;6(32):33733–42.

34. Minn I, Koo SM, Lee HS, et al. [64Cu]XYIMSR-06: a dual-motif CAIX ligand for PET imaging of clear cell renal cell carcinoma. Oncotarget 2016;7(35):56471–9.

35. Turkbey B, Lindenberg ML, Adler S, et al. PET/CT imaging of renal cell carcinoma with (18)F-VM4-037: a phase II pilot study. Abdom Radiol (NY) 2016;41(1):109–18.

36. Shuch BM, Pantuck AJ, Bernhard JC, et al. Results from phase 3 study of 89Zr-DFO-girentuximab for PET/CT imaging of clear cell renal cell carcinoma (ZIRCON). J Clin Oncol 2023;41(6_suppl):LBA602.

37. Rowe SP, Gorin MA, Solnes LB, et al. Correlation of (99m)Tc-sestamibi uptake in renal masses with

mitochondrial content and multi-drug resistance pump expression. EJNMMI Res 2017;7(1):80.

38. Rowe SP, Gorin MA, Gordetsky J, et al. Initial experience using 99mTc-MIBI SPECT/CT for the differentiation of oncocytoma from renal cell carcinoma. Clin Nucl Med 2015;40(4):309–13.

39. Gorin MA, Rowe SP, Baras AS, et al. Prospective evaluation of (99m)Tc-sestamibi SPECT/CT for the diagnosis of renal oncocytomas and Hybrid oncocytic/Chromophobe tumors. Eur Urol 2016;69(3): 413–6.

40. Rowe SP, Javadi MS, Allaf ME, et al. Characterization of indeterminate renal masses with molecular imaging: how do we turn potential into reality? EJNMMI Res 2017;7(1):34.

41. Rosenberg J, Sridhar SS, Zhang J, et al. EV-101: a phase I study of single-agent enfortumab vedotin in patients with nectin-4-positive solid tumors, including metastatic urothelial carcinoma. J Clin Oncol 2020;38(10):1041–9.

42. Taguchi S, Nakagawa T, Uemura Y, et al. Validation of major prognostic models for metastatic urothelial carcinoma using a multi-institutional cohort of the real world. World J Urol 2016;34(2):163–71.

43. Rosenberg JE, O'Donnell PH, Balar AV, et al. Pivotal trial of enfortumab vedotin in urothelial carcinoma after platinum and anti-programmed death 1/programmed death ligand 1 therapy. J Clin Oncol 2019;37(29):2592–600.

44. Tagawa ST, Balar AV, Petrylak DP, et al. TROPHY-U-01: a phase II open-label study of sacituzumab govitecan in patients with metastatic urothelial carcinoma Progressing after platinum-based chemotherapy and checkpoint inhibitors. J Clin Oncol 2021;39(22): 2474–85.

45. Yu EY, Petrylak DP, O'Donnell PH, et al. Enfortumab vedotin after PD-1 or PD-L1 inhibitors in cisplatin-ineligible patients with advanced urothelial carcinoma (EV-201): a multicentre, single-arm, phase 2 trial. Lancet Oncol 2021;22(6):872–82.

46. Hoimes CJ, Flaig TW, Milowsky MI, et al. Enfortumab vedotin Plus pembrolizumab in Previously Untreated advanced urothelial cancer. J Clin Oncol 2023;41(1): 22–31.

47. O'Donnell PH, Milowsky MI, Petrylak DP, et al. Enfortumab vedotin with or without pembrolizumab in cisplatin-ineligible patients with Previously Untreated locally advanced or metastatic urothelial cancer. J Clin Oncol 2023;41(25):4107–17.

48. Duan X, Xia L, Zhang Z, et al. First-in-human study of the radioligand 68Ga-N188 targeting nectin-4 for PET/CT imaging of advanced urothelial carcinoma. Clin Cancer Res 2023;29(17):3395–407.

49. Brahmer JR, Tykodi SS, Chow LQ, et al. Safety and activity of anti-PD-L1 antibody in patients with advanced cancer. N Engl J Med 2012;366(26): 2455–65.

50. Rui X, Gu TT, Pan HF, et al. Evaluation of PD-L1 biomarker for immune checkpoint inhibitor (PD-1/PD-L1 inhibitors) treatments for urothelial carcinoma patients: a meta-analysis. Int Immunopharmacol 2019;67:378–85.

51. Zhao X, Bao Y, Meng B, et al. From rough to precise: PD-L1 evaluation for predicting the efficacy of PD-1/PD-L1 blockades. Front Immunol 2022;13: 920021.

52. Hegi-Johnson F, Rudd SE, Wichmann C, et al. ImmunoPET: IMaging of cancer imMUNOtherapy targets with positron Emission Tomography: a phase 0/1 study characterising PD-L1 with (89)Zr-durvalumab (MEDI4736) PET/CT in stage III NSCLC patients receiving chemoradiation study protocol. BMJ Open 2022;12(11):e056708.

53. Mulgaonkar A, Elias R, Woolford L, et al. Immuno-PET imaging with 89Zr-labeled Atezolizumab Enables in Vivo evaluation of PD-L1 in Tumorgraft models of renal cell carcinoma. Clin Cancer Res 2022;28(22):4907–16.

54. Kumar D, Lisok A, Dahmane E, et al. Peptide-based PET quantifies target engagement of PD-L1 therapeutics. J Clin Invest 2019;129(2):616–30.

55. Mishra A, Kumar D, Gupta K, et al. Gallium-68-labeled peptide PET quantifies tumor Exposure of PD-L1 therapeutics. Clin Cancer Res 2023;29(3): 581–91.

56. Zhou X, Jiang J, Yang X, et al. First-in-Humans evaluation of a PD-L1-binding peptide PET radiotracer in non-small cell Lung cancer patients. J Nucl Med 2022;63(4):536–42.

57. Krutzek F, Kopka K, Stadlbauer S. Development of radiotracers for imaging of the PD-1/PD-L1 Axis. Pharmaceuticals 2022;15(6).

58. Komohara Y, Ohnishi K, Takeya M. Possible functions of CD169-positive sinus macrophages in lymph nodes in anti-tumor immune responses. Cancer Sci 2017;108(3):290–5.

59. Chang SS, O'Keefe DS, Bacich DJ, et al. Prostate-specific membrane antigen is produced in tumor-associated neovasculature. Clin Cancer Res 1999; 5(10):2674–81.

60. Milowsky MI, Nanus DM, Kostakoglu L, et al. Vascular targeted therapy with anti-prostate-specific membrane antigen monoclonal antibody J591 in advanced solid tumors. J Clin Oncol 2007;25(5):540–7.

61. Rowe SP, Gorin MA, Allaf ME, et al. Photorealistic 3-Dimensional Cinematic Rendering of clear cell renal cell carcinoma from Volumetric computed tomography data. Urology 2018;115:e3–5.

62. Rowe SP, Gorin MA, Hammers HJ, et al. Imaging of metastatic clear cell renal cell carcinoma with PSMA-targeted (1)(8)F-DCFPyL PET/CT. Ann Nucl Med 2015;29(10):877–82.

63. Raveenthiran S, Esler R, Yaxley J, et al. The use of (68)Ga-PET/CT PSMA in the staging of primary

and suspected recurrent renal cell carcinoma. Eur J Nucl Med Mol Imaging 2019;46(11):2280–8.

64. Rowe SP, Gorin MA, Hammers HJ, et al. Detection of 18F-FDG PET/CT occult lesions with 18F-DCFPyL PET/CT in a patient with metastatic renal cell carcinoma. Clin Nucl Med 2016;41(1):83–5.

65. Parghane RV, Basu S. (18)F-FDG PET/CT vs. (68) Ga-PSMA-11 PET/CT in evaluation of distant metastatic disease in recurrent Renal Cell Carcinoma. J Nucl Med Technol 2023;51(3):261–2.

66. Salas Fragomeni RA, Amir T, Sheikhbahaei S, et al. Imaging of Nonprostate cancers using PSMA-targeted radiotracers: Rationale, current state of the Field, and a Call to Arms. J Nucl Med 2018; 59(6):871–7.

67. Yin Y, Campbell SP, Markowski MC, et al. Inconsistent detection of sites of metastatic non-clear cell renal cell carcinoma with PSMA-targeted [(18)F] DCFPyL PET/CT. Mol Imaging Biol 2019;21(3): 567–73.

68. Rowe SP, Pomper MG. Molecular imaging in oncology: current impact and future directions. CA Cancer J Clin 2022;72(4):333–52.

69. Rowe SP, Gorin MA, Pomper MG. Imaging of prostate-specific membrane antigen with small-molecule PET radiotracers: from the Bench to advanced clinical applications. Annu Rev Med 2019;70:461–77.

70. Rowe SP. Artificial intelligence in molecular imaging: at the crossroads of revolutions in medical diagnosis. Ann Transl Med 2021;9(9):817.

PET/Computed Tomography Transformation of Oncology Ovarian Cancers

Elaine Yuen Phin Lee, BMedSci, BMBS (UK), MD (HK), FRCR[a],*,
Pun Ching Philip Ip, MB ChB (UK), FRCPath, FHKCPath, FHKAM (Pathology)[b],
Ka Yu Tse, MBBS (HK), MMedSc (HK), FHKCOG, FRCOG, Cert RCOG (Gynae Onc),
FHKAM (Obstetrics and Gynaecology)[c],
Shuk Tak Kwok, MBBS (HK), MRCOG, FHKCOG[d],
Wan Kam Chiu, MB ChB (HK), FHKAM (Obstetrics and Gynaecology)[e],
Grace Ho, MB ChB (HK), FRCR, FHKCR, FHKAM (Radiology)[f]

KEYWORDS

• Ovarian cancer • FDG • PET/CT • Recurrence detection • Disease staging • Cytoreduction

KEY POINTS

- Fluorine-18-fluorodeoxyglucose (FDG) PET/computed tomography (CT) is most useful in detecting recurrent disease in ovarian cancer.
- FDG PET/CT is able to identify extra-abdominal disease that may upstage the disease in ovarian cancer.
- Metabolic response on FDG PET/CT is associated with treatment response and better prognosis.

INTRODUCTION

The introduction of fluorine-18-fluorodeoxyglucose (FDG) PET has revolutionized the field of oncology. FDG PET offers metabolic information, but lacks the anatomic information that is required for accurate disease localization and to address areas or diseases that are non-FDG avid. Due to this limitation, during the early adoption of FDG PET, patients often required to undergo 2 separate imaging examinations, FDG PET and a diagnostic computed tomography (CT) for disease evaluation. When Beyer and Townsend and colleagues introduced the first hybrid imaging by combining PET and CT, this made extraordinary impact on the practice of oncology and medicine at large.[1,2]

Other cancers were quick to adopt FDG PET/CT in the clinical management algorithms, but gynecological cancers were slower in incorporating FDG PET/CT as part of the diagnostic pathway. Gynecological cancers are heterogenous with the 2 major types being ovarian cancers and uterine cancers, the latter included endometrial and cervical cancers. Ovarian cancer (OC) accounts for more death than any other gynecological cancers. Herein, this review will evaluate the evolution and

[a] Department of Diagnostic Radiology, School of Clinical Medicine, University of Hong Kong, Room 406, Block K, Queen Mary Hospital, 102 Pokfulam Road, Hong Kong SAR, China; [b] Department of Pathology, School of Clinical Medicine, University of Hong Kong, Room 019, 7/F, Block T, Queen Mary Hospital, 102 Pokfulam Road, Hong Kong SAR, China; [c] Department of Obstetrics and Gynaecology, School of Clinical Medicine, University of Hong Kong, 6/F, Professorial Block, Queen Mary Hospital, 102 Pokfulam Road, Hong Kong SAR, China; [d] Department of Obstetrics and Gynaecology, 6/F, Professorial Block, Queen Mary Hospital, 102 Pokfulam Road, Hong Kong SAR, China; [e] Department of Obstetrics and Gynaecology, United Christian Hospital, 5/F, Block S, Kwun Tong, Kowloon, Hong Kong, China; [f] Department of Radiology, Queen Mary Hospital, 102 Pokfulam Road, Hong Kong SAR, China
* Corresponding author.
E-mail address: eyplee77@hku.hk

PET Clin 19 (2024) 207–216
https://doi.org/10.1016/j.cpet.2023.12.007

impact of FDG PET/CT in the clinical management of OC, review the effect of new therapeutic options on the practice of FDG PET/CT, and finally discuss the new advances in PET/CT that will bring about opportunities in OC management.

Diagnostic Roles

Tumor characterization

It was recognized that many ovarian tumors were FDG avid, providing information on tumor characterization, especially in differentiating benign from malignant ovarian tumors. The first report of application of FDG PET in OC demonstrated high positive predictive value (PPV 86%) and negative predictive value (NPV 76%) in 51 patients.[3] As experience accumulated, it was noted that false-negative results could arise from early stage OC or borderline tumors, while false-positive cases might be due to inflammatory adnexal masses like tubo-ovarian abscess, benign pelvic diseases, for example, endometrioma and functional cysts.[4] These resulted in low sensitivity of FDG PET in tumor characterization compared to ultrasound and MRI, 58% vs. 92% and 83%, respectively; while maintaining high specificity at 76% to 80%.[4,5] The advent of FDG PET/CT overcomes some of these pitfalls by having the anatomic information from CT, for example corpus luteal cyst has typical hyperattenuating thickened wall in a premenopausal lady (**Fig. 1**), which could avoid unnecessary further investigation; the hyperattenuating fluid-filled adnexal mass with possible fluid-fluid level or gas, with or without the presence of pyosalpinx indicating tubo-ovarian abscess can prompt early antimicrobial treatment (**Fig. 2**). As a result, the sensitivity and specificity improved to 87% and 100%, respectively, with FDG PET/CT.[6] The diagnostic performance saw further improvement when clinical risk algorithm was considered.[7] Subsequent studies demonstrated that maximum

standardized uptake value (SUVmax) could differentiate benign or borderline ovarian tumors from OC using different cut-off values with high sensitivity and specificity.[8–10] Nevertheless, there was no uniform cut-off value of SUVmax that could reliably characterize the different ovarian masses.

Ovarian masses are commonly first detected through ultrasound or clinical examination. The introduction of The Ovarian-Adnexal Reporting and Data System (O-RADS) for ultrasound and MRI allow uniform evaluation of ovarian masses and risk-stratification to inform appropriate diagnostic pathways and clinical management.[11,12] These have largely replaced the need for FDG PET/CT in tumor characterization of indeterminate ovarian masses and these patients should be appropriately referred for ultrasound or MRI assessment instead (**Fig. 3**).

Disease staging

According to the Global Cancer Statistics 2020, there was an incidence of 313,959 cases of OC with mortality of 207,252 cases.[13] The lack of symptoms in early stage OC often results in late presentation with poor 5-year survival rate.[14] CT is commonly used to stage OC. At the turn of the millennium, in a small cohort of patients, the addition of FDG PET could increase the accuracy of staging of OC from 53% (CT alone) to 87% (consensus reading of FDG PET and CT).[15] Subsequent studies confirmed that FDG PET/CT was concordant with surgical staging in 75% to 78% of the cases and FDG PET/CT was able to identify unexpected extra-abdominal nodal metastases in 15.8% of the patients.[16,17] FDG PET/CT was superior in detecting extra-abdominal disease (**Fig. 4**) but insensitive to small lesion below 5 mm with difficulty in the epigastrium and subdiaphragmatic surfaces.[18–20] Interestingly, the identification of extra-abdominal disease had not led to a difference in

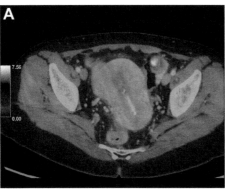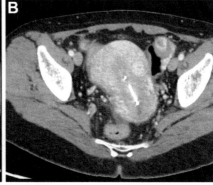

Fig. 1. (*A*) Axial fused fluorine-18-fluorodeoxyglucose (FDG) PET/computed tomography (FDG PET/CT) showed focal hypermetabolic activity in the left adnexa. (*B*) Axial CT showed the corresponding corpus luteal cyst with typical intense rim of enhancement around its wall on CT.

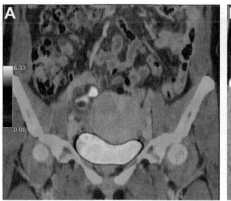 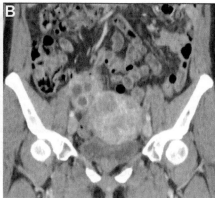

Fig. 2. (*A*) Coronal fused FDG PET/CT showed focal rims of uptake in the right adnexa. (*B*) Coronal CT showed that the uptake corresponded tubular multilocular right tubo-ovarian mass with thick enhancing wall, in keeping with tubo-ovarian abscess with formation of pyosalpinx.

disease outcome in terms of progression-free survival (PFS) and overall survival (OS).[20] Therefore, despite improvement in staging accuracy and potentially disease upstaging, the prognosis of primary OC remains with the ability of achieving complete cytoreduction at upfront or interval debulking surgery. FDG PET/CT could not replace surgical staging, especially when it could miss

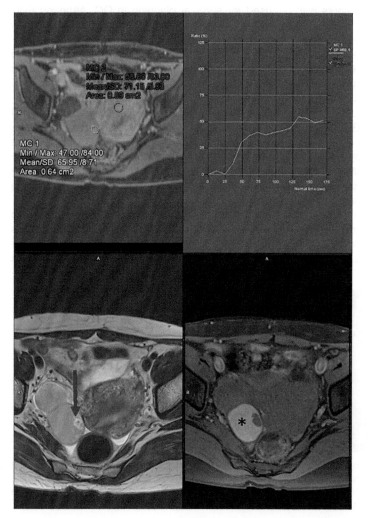

Fig. 3. A complex right ovarian mass with intralesional solid nodule (red *arrow*) that showed intermediate-risk time-intensity curve (*yellow curve*) on dynamic contrast-enhanced MRI. It had content with T1 shortening on fat-suppressed T1W sequence indicating the presence of mucin or blood (*). It carried a MRI O-RADS risk score of 4 and subsequently histologically proven to the serous borderline tumor with haemorrhage.

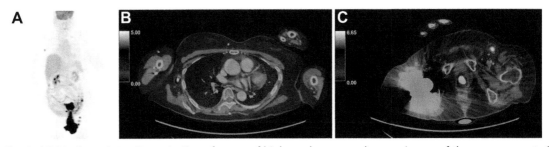

Fig. 4. (A) Maximum intensity projection of a case of high-grade serous adenocarcinoma of the ovary presented with metastatic disease on FDG PET/CT. (B) Axial fused FDG PET/CT showed hypermetabolic right axillary nodal metastasis. (C) Axial fused FDG PET/CT showed hypermetabolic left inguinal nodal metastasis.

sub-centimetre metastatic disease and performed poorly in detection of peritoneal metastasis in the right upper quadrant and small bowel mesentery.[19]

Recurrence detection

The earliest indication for use of FDG PET in OC was to detect recurrent disease. A study in 1993 showed that findings on FDG PET were correlated with surgical findings in recurrent tumors larger than 1 cm but it failed to identify 5 patients with microscopic disease.[21] A wealth of follow-up studies including those using FDG PET/CT showed the superiority of FDG PET/CT in recurrence detection, especially in the context of rising CA-125 but negative conventional imaging.[22–25] Furthermore, the findings on FDG PET/CT impacted clinical management in 44% to 58% of the cases.[24,26] Meta-analysis also supported the use of FDG PET/CT in detection of recurrence in OC[27] with level I evidence and grade A recommendation by European Association of Nuclear Medicine (EANM) guideline.[28] FDG PET/CT altered the original plan for pelvic exenteration in recurrent gynecological cancers in 38%, either due to identification of metastatic or unresectable disease, potentially reducing the number of futile attempts.[29] Nevertheless, similar to disease staging, sensitivity of FDG PET/CT is limited by size of the lesion, in that lesion smaller than 0.5 cm could be missed.[30]

Treatment Planning and Monitoring

Surgical planning and prediction of outcome of cytoreduction

The primary route of disease spread for OC is peritoneal dissemination. Conventionally, CT has been used for surgical planning in OC. Although FDG PET/CT improves disease staging by notably detecting extra-abdominal metastases, it has comparable diagnostic capability as CT in evaluating the abdominopelvic cavity with no difference in detecting upper abdominal sites that required extensive surgical procedures and multidisciplinary involvement.[19,31] FDG PET/CT has reduced sensitivity in areas where high background physiologic uptake are expected, for example, near the urinary bladder or bowel (**Fig. 5**), and when infiltrative pattern of peritoneal carcinomatosis is encountered. The meta-analysis conducted by Cochrane identified only 2 FDG PET/CT studies that evaluated tumor resectability and concluded that there was insufficient evidence to support routine use of FDG PET/CT in this clinical context, despite showing high specificity.[32] Risum and colleagues

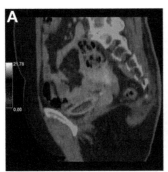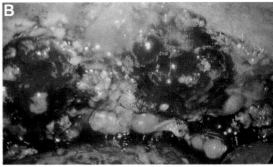

Fig. 5. (A) Sagittal fused FDG PET/CT did not demonstrate focal uptake in the pelvic peritoneal space, none at the fundus of the urinary bladder, the uterovesical pouch, nor the rectouterine pouch. (B) At interval debulking surgery, there was disease plaque against the fundus of the urinary bladder extending to the uterovesical pouch, missed on FDG PET/CT due to the intense FDG excretion in the urinary bladder masking the uptake from tumor deposits.

found that large bowel mesenteric implant was the only independent predictor of incomplete cytoreduction in a cohort of 54 patients with advanced OC. Nevertheless, among the 33 patients with large bowel mesenteric implant, 18% managed to achieve complete cytoreduction. Therefore, the group cautioned relying on this FDG PET/CT finding to exclude patient from primary cytoreductive surgery.[33] Metabolic tumor volume (MTV) and total lesion glycolysis (TLG) but not SUVmax were associated with optimal debulking (residual disease less than 1 cm) indicating that the tumor burden was an important determinant of the ability to achieve complete cytoreduction.[34] Other predictors that have been suggested included number of peritoneal avid sites[35] and modified peritoneal cancer index score.[36] More recently, a FDG PET/CT model was developed and validated using 325 patients with advanced OC; it included the number of metastatic lesions and MTV of the upper abdominal disease that could predict complete cytoreduction with high accuracy offering an area under the receiver operating characteristic curve (AUC) of 0.771 in the validation cohort.[37] By large, FDG PET/CT studies predicting complete cytoreduction suffer from small sample size, single-center study and lack large-scale external validation, therefore the above results should be interpreted with caution and the ability of FDG PET/CT in predicting outcome of cytoreduction remains unclear.

Treatment response assessment

The metabolic changes precede anatomic changes, allowing for early identification of non-responders from responders to therapeutic interventions,[38] making FDG PET/CT an ideal tool in treatment response assessment. Metabolic responses on sequential FDG PET, even after 1 cycle of neoadjuvant chemotherapy in advanced OC, were correlated with OS, which was superior than clinical and biochemical responses.[39] A normalization or reduction in SUVmax as early as after 1 cycle of neoadjuvant chemotherapy was correlated with histopathological response and PFS[40,41] (Fig. 6). Similarly, the reduction in MTV was also prognostic of PFS and OS.[42] Subsequently, it was found the PET Response Criteria in Solid Tumors (PERCIST) and European Organization for Research and Treatment of Cancer (EORTC) criteria were more discriminative than MTV and TLG in determining PFS and OS. Despite the notion that metabolic tumor burden could be useful in OC, both MTV and TLG using various thresholds could not predict PFS or OS in this study.[43] Contrary to above, Hyninnen and colleagues noted that residual active sites on the end-of-treatment FDG PET/CT did not affect disease prognosis.[44] Overall, majority of the studies favor a positive correlation between metabolic response and treatment response, hence disease prognosis. However, there was significant variation in the metabolic metrics and thresholds used. Currently, it is undecided which metabolic metric is superior in monitoring treatment response and practice is largely dependent on local preference, ease of use, and practicality.

New Advancements and Novel Tracers

New therapies in ovarian cancer

Almost all patients will experience disease relapse and develop resistance to platinum-based chemotherapy. The success of poly(ADP-ribose) polymerase (PARP) inhibitors has transformed the management of these patients, being initially used

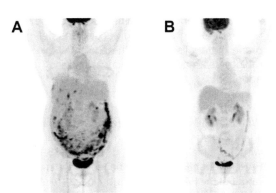
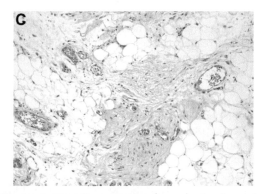

Fig. 6. (A) FDG PET/CT before neoadjuvant chemotherapy. Maximum intensity projection showed extensive metastatic disease in the peritoneum including small bowel serosal disease at presentation in a patient with high-grade serous adenocarcinoma of the ovary. (B) FDG PET/CT after 3 cycles of neoadjuvant chemotherapy showed complete metabolic response. The patient went on to achieve complete tumor debulking at interval debulking surgery and corresponded to CRS 3 in the resected omentum, indicating no residual disease on the omentectomy specimen. (C) Omentectomy specimen showed absence of viable tumor cells or inflammation (H&E ×10). CRS: chemotherapy response score.

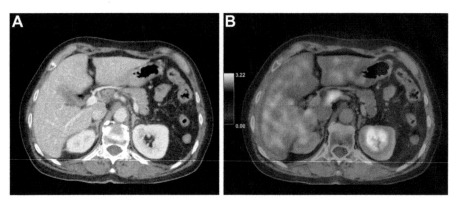

Fig. 7. (*A*) Axial contrast-enhanced CT upper abdomen showed a necrotic porta hepatis lymph node in a patient with ovarian cancer who had been on 16 months of niraparib as maintenance therapy. (*B*) Corresponding fused axial FDG PET/CT demonstrated focal hypermetabolic activity in the necrotic porta hepatis lymph node, suspicious of recurrent disease. This was subsequently biopsied through endoscopic ultrasound approach and confirmed to be recurrent ovarian cancer. The patient was re-challenged with platinum-based chemotherapy.

as maintenance therapy and transitioning to first-line setting.[45,46] Initial study showed promising results of FDG PET/CT in identifying responders to olaparib after 1 cycle of therapy.[47] FDG PET/CT is also useful in identifying PARP inhibitors (PARPi) failure (**Fig. 7**).

OC is thought to be immunoreactive tumor but the interim analysis from phase II KEYNOTE-100 study only demonstrated an objective response rate (ORR) of 8% with pembrolizumab as mono-therapy in recurrent advanced OC.[48] Combination therapies are being explored to investigate the potential synergic power of different immunomod-ulators.[49] A recent single-arm, phase 2 non-randomized clinical trial in 40 patients showed the synergistic power of pembrolizumab, bevaci-zumab, and cyclophosphamide in producing an ORR of 47.5% and median PFS of 10 months in recurrent OC.[50] Hence, it is conceivable that we may see more use of immune checkpoint inhibi-tors in recurrent OC. These may result in imaging features related to the interference with the im-mune checkpoints for T-cells and the most cited phenomenon of pseudo-progression was noted during the early use of immune checkpoint inhibi-tors, representing inflammatory reaction and heightened immunity to the cancer cells.[51,52]

Treating platinum-resistant OC is challenging with limited treatment options and poor response rates. Antibody-drug conjugate, mirvetuximab soravtan-sine that targets folate receptor alpha offers new hope for these patients as shown in SORAYA study. In patients with high folate receptor alpha expres-sion who received up to 3 previous lines of therapy, mirvetuximab soravtansine was able to produce an ORR of 32.4% with a median duration response of 6.9 months.[53] However, at present, it is unknown how the use of mirvetuximab soravtansine could

affect the practice of FDG PET/CT and more data are required to enhance our knowledge in coming years.

Advances in PET/Computed Tomography

Non-FDG radiotracers

One of the earliest studies evaluating non-FDG radiotracer in gynecological cancers utilized C11-methionine in 18 patients with OC, showing similar diagnostic efficacy as FDG PET with limitation of liver lesions due to the high background tracer accumulation in the liver.[54] As the half-life of C11-methionine is short, 20.4 min, on-site cyclo-tron is needed for its use and making accessibility more challenging.[55] Therefore, without additional benefit over FDG PET, the authors have not observed clinical integration of C11-methionine PET in mainstream assessment of OC. Similar work based on C11-choline PET was applied in recurrent OC in assessing accelerated cell mem-brane metabolism,[56] but the short half-live of the radiotracer made it impractical for easy clinical adoption.

Fibroblast activation protein (FAP) is overex-pressed by cancer- associated fibroblasts (CAF). With the FAP-ligands, we are able to visualize ma-lignant tissue and its stromal microenvironment with upregulation of CAF.[57,58] Gallium 68–labelled FAP inhibitor (FAPI) PET is based on the molecular target of the FAP. Its biodistribution correlated with FAP tissue expression and strong FAP expression was observed in many cancers, including gyneco-logical cancers with high tumour-to-background ratio when compared with FDG.[59,60] Although FAPI accumulation can be affected by hormone-sensitive organs like endometrium and breast in premenopausal ladies, no significant difference was observed in the ovaries.[60] Early results from FAPI PET/CT are promising but further research is required to clearly define its role in gynecological cancers over FDG PET/CT.

Theragnostic

With the increasing application of targeted and novel therapy agents as alluded earlier, radiotracer can be tagged to the specific therapy target to provide potential information on target delivery, biodistribution, and target expression on tumors. The theragnostic work in OC remains in its infancy with preliminary but promising results observed in-vivo and in-vitro.[61–65] Many of these may provide hopeful targets for further clinical trials by selecting the appropriate cohorts for testing to maximize the therapeutic potential.

Total body PET/Computed Tomography

The current PET/CT system has come a long way since the early PET systems with improved sensitivity and spatial resolution. These were achieved through use of detectors with higher detection efficiency, integration of a fully 3D system, introduction of time-of-flight measurements, and increase the axial length of the PET system, coupled with switch from large conventional photomultiplier tubes to small solid state detectors.[66] The more recent exciting development is the introduction of total body PET/CT with an impressive axial field of view (FOV) of 106 to 194 cm, allowing image of the whole-body with 1 bed position.[67] The EXPLORER Consortium (a collaboration between the University of California, CA, USA and United Imaging Healthcare based in Shanghai, China) developed the first human total body PET/CT system called the uEXPLORER PET/CT and became operational since mid-2018.[68] Another system, PennPET Explorer, was developed at the University of Pennsylvania, USA, around the same time.[69] Now, we have the commercially available total body PET/CT system offered by Siemens Healthineers, Siemens Biograph Vision Quadra PET/CT with an axial FOV of 106 cm. It has demonstrated better sensitivity, image quality, and lesion quantification.[70,71] The total body PET/CT offers opportunities in imaging of OC by offering global assessment with increased sensitivity and the possibility of dynamic imaging, which was not possible in the past unless in research setting. The ability of performing dual-phase or dynamic imaging will alleviate some of the challenges faced by the current PET/CT system in differentiating physiologic or benign uptake from malignant lesions. Furthermore, one of the major drawback of FDG PET/CT in OC assessment is the inability to detect small volume or miliary disease spread in the peritoneal cavity; but with total body PET/CT, the increased sensitivity and dynamic imaging capability, we may be able to overcome this pitfall. The shorten acquisition time for a whole-body assessment could potentially reduce patient discomfort, motion artifacts, increase patient throughput, and reduce radiation exposure by allowing less radiotracer to be injected for the same quality images.[72]

SUMMARY

Over the last quarter of a century, the advancement and improvement of technology and hardware have enabled incorporation of FDG PET/CT in the diagnostic and management algorithms of OC. The multifaceted roles of FDG PET/CT are better defined after building on experiences and research findings. These will continue to evolve over time as new developments emerge in therapeutics and technology.

CLINICS CARE POINTS

- FDG PET/CT is most useful in detecting recurrent disease in ovarian cancer.
- FDG PET/CT is able to identify extra-abdominal disease that may upstage the disease in ovarian cancer.
- Metabolic response on FDG PET/CT is associated with treatment response and better prognosis.

DISCLOSURE

The authors have nothing to disclose.

ACKNOWLEDGMENT

Some of the images used in this review were produced from research work supported by the Health and Medical Research Fund, Hong Kong (HMRF 06171706).

REFERENCES

1. Beyer T, Townsend DW, Brun T, et al. A combined PET/CT scanner for clinical oncology. J Nucl Med 2000;41(8):1369–79.
2. Townsend D, Beyer T, Czernin J. 20 Years of PET/CT: a conversation with david Townsend and thomas beyer. J Nucl Med 2020;61(11):1541–3.
3. Hubner KF, McDonald TW, Niethammer JG, et al. Assessment of primary and metastatic ovarian cancer by positron emission tomography (PET) using 2-

[18F]deoxyglucose (2-[18F]FDG). Gynecol Oncol 1993;51(2):197–204.

4. Grab D, Flock F, Stöhr I, et al. Classification of asymptomatic adnexal masses by ultrasound, magnetic resonance imaging, and positron emission tomography. Gynecol Oncol 2000;77(3):454–9.

5. Fenchel S, Grab D, Nuessle K, et al. Asymptomatic adnexal masses: correlation of FDG PET and histopathologic findings. Radiology 2002;223(3):780–8.

6. Castellucci P, Perrone AM, Picchio M, et al. Diagnostic accuracy of 18F-FDG PET/CT in characterizing ovarian lesions and staging ovarian cancer: correlation with transvaginal ultrasonography, computed tomography, and histology. Nucl Med Commun 2007;28(8):589–95.

7. Risum S, Høgdall C, Loft A, et al. The diagnostic value of PET/CT for primary ovarian cancer–a prospective study. Gynecol Oncol 2007;105(1):145–9.

8. Kim C, Chung HH, Oh SW, et al. Differential diagnosis of borderline ovarian tumors from stage i malignant ovarian tumors using FDG PET/CT. Nucl Med Mol Imaging 2013;47(2):81–8.

9. Kitajima K, Suzuki K, Senda M, et al. FDG-PET/CT for diagnosis of primary ovarian cancer. Nucl Med Commun 2011;32(7):549–53.

10. Tanizaki Y, Kobayashi A, Shiro M, et al. Diagnostic value of preoperative SUVmax on FDG-PET/CT for the detection of ovarian cancer. Int J Gynecol Cancer 2014;24(3):454–60.

11. Andreotti RF, Timmerman D, Strachowski LM, et al. O-RADS US risk stratification and management system: a consensus guideline from the ACR ovarian-adnexal reporting and data system committee. Radiology 2020;294(1):168–85.

12. Thomassin-Naggara I, Poncelet E, Jalaguier-Coudray A, et al. Ovarian-adnexal reporting data system magnetic resonance imaging (O-RADS MRI) score for risk stratification of sonographically indeterminate adnexal masses. JAMA Netw Open 2020;3(1):e1919896.

13. Sung H, Ferlay J, Siegel RL, et al. Global cancer statistics 2020: GLOBOCAN estimates of incidence and mortality worldwide for 36 cancers in 185 countries. CA Cancer J Clin 2021;71(3):209–49.

14. Webb PM, Jordan SJ. Epidemiology of epithelial ovarian cancer. Best Pract Res Clin Obstet Gynaecol 2017;41:3–14.

15. Yoshida Y, Kurokawa T, Kawahara K, et al. Incremental benefits of FDG positron emission tomography over CT alone for the preoperative staging of ovarian cancer. AJR Am J Roentgenol 2004; 182(1):227–33.

16. Kitajima K, Murakami K, Yamasaki E, et al. Diagnostic accuracy of integrated FDG-PET/contrast-enhanced CT in staging ovarian cancer: comparison with enhanced CT. Eur J Nucl Med Mol Imag 2008; 35(10):1912–20.

17. Nam EJ, Yun MJ, Oh YT, et al. Diagnosis and staging of primary ovarian cancer: correlation between PET/CT, Doppler US, and CT or MRI. Gynecol Oncol 2010;116(3):389–94.

18. De Iaco P, Musto A, Orazi L, et al. FDG-PET/CT in advanced ovarian cancer staging: value and pitfalls in detecting lesions in different abdominal and pelvic quadrants compared with laparoscopy. Eur J Radiol 2011;80(2):e98–103.

19. Hynninen J, Kemppainen J, Lavonius M, et al. A prospective comparison of integrated FDG-PET/contrast-enhanced CT and contrast-enhanced CT for pretreatment imaging of advanced epithelial ovarian cancer. Gynecol Oncol 2013;131(2):389–94.

20. Fruscio R, Sina F, Dolci C, et al. Preoperative 18F-FDG PET/CT in the management of advanced epithelial ovarian cancer. Gynecol Oncol 2013; 131(3):689–93.

21. Karlan BY, Hawkins R, Hoh C, et al. Whole-body positron emission tomography with 2-[18F]-fluoro-2-deoxy-D-glucose can detect recurrent ovarian carcinoma. Gynecol Oncol 1993;51(2):175–81.

22. Nakamoto Y, Saga T, Ishimori T, et al. Clinical value of positron emission tomography with FDG for recurrent ovarian cancer. AJR Am J Roentgenol 2001; 176(6):1449–54.

23. Sebastian S, Lee SI, Horowitz NS, et al. PET-CT vs. CT alone in ovarian cancer recurrence. Abdom Imag 2008;33(1):112–8.

24. Mangili G, Picchio M, Sironi S, et al. Integrated PET/CT as a first-line re-staging modality in patients with suspected recurrence of ovarian cancer. Eur J Nucl Med Mol Imag 2007;34(5):658–66.

25. Thrall MM, DeLoia JA, Gallion H, et al. Clinical use of combined positron emission tomography and computed tomography (FDG-PET/CT) in recurrent ovarian cancer. Gynecol Oncol 2007;105(1):17–22.

26. Simcock B, Neesham D, Quinn M, et al. The impact of PET/CT in the management of recurrent ovarian cancer. Gynecol Oncol 2006;103(1):271–6.

27. Gu P, Pan LL, Wu SQ, et al. CA 125, PET alone, PET-CT, CT and MRI in diagnosing recurrent ovarian carcinoma: a systematic review and meta-analysis. Eur J Radiol 2009;71(1):164–74.

28. Delgado Bolton RC, Aide N, Colletti PM, et al. EANM guideline on the role of 2-[(18)F]FDG PET/CT in diagnosis, staging, prognostic value, therapy assessment and restaging of ovarian cancer, endorsed by the American College of Nuclear Medicine (ACNM), the Society of Nuclear Medicine and Molecular Imaging (SNMMI) and the International Atomic Energy Agency (IAEA). Eur J Nucl Med Mol Imag 2021;48(10):3286–302.

29. Kim SR, Lee YY, Brar H, et al. Utility of 18F-FDG-PET/CT imaging in patients with recurrent gynecological malignancies prior to pelvic exenteration. Int J Gynecol Cancer 2019;ijgc(2018):000091.

30. Sironi S, Messa C, Mangili G, et al. Integrated FDG PET/CT in patients with persistent ovarian cancer: correlation with histologic findings. Radiology 2004;233(2):433–40.

31. Schmidt S, Meuli RA, Achtari C, et al. Peritoneal carcinomatosis in primary ovarian cancer staging: comparison between MDCT, MRI, and 18F-FDG PET/CT. Clin Nucl Med 2015;40(5):371–7.

32. Roze JF, Hoogendam JP, van de Wetering FT, et al. Positron emission tomography (PET) and magnetic resonance imaging (MRI) for assessing tumour resectability in advanced epithelial ovarian/fallopian tube/primary peritoneal cancer. Cochrane Database Syst Rev 2018;10(10):CD012567.

33. Risum S, Høgdall C, Loft A, et al. Prediction of sub-optimal primary cytoreduction in primary ovarian cancer with combined positron emission tomography/computed tomography–a prospective study. Gynecol Oncol 2008;108(2):265–70.

34. Vargas HA, Burger IA, Goldman DA, et al. Volume-based quantitative FDG PET/CT metrics and their association with optimal debulking and progression-free survival in patients with recurrent ovarian cancer undergoing secondary cytoreductive surgery. Eur Radiol 2015;25(11):3348–53.

35. Tsoi TT, Chiu KWH, Chu MY, et al. Metabolic active peritoneal sites affect tumor debulking in ovarian and peritoneal cancers. J Ovarian Res 2020;13(1): 61.

36. Boria F, Chiva L, Carbonell M, et al. ^{18}F-fluorodeoxyglucose positron emission tomography/computed tomography (^{18}F-FDG PET/CT) predictive score for complete resection in primary cytoreductive surgery. Int J Gynecol Cancer. 2022:ijgc-2022-003883.

37. Kim J, Gil J, Kim SI, et al. Development and validation of 18F-FDG PET/CT-Based models for predicting successful complete cytoreduction during primary cytoreductive surgery for advanced ovarian cancer. Clin Nucl Med 2023;48(2):e51–9.

38. Avril NE, Weber WA. Monitoring response to treatment in patients utilizing PET. Radiol Clin North Am 2005;43(1):189–204.

39. Avril N, Sassen S, Schmalfeldt B, et al. Prediction of response to neoadjuvant chemotherapy by sequential F-18-fluorodeoxyglucose positron emission tomography in patients with advanced-stage ovarian cancer. J Clin Oncol 2005;23(30): 7445–53.

40. Vallius T, Peter A, Auranen A, et al. 18F-FDG-PET/CT can identify histopathological non-responders to platinum-based neoadjuvant chemotherapy in advanced epithelial ovarian cancer. Gynecol Oncol 2016;140(1):29–35.

41. Chung YS, Kim HS, Lee JY, et al. Early assessment of response to neoadjuvant chemotherapy with 18F-FDG-PET/CT in patients with advanced-stage ovarian cancer. Cancer Res Treat 2020;52(4):1211–8.

42. Vallius T, Hynninen J, Kemppainen J, et al. 18)F-FDG-PET/CT based total metabolic tumor volume change during neoadjuvant chemotherapy predicts outcome in advanced epithelial ovarian cancer. Eur J Nucl Med Mol Imag 2018;45(7):1224–32.

43. Aide N, Fauchille P, Coquan E, et al. Predicting tumor response and outcome of second-look surgery with (18)F-FDG PET/CT: insights from the GINECO CHIVA phase II trial of neoadjuvant chemotherapy plus nintedanib in stage IIIc-IV FIGO ovarian cancer. Eur J Nucl Med Mol Imag 2021;48(6):1998–2008.

44. Hynninen J, Laasik M, Vallius T, et al. Clinical value of (18)F-fluorodeoxyglucose positron emission tomography/computed tomography in response evaluation after primary treatment of advanced epithelial ovarian cancer. Clin Oncol 2018;30(8):507–14.

45. Ledermann J, Harter P, Gourley C, et al. Olaparib maintenance therapy in patients with platinum-sensitive relapsed serous ovarian cancer: a pre-planned retrospective analysis of outcomes by BRCA status in a randomised phase 2 trial. Lancet Oncol 2014;15(8):852–61.

46. Ray-Coquard I, Pautier P, Pignata S, et al. Olaparib plus bevacizumab as first-line maintenance in ovarian cancer. N Engl J Med 2019;381(25):2416–28.

47. Benard F, Roy F, Wilson D, et al. FDG PET early metabolic response to the PARP inhibitor olaparib (AZD2281) in BRCA-deficient or recurrent high-grade ovarian carcinoma and BRCA-deficient or triple-negative breast cancer. J Nucl Med 2012; 53(supplement 1):63.

48. Matulonis UA, Shapira-Frommer R, Santin AD, et al. Antitumor activity and safety of pembrolizumab in patients with advanced recurrent ovarian cancer: results from the phase II KEYNOTE-100 study. Ann Oncol 2019;30(7):1080–7.

49. Kandalaft LE, Odunsi K, Coukos G. Immune therapy opportunities in ovarian cancer. American Society of Clinical Oncology Educational Book 2020;40:e228–40.

50. Zsiros E, Lynam S, Attwood KM, et al. Efficacy and safety of pembrolizumab in combination with bevacizumab and oral metronomic cyclophosphamide in the treatment of recurrent ovarian cancer: a phase 2 nonrandomized clinical trial. JAMA Oncol 2021; 7(1):78–85.

51. Wolchok JD, Hoos A, O'Day S, et al. Guidelines for the evaluation of immune therapy activity in solid tumors: immune-related response criteria. Clin Cancer Res 2009;15(23):7412–20.

52. Russo L, Avesani G, Gui B, et al. Immunotherapy-related imaging findings in patients with gynecological malignancies: what radiologists need to know. Korean J Radiol 2021;22(8):1310–22.

53. Matulonis UA, Lorusso D, Oaknin A, et al. Efficacy and safety of mirvetuximab soravtansine in patients with platinum-resistant ovarian cancer with high folate receptor alpha expression: results

from the SORAYA study. J Clin Oncol 2023; 41(13):2436–45.

54. Yoshikawa K, Tanaka N, Hasebe M, et al. Comparison of C-11 methionine and FDG PET in detection and evaluation of ovarian tumor. *J Nucl Med,* 48 (supplement 2) 2007, 386P.

55. Isohashi K, Shimosegawa E, Kato H, et al. Optimization of [11C]methionine PET study: appropriate scan timing and effect of plasma amino acid concentrations on the SUV. EJNMMI Res 2013;3(1):27.

56. Torizuka T, Kanno T, Futatsubashi M, et al. Imaging of gynecologic tumors: comparison of (11)C-choline PET with (18)F-FDG PET. J Nucl Med 2003;44(7): 1051–6.

57. An Y, Liu F, Chen Y, et al. Crosstalk between cancer-associated fibroblasts and immune cells in cancer. J Cell Mol Med 2020;24(1):13–24.

58. Erdogan B, Webb DJ. Cancer-associated fibroblasts modulate growth factor signaling and extracellular matrix remodeling to regulate tumor metastasis. Biochem Soc Trans 2017;45(1):229–36.

59. Mona CE, Benz MR, Hikmat F, et al. Correlation of (68)Ga-FAPi-46 PET biodistribution with FAP expression by immunohistochemistry in patients with solid cancers: interim analysis of a prospective translational exploratory study. J Nucl Med 2022;63(7): 1021–6.

60. Dendl K, Koerber SA, Finck R, et al. 68)Ga-FAPI-PET/CT in patients with various gynecological malignancies. Eur J Nucl Med Mol Imag 2021;48(12): 4089–100.

61. Deng H, Liu W, Yang X, et al. Preliminary evaluation and in vitro cytotoxicity studies of [131I]I-trastuzumab in HER2 expressing ovarian cancer cells. J Radioanal Nucl Chem 2022;331(6):2451–60.

62. Juweid M, Swayne LC, Sharkey RM, et al. Prospects of radioimmunotherapy in epithelial ovarian cancer: results with iodine-131-labeled murine and humanized MN-14 anti-carcinoembryonic antigen monoclonal antibodies. Gynecol Oncol 1997;67(3):259–71.

63. Kurata S, Ushijima K, Kawahara A, et al. Assessment of 99mTc-MIBI SPECT(/CT) to monitor multidrug resistance-related proteins and apoptosis-related proteins in patients with ovarian cancer: a preliminary study. Ann Nucl Med 2015;29(7):643–9.

64. Lindenblatt D, Fischer E, Cohrs S, et al. Paclitaxel improved anti-L1CAM lutetium-177 radioimmunotherapy in an ovarian cancer xenograft model. EJNMMI Res 2014;4(1):54.

65. Lindner T, Altmann A, Krämer S, et al. Design and development of (99m)Tc-labeled FAPI tracers for SPECT imaging and (188)Re therapy. J Nucl Med 2020;61(10):1507–13.

66. Vandenberghe S, Moskal P, Karp JS. State of the art in total body PET. EJNMMI Phys 2020;7(1):35.

67. Katal S, Eibschutz LS, Saboury B, et al. Advantages and applications of total-body PET scanning. Diagnostics 2022;12(2):426.

68. Badawi RD, Shi H, Hu P, et al. First human imaging studies with the EXPLORER total-body PET scanner. J Nucl Med 2019;60(3):299–303.

69. Pantel AR, Viswanath V, Daube-Witherspoon ME, et al. PennPET explorer: human imaging on a whole-body imager. J Nucl Med 2020;61(1):144–51.

70. Alberts I, Hünermund JN, Prenosil G, et al. Clinical performance of long axial field of view PET/CT: a head-to-head intra-individual comparison of the biograph vision quadra with the biograph vision PET/CT. Eur J Nucl Med Mol Imag 2021;48(8): 2395–404.

71. Prenosil GA, Sari H, Fürstner M, et al. Performance characteristics of the biograph vision quadra PET/CT system with a long axial field of view using the NEMA NU 2-2018 standard. J Nucl Med 2022; 63(3):476–84.

72. Triumbari EKA, Rufini V, Mingels C, et al. Long axial field-of-view PET/CT could answer unmet needs in gynecological cancers. Cancers 2023;15(9):2407.

Positron Emission Tomography/Computed Tomography Transformation of Oncology: Musculoskeletal Cancers

Stephen M. Broski, MD

KEYWORDS

- PET/CT • Sarcoma • Staging • Prognostic • Soft tissue • Bone • Therapy response

KEY POINTS

- 18F-fluorodeoxyglucose (FDG) positron emission tomography/computed tomography (PET/CT) is beneficial in staging and restaging bone and soft tissue sarcomas by accurately delineating locoregional and distant metastatic disease.
- Numerous studies have demonstrated that the information provided by PET/CT has important prognostic implications for musculoskeletal malignancy.
- Several investigational non-FDG PET radiotracers have utility for evaluating musculoskeletal cancers.

INTRODUCTION

During the past 25 years, there has been a paradigm shift in the role of molecular imaging in musculoskeletal oncology, for both bone and soft tissue tumors. At the beginning of this period, clinical molecular imaging for musculoskeletal oncology consisted primarily of bone scintigraphy for the evaluation of osseous metastatic disease. PET was in its relative infancy and not yet widely available for clinical application. Since that time, PET has undergone a remarkable transformation, both technologically and clinically. Technical advancements have seen an evolution from PET-only systems to widespread adoption of integrated positron emission tomography/computed tomography (PET/CT) systems, continuous development of more sensitive PET detectors, increasingly sophisticated reconstruction techniques, and additional improvements in image quality and display, culminating in the most recent generation of whole-body PET/CT systems. These continual technical advancements, in turn, have driven clinical development and application. In musculoskeletal oncology, PET has evolved from playing a minor role to now being important in diagnosis, staging, and evaluating response to therapy for a wide spectrum of musculoskeletal tumors.

BONE AND SOFT TISSUE SARCOMAS

Musculoskeletal tumors are a highly heterogeneous group of tumors with differing histologic subtypes and biologic activity. The World Health Organization now recognizes more than 100 different histologic subtypes of soft tissue sarcoma (STS)[1] and more than 25 subtypes of bone sarcoma (BS).[2] Despite the numerous types of malignant bone and soft tissue lesions, these lesions are overall rare, accounting for only approximately 1% of adult cancers.[3] Therapy is typically multidisciplinary and includes surgery, radiation therapy, and both cytotoxic and targeted chemotherapy. In patients with localized disease, the goal is complete surgical excision of the tumor with wide margins, with adjuvant or neoadjuvant chemoradiotherapy dictated by tumor histology, size, and location. Despite advances in treatment, the prognosis for many sarcoma types remains guarded—for example, in STS, the 5-year relative survival for localized disease is 82%, for

Department of Radiology, Mayo Clinic, Mayo Building, 2nd Floor, 200 First Street SW, Rochester, MN 55905, USA

E-mail address: Broski.stephen@mayo.edu

PET Clin 19 (2024) 217–229

https://doi.org/10.1016/j.cpet.2023.12.008

locally advanced disease is 60%, and for sarcomas that are found metastatic at presentation, the 5-year relative survival is 17%. Primary BS has a slightly better prognosis, with 5-year survival rates of 84%, 71%, and 33% for localized, locally advanced, and metastatic disease, respectively.[4]

Two notable studies illustrate the evolution of PET/CT for sarcoma evaluation during the past several decades. In 2003, Ionnidis and Lau published a meta-analysis incorporating 15 studies that concluded that 18F-fluorodeoxyglucose (¹⁸F-FDG) PET has good discriminatory ability for differentiating benign and malignant soft tissue lesions, and may be helpful in tumor grading, but is inadequate for discriminating between low-grade malignant and benign soft tissue lesions. A 2019 systematic review by Lim and colleagues that included 34 high-quality studies concluded that PET/CT is an important contributor to sarcoma grading, prognostication, and evaluation of treatment response; helps differentiate between low-grade and high-grade sarcomas; and facilitates early identification of patients who will respond to adjuvant or neoadjuvant therapy.[5] Therefore, during the past 25 years, the focus has shifted from how PET/CT can differentiate between benign and malignant lesions to the role that PET/CT can play in diagnosis, prognostication, and therapy response assessment. This mirrors the impact that PET/CT has had on a variety of other tumor types, where PET/CT has repeatedly been shown to significantly alter patient management.

PET/CT GUIDELINES

The evolving role of PET/CT in patients with sarcoma has led to incorporation of PET/CT in the imaging guidelines and recommendations from several key medical societies and oncology networks. For example, the National Comprehensive Care Network (NCCN) guidelines recommend bone scan or PET/CT in the workup of symptomatic bone lesions with abnormal radiographs in patients aged 40 years or older and state that the standard staging workup for a suspected primary bone cancer should include chest imaging, appropriate imaging of the primary lesion, and bone scan or PET/CT (**Fig. 1**). Regarding specific BS types, PET/CT and/or bone scan is recommended for initial staging and surveillance of osteosarcoma (see **Fig. 1**) and Ewing sarcoma (**Fig. 2**), and PET/CT may also be considered for the workup of chordomas (**Fig. 3**).[6] Regarding STSs, the NCCN states that, in general, PET/CT may be useful for staging (**Figs. 4** and **5**), prognostication, and determining response to systemic therapy. They also specify that review of PET/CT before biopsy may allow targeting of metabolically active areas of tumor and prevent sampling areas of necrosis (see **Fig. 4**). Regarding specific STS types, the NCCN states that PET/CT may be useful to differentiate between well-differentiated and dedifferentiated abdominal and retroperitoneal liposarcoma; to stage rhabdomyosarcoma; to distinguish between benign and malignant peripheral nerve sheath tumors (**Fig. 6**); and to evaluate regional lymph nodes in tumors with nodal metastatic risk, including (but not limited to) angiosarcoma, clear cell sarcoma, epithelioid sarcoma, and rhabdomyosarcoma.[7]

DIAGNOSIS

Since its inception, there has been interest in using PET/CT for the diagnosis of sarcoma and to aid in differentiating benign and malignant mesenchymal tumors. The meta-analysis conducted by Ionnidis and Lau in 2003 included 441 soft-tissue lesions (227 malignant and 214 benign) and demonstrated that ¹⁸F-FDG PET has a good discriminatory ability in differentiating benign and malignant soft tissue lesions (87% sensitivity/79% specificity with a standardized uptake value [SUV] cutoff of 2.0%, and 70% sensitivity/87% specificity with an SUV cutoff of 3.0).[8] A later meta-analysis in 2015 that included 755 patients with 757 soft tissue lesions (451 malignant and 306 benign) demonstrated a mean sensitivity, specificity, positive predictive value, and negative predictive value for diagnosing soft tissue lesions of 96%, 77%, 86%, and 91%, respectively, with an overall accuracy of 88%; the specificity, positive predictive value, and accuracy were higher on PET/CT compared with PET-only studies.[9] One of the best-studied musculoskeletal oncologic applications of FDG PET is to differentiate benign from malignant peripheral nerve sheath tumors, which is of particular interest in patients with neurofibromatosis and elevated risk of malignant transformation (see **Fig. 6**). Several quantitative metabolic parameters, including maximum standardized uptake value (SUVmax), total lesion glycolysis (TLG), metabolic tumor volume (MTV), and a variety of metabolic ratios have been used to make this distinction with high accuracy.[10–13]

Multiple studies have demonstrated a significant correlation between tumor metabolism and grade, and in general, higher FDG uptake corresponds to higher grade of tumor.[14–16] SUV also has proven useful to accurately delineate different histologic grades of both bone and STSs.[15,17] Another significant advantage of sarcoma PET evaluation is that PET imaging may guide biopsy to target the most

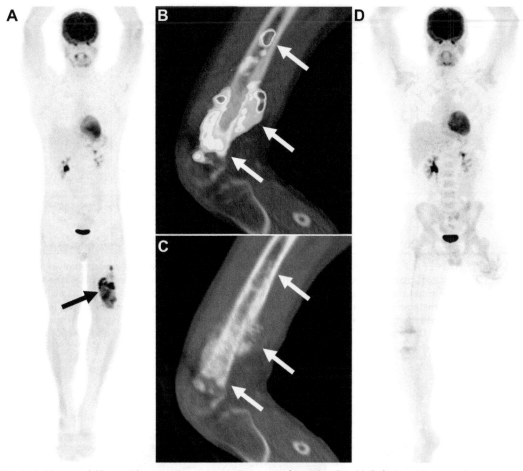

Fig. 1. A 15-year-old boy with an osteosarcoma originating from the distal left femur. Maximum intensity projection (MIP) (*A*), sagittal fused PET/CT (*B*), and sagittal CT (*C*) images from a staging ¹⁸F-FDG PET demonstrate a heterogeneously FDG-avid mass originating from the distal left femoral metadiaphysis with osteoid matrix, an associated soft tissue mass (*arrows, A–C*), and no evidence of metastatic disease. MIP image (*D*) from a restaging ¹⁸F-FDG PET/CT after a left lower extremity amputation demonstrates no evidence of locally recurrent or metastatic disease.

FDG-avid, highest-grade areas of tumor.[18,19] This can be especially important in large and/or high-grade sarcomas (see **Figs. 4** and **6**), which may be prone to nondiagnostic biopsy or undersampling given their significant heterogeneity.

Although metabolic activity on PET/CT may be useful to discriminate between benign and malignant lesions, and also between low-grade and high-grade tumors of the same histologic type, PET has less utility to delineate benign tumors from low-grade malignant tumors; this was noted in the earliest PET/CT studies and holds true 25 years later.[8,16,20,21] It should also be recognized that many benign musculoskeletal tumors may have intense FDG activity, such as giant cell tumor of bone,[22] tenosynovial giant cell tumor,[23] hibernoma,[24,25] and schwannoma,[26] whereas malignant tumors may demonstrate very low uptake, such as

myxoid liposarcoma,[21] and low-grade chondrosarcoma.[16,27] Careful evaluation of the morphologic features of these tumors on the CT component of PET/CT can be invaluable in diagnosis; for example, recognizing macroscopic fat within a hibernoma, or the osteolysis, nonsclerotic margins, and eccentric location extending to the subchondral bone in giant cell tumor of bone. The increased diagnostic accuracy of PET/CT compared with PET alone has been demonstrated in multiple studies.[28]

STAGING AND PROGNOSIS

Although BS and STS most frequently metastasize to the lungs[29] (see **Fig. 4**), some sarcomas (especially visceral and retroperitoneal) may develop hematogenous hepatic metastases (see **Fig. 5**), osseous metastases occur in approximately 10%

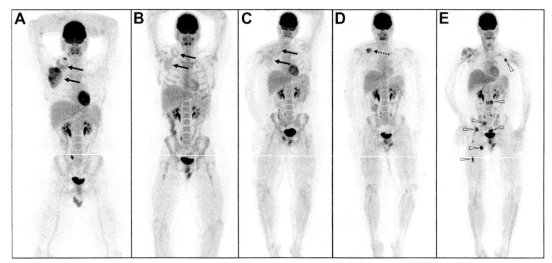

Fig. 2. Serial ^{18}F-FDG PET MIP images (*A–E*) in an 18-year-old male patient with Ewing sarcoma involving the right scapula and adjacent soft tissues. He was treated with chemoradiation and subsequent surgical resection after local recurrence. The initial staging examination (*A*) demonstrates a large, heterogeneously FDG avid mass (*arrows*), with excellent metabolic response to chemoradiotherapy on the ensuing two examinations (*arrows* in *B* and *C*). The patient subsequently developed local recurrence in the radiation field (*dashed arrow, D*), which was surgically resected. Unfortunately, the patient went on to develop multifocal nodal and osseous metastatic disease (*arrowheads, E*).

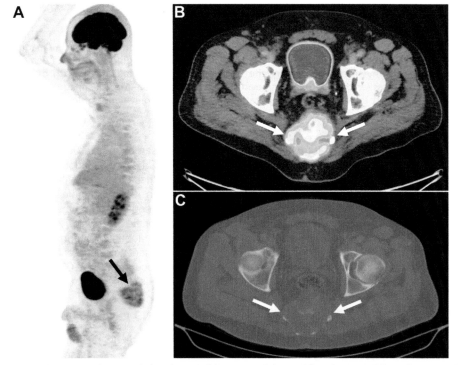

Fig. 3. A 70-year-old man with a sacral chordoma. Oblique MIP (*A*), axial fused PET/CT (*B*), and axial CT (*C*) images from a staging ^{18}F-FDG PET/CT examination demonstrate an FDG avid destructive mass originating from the sacrum and extending into the presacral space (*arrows*), and no evidence of metastatic disease.

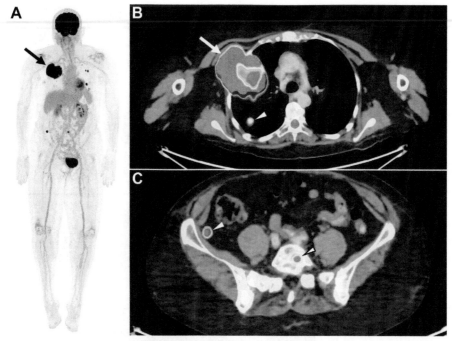

Fig. 4. A 71-year-old woman with an undifferentiated pleomorphic sarcoma originating within the right chest wall. MIP (*A*) and axial fused PET/CT (*B, C*) images from a staging ^{18}F-FDG PET/CT demonstrate an intensely FDG avid right chest wall mass with central necrosis (*arrows* in *A* and *B*) and multiple FDG avid metastases, including the right lung, lumbar spine, and right lower quadrant soft tissues (*arrowheads* in *B* and *C*).

of patients with STS[30] (see **Fig. 4**), myxoid liposarcomas have a predilection for bone and soft tissue metastases (especially in the spinal and paraspinal regions), and several STS including synovial sarcoma, rhabdomyosarcoma, and epithelioid sarcoma have a predilection for nodal metastases.[31,32] The combined functional metabolic and morphologic information provided by FDG PET/CT has been shown to result in superior sensitivity for detecting nodal metastatic disease (N-stage) compared with conventional imaging techniques, in both BS and STS.[33–35] PET/CT also has proven superiority in detecting distant metastases (M-stage)[34,35] and has been shown to upstage both patients with Ewing sarcoma and patients with osteosarcoma relative to conventional imaging.[36] In a retrospective study by Macpherson and colleagues, 957 consecutive FDG PET/CT scans were performed in 493 patients with a wide distribution of histologic subtypes of bone and STSs and were compared with CT and MRI for staging, restaging, and assessing treatment response. FDG PET led to upstaging in 12% (42 out of 344) of patients compared with CT and MRI by diagnosing metastatic lesions occult on conventional imaging.[37] Annovazzi and colleagues studied the diagnostic and clinical impact of FDG PET/CT in staging and restaging STSs of the trunk and extremities in 282 patients,

which included 345 consecutive FDG PET/CT scans performed for an initial staging (n = 171) or for a suspected disease relapse (n = 174). In this study, there were 80 cases with a documented change in management, 16.4% at staging, and 29.9% at restaging. Meanwhile, there was upstaging of disease in 58.8% of patients and downstaging of disease in 41.2% of patients.[38]

Baseline FDG activity in both STS and BS has been correlated with survival in several studies,[5,39–47] although there is still some debate regarding whether traditional metabolic measures, such as SUVmax and mean standardized uptake value (SUVmean), or volumetric metabolic measures, such as metabolic tumor volume (MTV) and TLG, are more useful in predicting survival. Notably, two larger meta-analyses have also confirmed the prognostic value that can be inferred from baseline FDG PET/CT in BS and STS.[48,49]

TREATMENT RESPONSE AND SURVEILLANCE

A deepening understanding of the genetic and molecular alterations driving various sarcoma types has allowed for the development of targeted, specific treatments such as tyrosine kinase inhibitors (imatinib, sunitinib, or pazopanib), trabectedin, platelet-derived growth factor (olaratumab), and

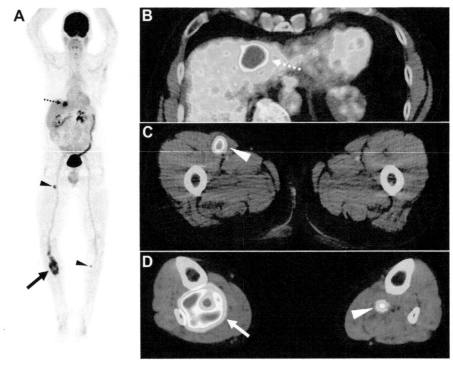

Fig. 5. A 63-year-old man with a right calf leiomyosarcoma. MIP (*A*) and axial fused PET/CT (*B–D*) images from a staging ¹⁸F-FDG PET/CT demonstrate an intensely FDG avid intramuscular leiomyosarcoma in the right calf (*arrows* in *A* and *D*), with FDG avid intramuscular metastases in the left calf and right thigh (*arrowheads* in *A*, *C*, and *D*), and an FDG hepatic metastasis (*dashed arrows* in *A* and *B*).

immunotherapy (ipilimumab or nivolumab).[50] The armamentarium of targeted treatment options for primary and metastatic disease, including various thermal ablation techniques (radiofrequency ablation, microwave ablation, high intensity focused ultrasound, and cryoblation) and targeted radiation therapy (stereotactic body radiotherapy and proton beam therapy), continues to grow. Given this wide range of treatment options, accurate determination of response to therapy for sarcoma has never been more important.

There are limitations in using morphologic assessment in determining sarcoma response to therapy. Some studies have shown poor correlation between changes in tumor size and histopathologic response,[51] and others have failed to demonstrate a significant association between size change and patient survival.[52,53] A tumor may increase in size secondary to spontaneous or treatment-related intralesional hemorrhage, even though the tumor may be positively responding to treatment (**Fig. 7**). It is also well-recognized that morphologic changes lag behind metabolic changes, and that some tumors may undergo significant necrosis without a substantial initial change in size. Along these lines, the Positron Emission Tomography Response Criteria in Solid

Tumors (PERCIST) guidelines have demonstrated superior predictive value in treatment response assessment compared with the Response Evaluation Criteria in Solid Tumors (RECIST) guidelines in patients with Ewing sarcoma.[54] In a study evaluating STS treated with combined regional hyperthermia and chemotherapy, PERCIST response was an independent predictor of progression-free survival, whereas changes in tumor size did not correlate with survival outcomes.[55] These studies highlight the benefits of using functional versus morphologic approaches in assessing therapy response.

The utility of FDG PET for assessing treatment response has been demonstrated for both STS[56] and BS.[57,58] Several metabolic measures have been shown to correlate better with histologic response as compared with changes in size on MRI.[46,51,59] Changes in volumetric metabolic indices may be more useful in assessing treatment response compared with SUVmax because multiple studies have shown better correlation of MTV and total lesion glycolysis (TLG) with tumor necrosis fraction as compared with SUVmax in patients with osteosarcoma.[46,59] A meta-analysis conducted by Hongtao and colleagues in 2012 comparing FDG PET/CT findings and histologic response in

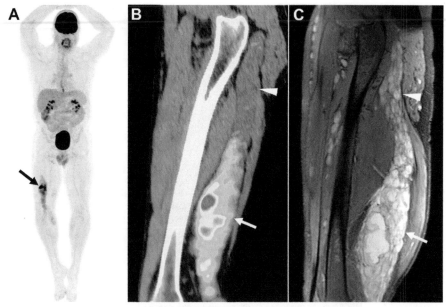

Fig. 6. A 38-year-old man with neurofibromatosis type 1 and concern for malignant transformation. ^{18}F-FDG PET MIP (*A*), sagittal fused PET/CT (*B*), and corresponding sagittal T2-weighted, fat-suppressed MRI (*C*) images demonstrate an extensive plexiform neurofibroma of the right sciatic nerve. There is no significant FDG uptake within the proximal aspect of the plexiform neurofibroma (*arrowheads* in *B* and *C*) but there is heterogeneous intense uptake distally (*arrows* in *A* and *B*) with corresponding fusiform enlargement on MRI (*arrow* in *C*). Subsequent biopsy targeting the region of greatest FDG uptake confirmed transformation to a malignant peripheral nerve sheath tumor.

178 patients with osteosarcoma undergoing neoadjuvant chemotherapy demonstrated that a change in the SUV on pretreatment and posttreatment PET/CT correlated with histologic response, with a posttherapy SUV of 2.5 or less and a posttherapy/pretherapy ratio of 0.5 or less to be predictive of histologic response to therapy.[57] Not only is baseline metabolic activity prognostic in BS and STS, but changes in SUV during therapy have also shown to confer prognosis.[60] Tateishi and colleagues demonstrated that a 60% or greater SUV reduction after completion of neoadjuvant therapy in STS was predictive of progression-free and overall survival.[61] Significant metabolic reduction on PET/CT has also been shown to be predictive of overall survival after only one cycle of chemotherapy in STS[62] and predictive of overall survival and progression-free survival after two cycles of chemotherapy in BS and STS.[63] Early differentiation of responders from nonresponders by PET/CT can facilitate prompt changes in therapeutic course for patients with nonresponding or progressive disease.

Sarcomas are also prone to local recurrence, and therefore surveillance imaging is an important part of patient management. Earlier studies showed FDG PET to have similar sensitivity and increased specificity compared with conventional imaging in recurrent osteosarcoma and Ewing sarcoma,[64] and equal accuracy in assessing locally recurrent and distant metastatic disease in pediatric patients with sarcoma.[65] A recent large meta-analysis including 31 studies of patients with Ewing sarcoma undergoing FDG PET/CT showed high sensitivity and specificity (89.9% and 92.6%, respectively) for detecting local recurrence after therapy[66] (see **Fig. 2**). Park and colleagues examined 152 patients with STS who underwent regular MRI and PET/CT for postoperative follow-up. Twenty patients were found to have locoregional recurrence after surgical excision, and the sensitivity and specificity of MRI versus PET/CT were 90.0% versus 95.0% and 97.7% versus 95.0%, respectively, although these differences did not reach statistical significance. The authors concluded that both modalities may be helpful in detecting local recurrence and differentiating recurrent tumor from posttherapy changes.[67] In our own practice, we have found the two modalities to often be complementary, especially in difficult cases. For example, PET/CT has proven utility for the evaluation of recurrent disease along metallic prostheses, which may be obscured by artifact on CT and MRI[37] (**Fig. 8**).

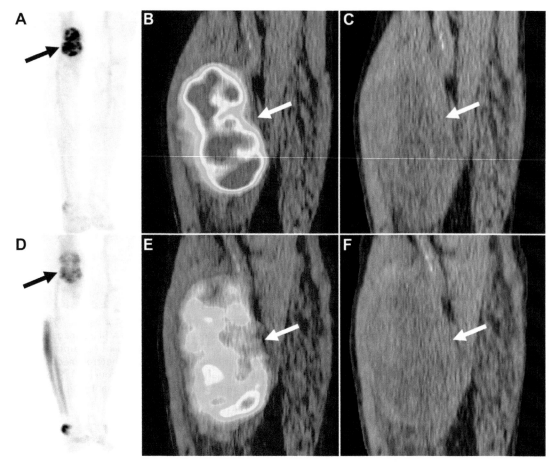

Fig. 7. A 67-year-old man with a high-grade pleomorphic sarcoma involving the distal right quadriceps muscula-ture treated with neoadjuvant chemotherapy. MIP (*A*), sagittal fused PET/CT (*B*), and sagittal CT (*C*) images from a staging ^{18}F-FDG PET/CT examination demonstrate a low attenuation FDG-avid soft tissue mass measuring approx-imately 9.5 × 6.0 × 5.0 cm with SUVmax of 12.5. Corresponding images from a posttherapy PET/CT (*D–F*) demon-strate increased size to 11.5 × 6.5 × 5.5 cm but decreased uptake with SUVmax of 6.4 (*arrows*). The findings are consistent with a partial metabolic response despite increased size.

FUTURE DIRECTIONS

Although the last 25 years has been a dynamic and exciting period for musculoskeletal oncologic PET/CT, the next 25 years hold even great prom-ise. A deeper understanding of the genetic and molecular underpinnings of sarcoma should continue to drive the development of radiotracers with increasing specificity, and open doors to new diagnostic and therapeutic options. The fibro-blast activation protein (FAP) has attracted partic-ular interest as a theranostic target. FAP is absent in normal adult tissues but is highly expressed on cancer-associated fibroblasts that infiltrate the stromal tumor microenvironment in most malig-nant tumors.[68] A series of recently developed FAP inhibitors (FAPIs), in particular gallium 68 (68Ga)–labeled FAP inhibitor (^{68}Ga-FAPI), have demonstrated favorable pharmacokinetic proper-ties and high uptake in a variety of tumor

types.[69,70] Of these tumor types, sarcoma has been found to be among the tumors with the high-est uptake (SUVmax >12).[71]

Koerver and colleagues characterized ^{68}Ga-FAPI uptake in 15 patients with a variety of sar-coma types, including liposarcoma (n = 5), undif-ferentiated pleomorphic sarcoma (n = 3), and leiomyosarcoma (n = 2). They found excellent tumor-to-background ratios (>7) for primary tu-mors, local recurrence, and metastatic disease.[72] A recent study by Gu and colleagues including 45 patients with a variety of STSs evaluated by both ^{18}F-FDG and ^{68}Ga-FAPI PET/CT demon-strated that ^{68}Ga-FAPI PET/CT detected more to-tal lesions (275 vs 186) and had higher sensitivity, specificity, PPV, NPV, and accuracy for the diag-nosis of recurrent lesions (*P* < .001) compared with ^{18}F-FDG PET/CT.[73] Another study including 47 patients with BS or STS, 43 of whom were

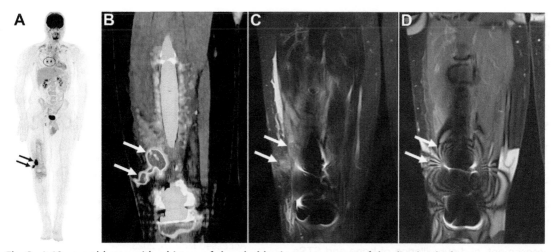

Fig. 8. A 19-year-old man with a history of chondroblastic osteosarcoma of the distal right femur, status postsurgical resection with custom total knee arthroplasty. MIP image (A) from a surveillance ^{18}F-FDG PET/CT examination demonstrates FDG avid local recurrence within the distal right thigh (arrows) and new pulmonary metastases (dashed oval). Coronal fused PET/CT image (B) demonstrates FDG-avid locally recurrent tumor along the lateral aspect of the arthroplasty femoral component (arrows). The locally recurrent tumor (arrows) is less clearly seen on the corresponding coronal fluid-sensitive MRI image (C) and completely obscured on the coronal T1-weighted fat-saturated postgadolinium MRI image (D) due to metallic susceptibility artifact.

also imaged by ^{18}F-FDG, demonstrated that 8 out of 43 (18.6%) patients were upstaged by ^{68}Ga-FAPI PET as compared with ^{18}F-FDG PET and that clinical management changed in 30% of patients after ^{68}Ga-FAPI PET imaging.[74] These early studies herald the tremendous diagnostic potential of FAPI PET/CT and, in particular, the possible application to low-grade sarcomas, which tend to have lower level FDG activity.

The dodecane tetraacetic acid (DOTA) chelator in the molecular structure also allows the coupling of FAPI molecules with therapeutic radioisotopes, including lutetium-177 (^{177}Lu) and yttrium-90 (^{90}Y) for therapeutic purposes,[70] making FAPI a suitable theranostic agent. A recent study examined ^{90}Y-FAPI-46 radioligand therapy in 16 patients with sarcoma with progressive disease who had exhausted approved therapies and found that ^{90}Y-FAPI-46-therapy was safe, and of the 12 evaluable patients with sarcoma, a partial response was observed in 1 patient (8%) and there was stable disease in 6 patients (50%).[75] The feasibility of additional FAPI-based therapeutic agents has been demonstrated in case reports or small series of patients with sarcoma, including ^{177}Lu-FAPI-46[76] and samarium 153 (^{153}Sm)-FAPI-46.[77]

Several additional alternative PET radiotracers have been explored for application in sarcoma during the past several decades. ^{18}F-FLT, which is a radiolabeled thymidine nucleoside analog and a marker for tumor proliferation, is perhaps the best studied of these non-FDG PET radiotracers. Cobben and colleagues evaluated ^{18}F-FLT PET in 19 patients with 20 STS lesions and found that fluorothymidine (FLT) PET detected all 20 lesions with high tumor to background contrast and that SUVmean and SUVmax were able to differentiate between low-grade and high-grade STSs. Further, there were significant positive correlations between ^{18}F-FLT SUVmax and both mitotic score and histologic grade.[78] ^{18}F-FLT has also been studied for sarcoma response assessment. In 20 patients with high-grade STS undergoing neoadjuvant chemotherapy, Benz and colleagues found that ^{18}F-FLT SUVmax significantly decreased after therapy (7.1 ± 3.7 vs 2.7 ± 1.6; P<.001), and changes in peak FLT uptake were correlated with both tumor size and tumor necrosis.[79]

Artificial intelligence and radiomics promises to revolutionize all areas of medicine, and PET/CT evaluation of sarcoma is no exception. Wolsztynki and colleagues developed a model-based approach to measuring intratumoral heterogeneity and metabolic gradients on FDG PET/CT in patients with sarcoma and found that combining texture and model-based variables can achieve better prognostic assessment than these variables alone.[80] Peng and colleagues developed a convolutional neural network radiomics model to predict the risk of distant metastases in patients with STS, using the multimodality information on both PET and CT in patients undergoing FDG PET/CT, and found that this model provided higher sensitivity, accuracy, and area under the curve in comparison to other state-of-the-art methods.[81] Additional predictive models developed from a combination of PET imaging features and clinical information,[82] and also from joint FDG PET and MRI texture features,[83] have shown utility in predicting the risk of pulmonary metastases in patients with STS.

SUMMARY

The past 25 years have seen significant growth in the role of PET/CT in musculoskeletal oncology. Substantiative advances in technical capability and image quality have been paralleled by increasingly widespread clinical adoption and implementation. It is now recognized that PET/CT is useful in diagnosis, staging, prognostication, response assessment, and surveillance of bone and STSs, often providing critical information in addition to conventional imaging assessment. As individualized, precision medicine continues to evolve for patients with sarcoma, PET/CT is uniquely positioned to offer additional insight into the biology and management of these tumors, and the growth of theranostics and potential application to musculoskeletal sarcomas provides an exciting avenue for future exploration.

CLINICS CARE POINTS

- In the past 25 years, there has been significant growth in the use of PET/CT in musculoskeletal oncology, driven by substantiative technical advances and widespread clinical adoption.
- At staging, FDG PET/CT is useful for delineating locoregional and distant metastatic disease. Baseline FDG uptake correlates with tumor grade, and FDG PET/CT is useful in directing biopsy to the highest-grade areas of tumor.
- FDG uptake, both at baseline and at restaging after therapy, offers important prognostic information and has been correlated with survival in multiple studies.
- Several non-FDG PET radiotracers have utility for evaluating musculoskeletal cancers. FAPI is of particular interest given its high tumor-to-background uptake in sarcoma and theranostic potential.

DISCLOSURE

The authors have no relevant financial disclosures or conflicts of interest.

REFERENCES

1. Bansal A, Goyal S, Goyal A, et al. WHO classification of soft tissue tumours 2020: an update and simplified approach for radiologists. Eur J Radiol 2021; 143:109937.
2. Hwang S, Hameed M, Kransdorf M. The 2020 World Health Organization classification of bone tumors: what radiologists should know. Skeletal Radiol 2023;52(3):329–48.
3. Hui JY. Epidemiology and etiology of sarcomas. Surg Clin North Am 2016;96(5):901–14.
4. SEER*Explorer: An interactive website for SEER cancer statistics Internet. Surveillance Research Program, National Cancer Institute. Available at: https://seer.cancer.gov/statistics-network/explorer/. Accessed May 15, 2023.
5. Lim HJ, Johnny Ong CA, Tan JW, et al. Utility of positron emission tomography/computed tomography (PET/CT) imaging in the evaluation of sarcomas: a systematic review. Crit Rev Oncol Hematol 2019; 143:1–13.
6. National Comprehensive Cancer Network. Bone Cancer (Version 3.2023). Available at: https://www.nccn.org/professionals/physician_gls/pdf/bone.pdf. Accessed May 15, 2023.
7. National Comprehensive Cancer Network. Soft Tissue Sarcoma (Version 2.2023). Available at: https://www.nccn.org/professionals/physician_gls/pdf/sarcoma.pdf. Accessed May 15, 2023.
8. Ioannidis JP, Lau J. 18F-FDG PET for the diagnosis and grading of soft-tissue sarcoma: a meta-analysis. J Nucl Med 2003;44(5):717–24.
9. Etchebehere EC, Hobbs BP, Milton DR, et al. Assessing the role of (1)(8)F-FDG PET and (1)(8)F-FDG PET/CT in the diagnosis of soft tissue musculoskeletal malignancies: a systematic review and meta-analysis. Eur J Nucl Med Mol Imaging 2016; 43(5):860–70.
10. Benz MR, Czernin J, Dry SM, et al. Quantitative F18-fluorodeoxyglucose positron emission tomography accurately characterizes peripheral nerve sheath tumors as malignant or benign. Cancer 2010;116(2): 451–8.
11. Broski SM, Johnson GB, Howe BM, et al. Evaluation of (18)F-FDG PET and MRI in differentiating benign and malignant peripheral nerve sheath tumors. Skeletal Radiol 2016;45(8):1097–105.
12. Chirindel A, Chaudhry M, Blakeley JO, et al. 18F-FDG PET/CT qualitative and quantitative evaluation in neurofibromatosis type 1 patients for detection of malignant transformation: comparison of early to delayed imaging with and without liver activity normalization. J Nucl Med 2015;56(3):379–85.
13. Salamon J, Veldhoen S, Apostolova I, et al. 18F-FDG PET/CT for detection of malignant peripheral nerve sheath tumours in neurofibromatosis type 1:

tumour-to-liver ratio is superior to an SUVmax cut-off. Eur Radiol 2014;24(2):405–12.

14. Benz MR, Dry SM, Eilber FC, et al. Correlation between glycolytic phenotype and tumor grade in soft-tissue sarcomas by 18F-FDG PET. J Nucl Med 2010;51(8):1174–81.

15. Tateishi U, Yamaguchi U, Seki K, et al. Glut-1 expression and enhanced glucose metabolism are associated with tumour grade in bone and soft tissue sarcomas: a prospective evaluation by [18F]fluorodeoxyglucose positron emission tomography. Eur J Nucl Med Mol Imaging 2006;33(6):683–91.

16. Subhawong TK, Winn A, Shemesh SS, et al. F-18 FDG PET differentiation of benign from malignant chondroid neoplasms: a systematic review of the literature. Skeletal Radiol 2017;46:1233–9.

17. Brenner W, Eary JF, Hwang W, et al. Risk assessment in liposarcoma patients based on FDG PET imaging. Eur J Nucl Med Mol Imaging 2006;33(11):1290–5.

18. Nanni C, Gasbarrini A, Cappelli A, et al. FDG PET/CT for bone and soft-tissue biopsy. Eur J Nucl Med Mol Imaging 2015;42(8):1333–4.

19. Hain SF, O'Doherty MJ, Bingham J, et al. Can FDG PET be used to successfully direct preoperative biopsy of soft tissue tumours? Nucl Med Commun 2003;24(11):1139–43.

20. Rakheja R, Makis W, Skamene S, et al. Correlating metabolic activity on F-18-FDG PET/CT with histopathologic characteristics of osseous and soft-tissue sarcomas: a retrospective review of 136 patients. Am J Roentgenol 2012;198(6):1409–16.

21. Lunn BW, Littrell LA, Wenger DE, et al. (18)F-FDG PET/CT and MRI features of myxoid liposarcomas and intramuscular myxomas. Skeletal Radiol 2018; 47(12):1641–50.

22. Costelloe CM, Chuang HH, Madewell JE. FDG PET/CT of primary bone tumors. AJR Am J Roentgenol 2014;202(6):W521–31.

23. Broski SM, Murdoch NM, Skinner JA, et al. Pigmented villonodular synovitis: potential pitfall on oncologic 18F-FDG PET/CT. Clin Nucl Med 2016; 41(1):e24–31.

24. Kim JD, Lee HW. Hibernoma: intense uptake on F18-FDG PET/CT. Nucl Med Mol Imaging 2012;46(3): 218–22.

25. Baffour FI, Wenger DE, Broski SM. (18)F-FDG PET/CT imaging features of lipomatous tumors. Am J Nucl Med Mol Imaging 2020;10(1):74–82.

26. Dewey BJ, Howe BM, Spinner RJ, et al. FDG PET/CT and MRI features of pathologically proven schwannomas. Clin Nucl Med 2021;46(4):289–96.

27. Schulte M, Brecht-Krauss D, Heymer B, et al. Grading of tumors and tumorlike lesions of bone: evaluation by FDG PET. J Nucl Med 2000;41(10): 1695–701.

28. Younis MH, Abu-Hijleh HA, Aldahamsheh OO, et al. Meta-analysis of the diagnostic accuracy of primary bone and soft tissue sarcomas by 18F-FDG-PET. Med Princ Pract 2020;29(5):465–72.

29. Burningham Z, Hashibe M, Spector L, et al. The epidemiology of sarcoma. Clin Sarcoma Res 2012; 2(1):14.

30. Vincenzi B, Frezza AM, Schiavon G, et al. Bone metastases in soft tissue sarcoma: a survey of natural history, prognostic value and treatment options. Clin Sarcoma Res 2013;3(1):6.

31. Kandathil A, Subramaniam RM. PET/Computed tomography and precision medicine: musculoskeletal sarcoma. Pet Clin 2017;12(4):475–88.

32. Sherman KL, Kinnier CV, Farina DA, et al. Examination of national lymph node evaluation practices for adult extremity soft tissue sarcoma. J Surg Oncol 2014;110(6):682–8.

33. Klem ML, Grewal RK, Wexler LH, et al. PET for staging in rhabdomyosarcoma: an evaluation of PET as an adjunct to current staging tools. J Pediatr Hematol Oncol 2007;29(1):9–14.

34. Tateishi U, Hosono A, Makimoto A, et al. Comparative study of FDG PET/CT and conventional imaging in the staging of rhabdomyosarcoma. Ann Nucl Med 2009;23(2):155–61.

35. Volker T, Denecke T, Steffen I, et al. Positron emission tomography for staging of pediatric sarcoma patients: results of a prospective multicenter trial. J Clin Oncol 2007;25(34):5435–41.

36. Kneisl JS, Patt JC, Johnson JC, et al. Is PET useful in detecting occult nonpulmonary metastases in pediatric bone sarcomas? Clin Orthop Relat Res 2006; 450:101–4.

37. Macpherson RE, Pratap S, Tyrrell H, et al. Retrospective audit of 957 consecutive (18)F-FDG PET-CT scans compared to CT and MRI in 493 patients with different histological subtypes of bone and soft tissue sarcoma. Clin Sarcoma Res 2018;8:9.

38. Annovazzi A, Rea S, Zoccali C, et al. Diagnostic and clinical impact of 18F-FDG PET/CT in staging and restaging soft-tissue sarcomas of the extremities and trunk: mono-institutional retrospective study of a sarcoma Referral center. J Clin Med 2020;9(8).

39. Andersen KF, Fuglo HM, Rasmussen SH, et al. Volume-based F-18 FDG PET/CT imaging markers provide supplemental prognostic information to histologic grading in patients with high-grade bone or soft tissue sarcoma. Medicine (Baltim) 2015; 94(51):e2319.

40. Benz MR, Tchekmedyian N, Eilber FC, et al. Utilization of positron emission tomography in the management of patients with sarcoma. Curr Opin Oncol 2009;21(4):345–51.

41. Choi ES, Ha SG, Kim HS, et al. Total lesion glycolysis by F-18-FDG PET/CT is a reliable predictor of prognosis in soft-tissue sarcoma. Eur J Nucl Med Mol I 2013;40(12):1836–42.

42. Costelloe CM, Macapinlac HA, Madewell JE, et al. 18F-FDG PET/CT as an indicator of progression-free and overall survival in osteosarcoma. J Nucl Med 2009;50(3):340–7.

43. Fuglo HM, Jorgensen SM, Loft A, et al. The diagnostic and prognostic value of (1)(8)F-FDG PET/CT in the initial assessment of high-grade bone and soft tissue sarcoma. A retrospective study of 89 patients. Eur J Nucl Med Mol Imaging 2012;39(9): 1416–24.

44. Hong SP, Lee SE, Choi YL, et al. Prognostic value of 18F-FDG PET/CT in patients with soft tissue sarcoma: comparisons between metabolic parameters. Skeletal Radiol 2014;43(5):641–8.

45. Hack RI, Becker AS, Bode-Lesniewska B, et al. When SUV Matters: FDG PET/CT at baseline correlates with survival in soft tissue and ewing sarcoma. Life 2021;11(9).

46. Byun BH, Kong CB, Lim I, et al. Early response monitoring to neoadjuvant chemotherapy in osteosarcoma using sequential (1)(8)F-FDG PET/CT and MRI. Eur J Nucl Med Mol Imaging 2014;41(8): 1553–62.

47. Chen L, Wu X, Ma X, et al. Prognostic value of 18F-FDG PET-CT-based functional parameters in patients with soft tissue sarcoma: a meta-analysis. Medicine (Baltim) 2017;96(6):e5913.

48. Kubo T, Furuta T, Johan MP, et al. Prognostic significance of (18)F-FDG PET at diagnosis in patients with soft tissue sarcoma and bone sarcoma; systematic review and meta-analysis. Eur J Cancer 2016; 58:104–11.

49. Li YJ, Dai YL, Cheng YS, et al. Positron emission tomography (18)F-fluorodeoxyglucose uptake and prognosis in patients with bone and soft tissue sarcoma: a meta-analysis. Eur J Surg Oncol 2016; 42(8):1103–14.

50. Rodriguez-Alfonso B, Simo-Perdigo M, Orcajo Rincon J. Functional image in soft tissue sarcomas: an update of the indications of (18)F-FDG-PET/CT. Rev Esp Med Nucl Imagen Mol (Engl Ed) 2020; 39(4):233–43.

51. Evilevitch V, Weber WA, Tap WD, et al. Reduction of glucose metabolic activity is more accurate than change in size at predicting histopathologic response to neoadjuvant therapy in high-grade soft-tissue sarcomas. Clin Cancer Res 2008;14(3): 715–20.

52. Miki Y, Ngan S, Clark JC, et al. The significance of size change of soft tissue sarcoma during preoperative radiotherapy. Eur J Surg Oncol 2010;36(7): 678–83.

53. Tanaka K, Ogawa G, Mizusawa J, et al. Prospective comparison of various radiological response criteria and pathological response to preoperative chemotherapy and survival in operable high-grade soft tissue sarcomas in the Japan Clinical Oncology Group study JCOG0304. World J Surg Oncol 2018;16(1): 162.

54. Koshkin VS, Bolejack V, Schwartz LH, et al. Assessment of imaging modalities and response metrics in ewing sarcoma: correlation with survival. J Clin Oncol 2016;34(30):3680–5.

55. Fendler WP, Lehmann M, Todica A, et al. PET response criteria in solid tumors predicts progression-free survival and time to local or distant progression after chemotherapy with regional hyperthermia for soft-tissue sarcoma. J Nucl Med 2015;56(4):530–7.

56. Benz MR, Czernin J, Allen-Auerbach MS, et al. FDG-PET/CT imaging predicts histopathologic treatment responses after the initial cycle of neoadjuvant chemotherapy in high-grade soft-tissue sarcomas. Clin Cancer Res 2009;15(8):2856–63.

57. Hongtao L, Hui Z, Bingshun W, et al. 18F-FDG positron emission tomography for the assessment of histological response to neoadjuvant chemotherapy in osteosarcomas: a meta-analysis. Surg Oncol 2012; 21(4):e165–70.

58. Kong CB, Byun BH, Lim I, et al. 1)(8)F-FDG PET SUVmax as an indicator of histopathologic response after neoadjuvant chemotherapy in extremity osteosarcoma. Eur J Nucl Med Mol Imaging 2013;40(5): 728–36.

59. Im HJ, Kim TS, Park SY, et al. Prediction of tumour necrosis fractions using metabolic and volumetric 18F-FDG PET/CT indices, after one course and at the completion of neoadjuvant chemotherapy, in children and young adults with osteosarcoma. Eur J Nucl Med Mol Imaging 2012;39(1):39–49.

60. Castillo-Flores S, Gonzalez MR, Bryce-Alberti M, et al. PET-CT in the evaluation of neoadjuvant/adjuvant treatment response of soft-tissue sarcomas: a comprehensive review of the literature. JBJS Reviews 2022;10(12). e22.00131.

61. Tateishi U, Kawai A, Chuman H, et al. PET/CT allows stratification of responders to neoadjuvant chemotherapy for high-grade sarcoma: a prospective study. Clin Nucl Med 2011;36(7):526–32.

62. Herrmann K, Benz MR, Czernin J, et al. 18F-FDG-PET/CT Imaging as an early survival predictor in patients with primary high-grade soft tissue sarcomas undergoing neoadjuvant therapy. Clin Cancer Res 2012;18(7):2024–31.

63. Eary JF, Conrad EU, O'Sullivan J, et al. Sarcoma mid-therapy [F-18] fluorodeoxyglucose positron emission tomography (FDG PET) and patient outcome. J Bone Jt Surg Am Vol 2014;96(2):152.

64. Franzius C, Daldrup-Link HE, Wagner-Bohn A, et al. FDG-PET for detection of recurrences from malignant primary bone tumors: comparison with conventional imaging. Ann Oncol 2002;13(1):157–60.

65. Arush MWB, Israel O, Postovsky S, et al. Positron emission tomography/computed tomography with (18)fluoro-deoxyglucose in the detection of local

recurrence and distant metastases of pediatric sarcoma. Pediatr Blood Cancer 2007;49(7):901–5.

66. Seth N, Seth I, Bulloch G, et al. 18) F-FDG PET and PET/CT as a diagnostic method for Ewing sarcoma: a systematic review and meta-analysis. Pediatr Blood Cancer 2022;69(3):e29415.

67. Park SY, Chung HW, Chae SY, et al. Comparison of MRI and PET-CT in detecting the loco-regional recurrence of soft tissue sarcomas during surveillance. Skeletal Radiol 2016;45(10):1375–84.

68. Hamson EJ, Keane FM, Tholen S, et al. Understanding fibroblast activation protein (FAP): substrates, activities, expression and targeting for cancer therapy. Proteomics Clin Appl 2014;8(5–6):454–63.

69. Hamacher R, Lanzafame H, Mavroeidi IA, et al. Fibroblast activation protein inhibitor theranostics: the case for use in sarcoma. PET Clin 2023;18(3): 361–7.

70. Mori Y, Dendl K, Cardinale J, et al. FAPI PET: fibroblast activation protein inhibitor use in oncologic and nononcologic disease. Radiology 2023;306(2): e220749.

71. Kratochwil C, Flechsig P, Lindner T, et al. 68)Ga-FAPI PET/CT: Tracer uptake in 28 different kinds of cancer. J Nucl Med 2019;60(6):801–5.

72. Koerber SA, Finck R, Dendl K, et al. Novel FAP ligands enable improved imaging contrast in sarcoma patients due to FAPI-PET/CT. Eur J Nucl Med Mol Imaging 2021;48(12):3918–24.

73. Gu B, Liu X, Wang S, et al. Head-to-head evaluation of [(18)F]FDG and [(68) Ga]Ga-DOTA-FAPI-04 PET/CT in recurrent soft tissue sarcoma. Eur J Nucl Med Mol Imaging 2022;49(8):2889–901.

74. Kessler L, Ferdinandus J, Hirmas N, et al. (68)Ga-FAPI as a diagnostic tool in sarcoma: data from the (68)Ga-FAPI PET prospective observational trial. J Nucl Med 2022;63(1):89–95.

75. Fendler WP, Pabst KM, Kessler L, et al. Safety and efficacy of 90Y-FAPI-46 radioligand therapy in

patients with advanced sarcoma and other cancer entities. Clin Cancer Res 2022;28(19):4346–53.

76. Assadi M, Rekabpour SJ, Jafari E, et al. Feasibility and therapeutic potential of 177Lu-fibroblast activation protein inhibitor-46 for patients with relapsed or refractory cancers: a preliminary study. Clin Nucl Med 2021;46(11):e523–30.

77. Kratochwil C, Giesel FL, Rathke H, et al. [(153)Sm] Samarium-labeled FAPI-46 radioligand therapy in a patient with lung metastases of a sarcoma. Eur J Nucl Med Mol Imaging 2021;48(9):3011–3.

78. Cobben DC, Elsinga PH, Suurmeijer AJ, et al. Detection and grading of soft tissue sarcomas of the extremities with (18)F-3'-fluoro-3'-deoxy-L-thymidine. Clin Cancer Res 2004;10(5):1685–90.

79. Benz MR, Czernin J, Allen-Auerbach MS, et al. 3'-deoxy-3'-[18F]fluorothymidine positron emission tomography for response assessment in soft tissue sarcoma: a pilot study to correlate imaging findings with tissue thymidine kinase 1 and Ki-67 activity and histopathologic response. Cancer 2012;118(12): 3135–44.

80. Wolsztynski E, O'Sullivan F, Keyes E, et al. Positron emission tomography-based assessment of metabolic gradient and other prognostic features in sarcoma. J Med Imaging 2018;5(2):024502.

81. Peng Y, Bi L, Kumar A, et al. Predicting distant metastases in soft-tissue sarcomas from PET-CT scans using constrained hierarchical multi-modality feature learning. Phys Med Biol 2021;66(24).

82. Deng J, Zeng W, Shi Y, et al. Fusion of FDG-PET image and clinical features for prediction of lung metastasis in soft tissue sarcomas. Comput Math Methods Med 2020;2020:8153295.

83. Vallieres M, Freeman CR, Skamene SR, et al. A radiomics model from joint FDG-PET and MRI texture features for the prediction of lung metastases in soft-tissue sarcomas of the extremities. Phys Med Biol 2015;60(14):5471–96.

Positron Emission Tomography/Computed Tomography Transformation of Oncology
Melanoma and Skin Malignancies

Sze-Ting Lee, MBBS, PhD, FRACP, FAANMS[a,b,c,d,e], Natalia Kovaleva, MBBS[a],
Clare Senko, MBBS, FRACP[c,f], Damien Kee, MBBS, FRACP[c,f,g],
Andrew M. Scott, MBBS, MD, FRACP, FAHMS, FAANMS[a,b,c,*]

KEYWORDS

• PET • FDG-PET • Melanoma • Cutaneous malignancies • Immunotherapy • PET radiomics

KEY POINTS

- Accurate staging of melanoma is important for detemination of best management, with significant impact on management change.
- FDG PET is recommended for staging and restaging of AJCC Stage III (regional nodal) and Stage IV (systemic) disease.
- FDG PET has a high sensitivity, specificity and accuracy in detection of recurrent melanoma.
- FDG PET has an important role in treatment monitoring and detection of immunotherapy treatment related side effects, guiding further management.
- FDG PET has a role in detection of nodal and distant metastases in high risk non-melanomatous cutaneous disease such as cSCC, Merkel cell carcinoma and basal cell carcinoma.

BACKGROUND

Skin cancers are the most common of all cancers, with the most aggressive cutaneous malignancies including malignant melanoma, cutaneous squamous cell carcinoma (cSCC), Merkel cell carcinoma, and advanced invasive basal cell carcinoma. Although melanoma accounts for only about 1% of skin cancers, it is the cause of the most skin cancer deaths, and will be the main focus of this review.

The rates of melanoma have been rising rapidly over the past few decades, but this varies by age.

Melanoma mortality rates declined rapidly over the past decade (2011–2020) due to treatment, by about 5% per year in adults less than 50 year old, and 3%/year in 50 and older.[1] An epidemiologic assessment of global cancer data estimates around 325,000 new melanoma cases and 57,000 deaths due to melanoma in 2020, with large geographic variations in incidence across countries and world regions, being highest in Australia. If 2020 rates remain stable, the global burden from melanoma is estimated to increase to 510,000 new cases and 96,000 deaths by 2040.[2]

[a] Department of Molecular Imaging and Therapy, Austin Health, Heidelberg, Australia; [b] Department of Medicine, University of Melbourne, Melbourne, Australia; [c] Olivia Newton-John Cancer Research Institute, and La Trobe University, Heidelberg, Australia; [d] Department of Surgery, University of Melbourne, Melbourne, Australia; [e] School of Health and Biomedical Sciences, RMIT University, Melbourne, Australia; [f] Department of Medical Oncology, Olivia Newton-John Cancer and Wellness Centre, Austin Health, Heidelberg, Australia; [g] Department of Medical Oncology, Peter MacCallum Cancer Center, Melbourne, Australia
* Corresponding author. Department of Molecular Imaging and Therapy, Austin Health, 145 Studley Road, Heidelberg, Victoria 3084, Australia.
E-mail address: andrew.scott@onjcri.org.au

PET Clin 19 (2024) 231–248
https://doi.org/10.1016/j.cpet.2023.12.009

There are genetic and environmental risk factors which have led to wide variations in melanoma incidence among different geographic areas and ethnic groups. The most well-known risk factor for melanoma is due to phenotypic features associated with a 2-fold to 4-fold increased risk of melanoma. The other risk factors include atypical nevi, intermittent exposure to sunlight and sunburn occurring during adolescence or childhood, ultraviolet exposure from tanning beds (especially prior to age 35 years and for >10 lifetime sessions), methoxsalen and UV-A radiation for psoriasis treatment, and other skin conditions immunosuppression due to lymphoma, human immunodeficiency virus or transplant, personal history of basal cell or squamous cell carcinoma, and several drugs.[3–7] Approximately 10% of melanoma cases are familial, with several melanoma-subordinate hereditary syndromes, and germline mutations in the *BAP-1, BRCA1,* BRCA2, *TP53* germline mutations in Li-Fraumeni syndrome and *PTEN* gene mutations in Cowden syndrome. Testing for hereditary melanoma and/or genetic counseling should be considered in those with multiple primary melanomas, earlier age diagnosis, and family history.[8]

Surgery remains the mainstay treatment for most patients with melanoma and is curative in the majority of patients with early-stage disease. For patients with advanced melanoma, the last decade has witnessed dramatic improvements in outcomes secondary to parallel advances in genomic and immune based treatments. The discovery that the majority of melanomas are dependent on oncogenic activation of the mitogen-activated protein kinase cell growth pathway, led to the development of selective BRAF-inhibitors and MEK-inhibitors, that are highly active in melanomas with BRAF V600-mutations (40%–60%). Melanomas are also highly-immunogenic and are among the most responsive cancers to treatments developed against immune-checkpoints that can overcome immune tolerance, leading to durable responses that last well beyond completion of therapy.[9]

The most common melanoma is cutaneous melanoma, with less than 5% of primary melanoma arising from non-cutaneous sites such as mucosal (eg, sinus, nasopharynx, respiratory, esophagus, gastrointestinal, and genitourinary tracts), meninges and choroidal layer of the eye, with a common ectodermal origin in these tumors.[10] Mucosal melanomas are more aggressive possibly due to delayed diagnosis with metastases. Uveal melanomas are separate entity, and is the most common primary intraocular cancer in adults, while 5-year local tumor control is around 90%, liver metastasis occurs in greater than 50% of patients, with bone and lung metastases present.

STAGING SYSTEMS FOR MELANOMA

The American Joint Committee on Cancer (AJCC) melanoma staging system is typically used for risk stratification.[11] Clinical staging is based on the primary lesion (T), clinical and radiological nodal (N), and distant metastases (M). The major prognostic features are in **Box 1**. The most common sites for metastases are cutaneous, lung, liver, and brain, although any site in the body may be affected. Patterns of spread are dependent on tumor site and thickness, with around one-third of melanomas from lower extremities metastasizing locally to satellite/in-transit metastases, whereas one-thirds of melanomas from the trunk and upper extremities disseminate directly to distant sites.[12]

BRAF and NRAS mutant melanomas present with higher stage primary tumors, hence worse prognosis, with a trend toward increased mortality in those with mutations plus $\geq$ T2b primary tumors.[13]

TREATMENTS FOR LOCAL AND REGIONAL MELANOMA

Surgical excision with clear margins is the gold-standard treatment for primary cutaneous melanoma, and is essential for histologic confirmation of diagnosis, accurate and complete micro-staging to guide further treatment, minimization of local recurrence, with recommended margins dependent on tumor thickness. Sentinel lymph node biopsy (SLNB) is generally recommended in cutaneous melanoma with a primary thickness greater than 1.0 mm or in ulcerated tumors 0.8 to 1.0 mm thick or elevated mitoses,[14] with a role in prognostication and appropriate management.[11] The landmark MSLT-II trial recommended observation instead of completion nodal dissection

---

Box 1
Major prognostic features for melanoma

Major Prognostic Features

Breslow thickness

Ulceration of primary tumor

Mitotic rate of primary tumor

Extent of local and regional nodal involvement (N)

Presence of distant metastases (M) - separate for central nervous system

Others: LDH, growth phases, regression, angio-lymphatic invasion, perineural invasion, genetic

(CLND) in positive SLNB following wide local excision, with CLND performed in recurrences. Observation includes ultrasound of the involved lymph node basin every 4 months for years 1 to 2, every 6 months for years 3 to 5, and then annually.[15]

ADJUVANT THERAPY OF MALIGNANT MELANOMA

Although surgical excision of cutaneous melanoma in early-stage disease is most often curative, patients with resected stage IIB–IV remain at high risk for recurrence and death and may benefit from adjuvant systemic therapy. Similar to high-dose interferon, adjuvant therapy with ipilimumab was associated with significant improvements in relapse free and overall survival, but was highly toxic, and has been superseded by newer therapies.[16] In resected stage IIIB-IV melanoma, these include anti-PD1 inhibitors, nivolumab and pembrolizumab, and the targeted therapy combination, dabrafenib and trametinib, which is active only in BRAF-mutant melanoma. These drugs significantly reduce risk of recurrence when compared to ipilimumab (nivolumab, HR 0.70) or placebo (pembrolizumab, HR 0.56; dabrafenib and trametinib, HR 0.47); although evidence of a statistically significant improvement in overall survival is still pending.[17–19] For resected stage IIB-IIC melanoma, a similar relative risk reduction for recurrence has been observed for pembrolizumab (HR 0.65) and nivolumab (HR 0.42).[20,21] Again, the overall survival data are immature. Generally, these drugs are better tolerated than those they replace; however, the anti-PD1 inhibitors remain associated with a small potential risk of long-term immune-related toxicities that needs to be considered when evaluating overall patient benefit, particularly in more susceptible patients or at lower risk or recurrence.

Looking ahead, a neoadjuvant immunotherapy approach may become preferable. Initiating treatment before surgery will potentially allow better priming of the immune system as the melanoma affected lymph nodes remain in situ.[22] Early pilot and larger phase II trials have shown promising outcomes, with the added benefit of allowing pathologic evaluation of responses that may predict future recurrence risk, allowing adaption of subsequent treatment or the intensity of observation.

TREATMENT OF METASTATIC MALIGNANT MELANOMA

Similar to adjuvant therapy for melanoma, the treatment of patients with advanced disease has been dramatically transformed with the development of immune checkpoint therapy (developed against CTLA-4, PD1/PD-L1 and LAG3) and in patients with advanced BRAF V600-mutant melanoma, the combination of a BRAF and MEK-inhibitor. Presently, 3 BRAF and MEK inhibitor combinations have gained approval: dabrafenib and trametinib, vemurafenib and cobimetinib, and encorafenib and binimetinib.[18,19,23,24] These combinations exhibit a notably high response rate, often leading to swift clinical improvement, manifested by a reduction in FDG-uptake within 15 days of treatment initiation.[25] However, despite their initial dramatic activity, a critical limitation of these targeted therapies is the eventual emergence of secondary resistance, with 2-year and 5-year progression-free survival rates ranging between 31% to 37% and 14% to 23%, respectively.

In contrast, immune checkpoint therapy exhibits generally lower initial activity. However, in many cases, it can lead to durable responses persisting long after treatment cessation and the raising the potential for cure. Ipilimumab, a monoclonal antibody targeting CTLA-4, stands out as the first drug to demonstrate improved overall survival in advanced melanoma. Although the response rates are low (between 10%–20%), they are associated with a persistent overall survival plateau beginning at 3-year of 21% that extends out to beyond 10-year of follow-up.[26] Anti-PD1 antibodies, pembrolizumab and nivolumab, have superior response rates (33%–44%) and long-term overall survival (3-year OS, 51%–52%) along with significantly lower rates of adverse events.[27,28] However, the combination of both ipilimumab and nivolumab has the highest response rate (58%) and 3-year overall survival (58%), albeit with a substantially higher incidence of high-grade adverse events (59% vs 21%).[29] This combined approach is most beneficial in patients with BRAF mutations, asymptomatic brain involvement, and elevated lactate dehydrogenase. A newer combination of nivolumab plus relatlimab (which targets LAG3) has also demonstrated higher efficacy compared to nivolumab alone, with a 1-year progression-free survival of 48% versus 36%, and a much lesser increase in toxicity (19% vs 10%).

INVESTIGATIONS FOR PRIMARY MELANOMA
Lymphoscintigraphy

In early-stage melanoma (AJCC stage I–II), SLNB is still the standard of care for staging the regional draining lymph nodes particularly in patients presenting with an intermediate Breslow thickness lesion (1–4 mm).[30] SLNB is the single most important prognostic factor for disease recurrence and survival. Around 30% AJCC stage I–II patients are upstaged to stage III after SLNB.[31] Single-photon emitted computed tomography/computed tomography (CT) provides anatomic correlation of the lymphoscintigram to improve accuracy and excluding false-positive results, compared to planar imaging.[32]

[^{18}F] Fludeoxyglucose Positron Emission Tomography

In patients with AJCC stage I to II melanoma, multiple studies with fludeoxyglucose positron emission tomography (FDG-PET)/CT, have shown a poor sensitivity for detection of metastatic disease in draining nodes. FDG-PET has a low sensitivity for detecting SLN metastases, given the relative small size of nodal disease, in stage I–II disease.[33,34] The micrometastases in involved nodes is a major factor in disease detection, as most metastatic melanoma sites are FDG-avid. However, PET sensitivity for SLN was 23% for less than 5 mm, 83% for 6 to 10 mm, and 100% for greater than 10 mm nodes.[35] A meta-analysis of greater than 10,000 patients for lymph node detection in staging and surveillance showed ultrasound with the highest specificity and positive predictive value, compared to diagnostic CT and FDG-PET.[36]

AJCC stage III patients are at higher risk of presenting with systemic metastases, therefore accurate staging is important to guide therapy, with FDG-PET more accurate than conventional imaging in identifying metastases, with prognostic impact (**Fig. 1**).[37–40] A meta-analysis of greater than 10,000 patients showed that FDG-PET/CT is superior to CT alone for detection of extracerebral metastases (sensitivity 86% and specificity 91%).[36]

Patients with known or suspected AJCC stage IV disease benefit from FDG-PET staging which can impact on initial treatment (**Figs. 2, 3**; and **Table 1**).[32,41] The majority of melanoma metastases are FDG-avid, provided lesions are less than 5 to 6 mm in size. The exceptions are brain metastases, which may be difficult to identify due to physiologic gray-matter FDG uptake (**Fig. 4**), and hepatic metastases of uveal melanoma which have been shown to be negative on FDG-PET in up to 59% (unrelated to GLUT-1 expression).[42] A meta-analysis in staging of stage III and IV disease reported sensitivity and specificity for FDG-PET was 68% to 87% and 92% to 98%, respectively.[43]

Melanoma patients should have whole-body PET imaging, including arms/legs in patients whose primary lesions arise on extremities (**Fig. 5**). Reported studies have shown the value of whole-body imaging in melanoma patients, where primary lesions were in the limbs. A retrospective study of 153 patients, showed abnormal PET findings in the legs in 53 patients (35%), of which 72% also had distant metastases.[44] Published guidelines support the use of whole-body PET with extremities in patients with primary melanoma of the arms or legs and full images of the head in patients with primary scalp melanoma.[45] False-negative results can occur with small skin and brain metastases, and lesions adjacent to the heart, kidneys, or urinary bladder. Furthermore, while PET is more specific in the diagnosis of melanoma pulmonary metastases, chest CT is more sensitive. FDG-PET/CT provides an improved technique for assessing pulmonary disease, although it should be performed in conjunction with brain MR imaging to optimally identify brain metastases.

Investigations for recurrent metastatic melanoma

Identifying metastatic disease is critically important in melanoma patients, as the median survival after the appearance of distant metastases is approximately 6 months, with treatment decisions often based on the site and extent of disease, which may include surgery or radiotherapy.[46] Conventional investigations of CT, brain MRI ± bone scan have limited sensitivity and specificity for the detection of melanoma metastases and have been estimated in patients with stage II–IV melanoma to have a sensitivity and specificity of 57% to 81% and 45% to 87% respectively, on the basis of single melanoma lesions.[47]

In a meta-analyses, the reported sensitivity, specificity, and accuracy of FDG-PET in detecting recurrent melanoma ranges from 70% to 100%.[48] PET is particularly sensitive and specific for detecting soft tissue and lymph node metastases that are not assessable by clinical examination and have not been demonstrated by CT (**Fig. 6**). FDG-PET has also been shown to detect disease up to 6 months earlier than conventional techniques, with superior accuracy for the detection of both locoregional and distant metastases.[38,49] In a prospective, multicenter study of FDG-PET in 134 patients with known or suspected recurrent metastatic melanoma, PET identified an additional 189 lesions in 55.2% of patients, principally in soft tissue, bone, and nodal sites.[50] Most false negative PET in recurrent disease are less than 1 cm and are mainly pulmonary, hepatic or intracranial. PET should complement rather than replace CT or MRI scanning in patients with suspected recurrent disease. Most CT false negatives are located in the abdomen, suggesting that PET can especially assist in the restaging of this region.

FDG-PET/CT is superior to PET alone in the assessment of metastatic melanoma, with improved detection of nodal spread and distant metastases

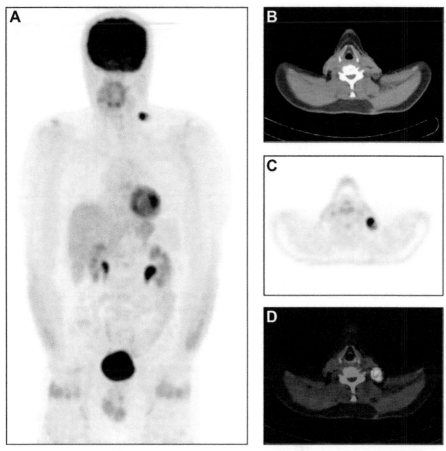

Fig. 1. FDG-PET/CT of a left cervical nodal metastatic melanoma in a patient with surgically resected left upper back primary cutaneous melanoma. Maximum intensity projection (*A*), axial CT (*B*), axial PET (*C*), axial fused PET/CT (*D*).

(**Fig. 7**); however the use of contrast-enhanced CT as part of the FDG-PET/CT study has shown that nodal detection was poor (38% vs 23% for CT), and detection of systemic metastases was slightly improved, although no statistically significant difference was seen.[51,52] Changes in treatment were implemented in 64% of patients due to imaging findings, indicating the potential clinical value of combined FDG-PET/CT and organ-specific MRI in melanoma patients.[53]

Monitoring treatment response of metastatic melanoma

Whole-body FDG-PET can also play a useful role in the treatment monitoring of metastatic melanoma. This is particularly relevant in patients with unresectable regional or distant metastatic disease who are enrolled in immunotherapy, chemotherapy, or biologic therapy protocols. PET has been shown to accurately detect early metabolic response to conventional and experimental therapies in patients with metastatic melanoma (**Fig. 8**). Therefore, the timely incorporation of whole-body PET into clinical trial protocols may help improve the efficacy of treatment regimens including dosage and scheduling optimization.

The utility of FDG-PET in assessing treatment response to treatment (including chemoimmunotherapy) have been widely published.[54–56] FDG-PET/CT is commonly used in evaluating melanoma treatment response to immunotherapy, with increasing evidence over the last decade. In patients treated with anti-PD1 based mono-or dual-therapy, most patients with a partial response on CT had complete metabolic response on PET, with sustained response at 1 year follow up. This has implications on using PET to predict long-term benefit and help guide duration of therapy.[57] Patients treated with first line combination ipilimumab and nivolumab, whole body metabolic tumor volume (wbMTV) was measured pre-treatment and post-treatment, showing progressive metabolic

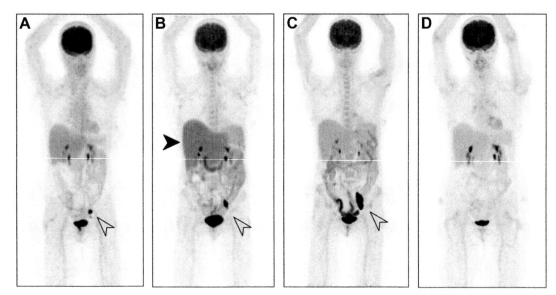

Fig. 2. Maximum intensity projection FDG-PET staging scan of patient with low rectal melanoma primary, demonstrating left external iliac nodal metastasis (*A white arrow*). Maximum intensity projection restaging PET scans demonstrating progression of the left iliac nodal mass while on Ipilimumab/Nivolumab immunotherapy (*B, C*), complicated by immune-mediated hepatitis demonstrated by hepatomegaly and increased hepatic FDG activity (*black arrow*) (*B*). Subsequent complete metabolic response after radiotherapy to the left iliac nodal mass, and resolution of immune-mediated hepatitis (*D*).

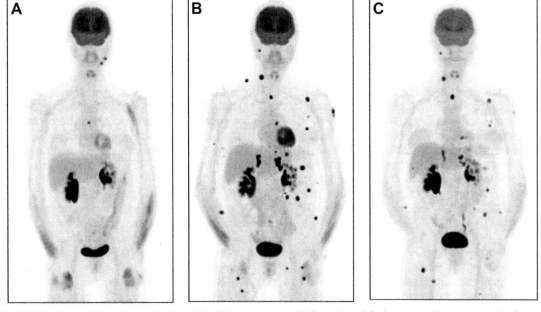

Fig. 3. Maximum intensity projection FDG-PET images at initial staging (*A*) demonstrating metastatic disease involving one sternal skeletal lesion and 2 submandibular lymph nodes. (*B*) Restaging FDG-PET scan after Nivolumab immunotherapy demonstrating resolution of the sternal and submandibular sites of disease but marked progression with multiple subcutaneous, intramuscular and nodal metastases above and below the diaphragm as well as bilateral adrenal and multiple intraperitoneal metastatic deposits. (*C*) Restaging PET/CT scan after commencing Encorafenib and Binimetinib therapy demonstrating partial metabolic response.

Table 1	
Role of FDG-PET in melanoma	
Staging	
AJCC Stage I–II	Not routinely recommended, unless high risk (intermediate-high-risk or high-risk primary lesions, multiple melanomas or unusual gene signatures in melanoma lesions.[29,34]
AJCC Stage III (regional nodal)	Recommended.[34,40]
AJCC Stage IV (systemic)	Recommended.[42,44]
Restaging	
Recommended, complement with CT or MRI scanning in patients with suspected recurrent disease in lungs, liver and brain.	

disease was associated with statistically significant higher baseline wbMTV.[58] Melanoma lesions had higher SUV_{max} (SUV_{max} 18) compared to inflammatory lesions (SUV_{max} 7.1), and those with similar SUV_{max} at baseline and post-treatment were more suspicious than those that were altered, unless the lesion was subjected to partial volume effect. Conversely, a negative FDG-PET showed sustained disease remission at 6 to 10 months, hence could identify those who may stop treatment, especially in the presence of toxicities.[59] A meta-analysis showed that baseline SUV_{peak}, MTV, and total glycolytic volume were promising predictors of the final response in patients with metastatic melanoma treated with immunotherapy. Furthermore, the presence of PET-detectable immune related adverse event (irAE) was also associated with therapy response.[60]

There are 2 treatment response criteria guidelines for PET which are typically used: the EORTC and PERCIST criteria. However, there have been numerous other criteria which take into account immune responses (eg, irRC, iRECIST, irRECIST, imRECIST, PECRIT, PERCIMT, imPERCIST, iPERCIST) which focus on the combination of morphologic (change in diameter) and metabolic response (reduction in SUV).[61] For melanoma the PERCIMT criteria were introduced. The most remarkable change in these criteria is that the appearance of up to 4 new lesions, depending on their size, can be accepted to define clinical benefit and support treatment continuation.[62] The categories are outlined in **Table 2**.

However, given that both melanoma and immune infiltrates are FDG-avid, it is prudent to differentiate true progression from "pseudoprogression".[63] The other categories in treatment pitfalls are summarized in **Table 3**. These unique immune-related inflammatory responses seen on FDG-PET can be identified with experience, and follow-up scanning will assess temporal change prior to confirming disease progression.

Earlier detection of clinically relevant irAEs which may precede clinical diagnosis has also been observed, which most commonly involved endocrinopathies (36%) and enterocolitis (35%) (**Figs. 9–11**).[64,65] These atypical immune responses have been associated with improved survival compared to those patients who would have been misclassified as having progressive disease by traditional classifications such as the WHO or RECIST.[66] Immune flare response has more frequently observed with anti-CTLA-4 compared to anti-PD1 agents, congruent with the higher incidence of autoimmune side effects seen with anti-CTLA4 agents. These tend to occur relatively early after introduction of treatment and are often associated with increased splenic activity. Since anti-PD1/PDL1 agents are thought to activate established antitumor cytotoxic T-cells

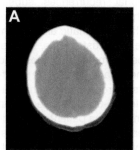 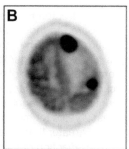 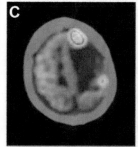 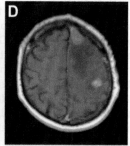

Fig. 4. FDG-PET/CT of brain metastases from melanoma axial images showing the 2 intensely FDG-avid lesions within the left frontal lobe and left parietal lobe with surrounding decreased FDG uptake in an area of perilesional edema. Axial CT (*A*), axial PET (*B*), axial fused PET/CT (*C*), corresponding axial T1+C MRI image (*D*).

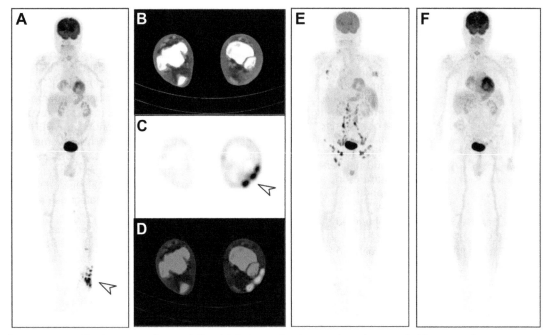

Fig. 5. FDG-PET/CT demonstrating multifocal left lower leg in-transit melanoma (*white arrows*) recurrence on pembrolizumab - Maximum intensity projection (*A*), axial CT (*B*), axial PET (*C*), axial fused PET/CT (*D*). Restaging FDG-PET/CT demonstrating complete response to ipilimumab with immune mediated widespread adenopathy on Maximum intensity projection (*E*). Sustained complete metabolic response is seen on subsequent PET/CT study with resolution of immune mediated adenopathy - Maximum intensity projection (*F*).

to facilitate rapid cell killing, the most common response is a progressive reduction FDG-avidity and MTV, similar to chemotherapy response, over a longer timeframe. With early imaging, progression on anti-PD1/PDL1 agents is very seldom a manifestation of immune flare response unless the patient is on a combination with anti-CTLA4 treatment.[67]

Management impact of fludeoxyglucose positron emission tomography/computed tomography in metastatic melanoma

FDG PET has been found to result in a change in management in 49% of patients, impacting surgery, chemotherapy or radiotherapy plans.[68] A meta-analysis reported that FDG-PET/CT was associated with 15% to 64% of management change strategies for AJCC stage III and IV melanoma.[69] This showed that FDG-PET performed at initial diagnosis for patients with confirmed stage III melanoma conferred survival benefits for patients who were negative for disseminated disease and those with upstaged disease due to distant metastases, which was attributed to early detection of occult subclinical metastases and subsequent modifications in treatment decisions. The 5-year melanoma-specific survival rates for patients with negative findings for distant metastasis

and for those with positive findings were 47.6% and 16.9%, respectively.

Surveillance for metastatic melanoma

Surveillance follow-up of patients with melanoma is guided by risk factors, patient history, and institutional guidelines. The natural history of melanoma and the likelihood of recurrent disease provide guidance about the frequency and duration of follow-up required. In patients with stage I–II melanoma, recurrences occur within 2 to 3 years after initial diagnosis (**Fig. 12**).[56] In stage IV patients, metastatic recurrence usually occurs within 2 years. Melanoma patients with asymptomatic and locoregional recurrences subsequently treated have shown an improved survival compared to those with symptomatic and distant recurrences.[53] The type of metastases (ie, visceral vs non-visceral), number of metastatic sites, and temporal evolution of metastatic burden are significant prognostic factors in treated melanoma patients.[54] Thus, regular follow-up is required for at least 2 years for most melanoma patients, extending to greater than 5 years for long-term survivors.

The selection of follow-up investigations in melanoma patients includes blood tests (serum LDH ± S-100B) and imaging. In asymptomatic melanoma patients, CT and MRI are of limited

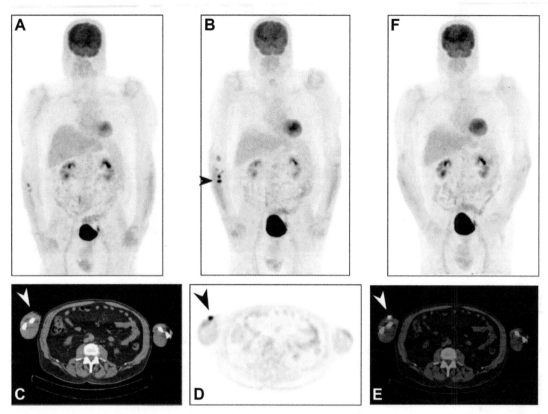

Fig. 6. FDG-PET/CT images demonstrating a right forearm in transit melanoma recurrence (*black arrows* in *B, D* and *white arrows* in *C, E*). Baseline maximum intensity projection image (*A*), after 12 months of adjuvant Nivolumab maximum intensity projection (*B*), axial CT (*C*), axial PET (*D*), axial fused PET/CT (*E*), with complete metabolic response after surgical resection and radiotherapy (*F*).

value for detecting nodal and visceral metastases,[70] whereas PET detection of occult metastases is estimated at 34%, thereby avoiding futile and cost-prohibitive interventions.[71] A cost-effectiveness study for surveillance of melanoma patients with suspected pulmonary metastases showed, FDG-PET/CT was less costly and resulted in 20% less futile surgeries and a potential 10-year survival benefit.[72] The likelihood of PET detecting recurrent disease is higher in patients with symptoms and recent treatment of metastatic disease.

Most importantly, a structured follow-up to detect relapses and secondary primary melanomas should be established as early as possible. Whilst there is no evidence to support the frequency and extent of PET scans, a stage-based follow-up scheme is proposed. A meta-analysis of 1047 articles contributed to guidelines for surveillance, which include life-long annual skin surveillance (preferably by experienced dermatologist), routine laboratory investigations, regional lymph node ultrasound (in stage IB or higher), and FDG-PET/CT or CT/MRI (in stage IIC or higher).[73]

Other cutaneous malignancies

cSCC is the second most common skin malignancy after basal cell carcinoma, and locoregional nodal involvement is found in 10% to 25% of patients with high risk features.[74,75] Distant metastases are found in less than 5% of cSCC patients. FDG-PET has been reported to have moderate sensitivity for detection of primary lesions and is usually dependent on size of lesion, but has a sensitivity of 91% to 100% and specificity of 81% to 90% for nodal involvement.[74,75] FDG-PET has improved sensitivity for detection of distant metastases, and may change in management in 26.1% of cases.[75] National Comprehensive Cancer Network guidelines support the use of FDG-PET at the clinician's discretion to rule out distant disease in patients with nodal involvement and for radiotherapy treatment planning. FDG-PET may also be useful in evaluation of

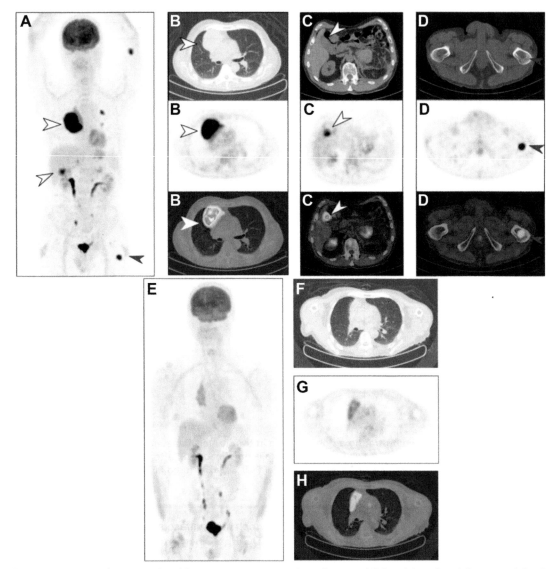

Fig. 7. FDG-PET/CT demonstrating biopsy proven metastatic melanoma (*A*) involving the right upper lobe (*B*, *white arrows*), multiple smaller bilateral lung lesions, lytic lesions within the left 6th rib and proximal left femur (*D*, *red arrows*) and a soft tissue mass within the gall bladder (*C*, *white arrows*) and a small left adrenal metastasis. (*E–H*) Restaging FDG-PET/CT scan after Ipilimumab and Nivolumab immunotherapy demonstrate a chronic inflammatory process in the anteromedial right upper lobe and complete response at all other sites, with the chronic inflammatory right upper lobe activity remaining stable on FDG-PET/CT imaging over 2 years.

response following treatment of metastatic disease with immune checkpoint inhibitors.[76]

Merkel cell carcinoma is a rare skin cancer, with locoregional nodal metastases found in 15% to 32% of cases but only a small number (7%–8%) having distant metastatic disease at initial presentation.[77] FDG-PET/CT has been shown to have a sensitivity of 82% to 95% and specificity of 88% to 96% for detecting spread of disease, with upstaging in 16% to 26% and change in management in up to 27.6% of patients.[77–79] It may also

have a role in the evaluation of patients with Merkel cell carcinoma after treatment with immune checkpoint inhibitors.[78]

Basal cell carcinomas are slow growing neoplasms principally found on sun exposed areas of the head and neck (85%–93% cases), and along with cSCC account for around 95% of nonmelanoma skin cancers.[80] BCCs may spread to subcutaneous tissues, and while distant spread is unusual metastases are typically FDG-avid (**Fig. 13**). FDG-PET may be used for evaluation of

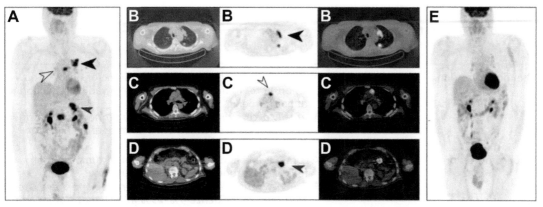

Fig. 8. Staging FDG-PET/CT. Maximum intensity projection (*A*), with multiple left pulmonary metastases (*B, black arrow*), mediastinal prevascular nodal metastasis (*C, white arrow*); and small bowel metastases (*D, red arrow*); with complete metabolic response on restaging PET/CT after Pembrolizumab immunotherapy - Maximum intensity projection image (*E*).

response to therapy in patients with advanced basal cell carcinoma.[81]

FUTURE DIRECTIONS

Whilst FDG PET is widely accepted in the management of patients with malignant melanoma and other high risk cutaneous malignancies, it is subjected to pitfalls which have resulted in the investigation of newer PET radiotracers in various clinical scenarios.

The exploration of novel biomarkers and imaging techniques with more sensitivity and specificity to melanoma cells have been investigated. These include markers of PD-1/PD-L1 inhibitors (^{89}Zr-DFO-6E11, ^{64}Cu-atezolizumab, ^{68}Ga-NOTA-Nb109); fibroblasts in tumor microenvironment such as fibroblast activation protein; melanin (^{18}F-5-FPN, ^{18}F-DMPY2, ^{18}F-ICF-1006); benzamides (^{123}I-BZA(2), 4-^{11}C-MBZA, ^{18}F-MEL050); β-integrin found in tumor vasculature (^{18}F-Galacto RGD); and MEK (^{124}I-trametinib).[82] ^{18}F-fluorothymidine (^{18}F-FLT) PET for cell proliferation has been investigated in stage III disease with a sensitivity of 88% and specificity of 60% for metastatic disease when compared with histopathology.[83] ^{18}F-fluoro-L-DOPA (^{18}F-DOPA) has been shown to be incorporated into melanin, representing an indicator of melanogenesis,[84] and could potentially increase the accuracy of PET for managing patients with treated metastases and negative FDG-PET.[85] Several preclinical studies have also investigated melanin-specific PET probes like ^{18}F-6-fluoro-N-[2-(diethylamino)ethyl]pyridine-3-carboxamide,[86] and ^{18}F-N-(2-(diethylamino)ethyl)-6-fluoronicotinamide,[87] for detection of regional melanoma metastases.

Advancements in PET scanner technology could potentially change the landscape of the detection of melanoma, nodal and metastatic disease, with a resultant change in management. Novel PET parameters such as maximum standardized uptake value (SUV$_{max}$), total metabolic volume (TMV), total lesion glycolysis (TLG) have been investigated in other tumor types and shown to be prognostic. In advanced melanoma, SUV$_{max}$ and TMV have been shown to be predictive in monitoring immunotherapy, with strong negative predictive power at

Table 2
FDG PET treatment response criteria based on PERCIMT[61]

Response	Definition
Complete Metabolic Response (CMR)	Disappearance of all metabolically active lesions
Partial Metabolic Response (PMR)	Disappearance of some but not all metabolic lesions and no new lesions
Stable Metabolic Disease (SMD)	Neither PMD nor PMR/CMR
Progressive Metabolic Disease (PMD)	4 or more new lesions (<1 cm in diameter), *or* 3 or more new lesions (>1 cm), or 2 or more new lesions (>1.5 cm in diameter)

Table 3
Immune response pitfalls[63]

Response	Definition
Pseudoprogression	Initial enlargement in total tumor volume or onset of new lesions after initiating treatment followed by reduction in tumor burden.[64] *Normally occurs within 4–6 wk after treatment and classified as early or delayed based on: before or after 12 wk of therapy.*
Hyperprogression	A considerable and early enlargement of tumor burden following introduction of immunotherapy. *Frequency varies depending on tumor type and agent used, with rates of incidence 4%–29% in different studies and publications. Consider in patients with high-risk factors (elderly, numerous metastatic lesions, and history of prior irradiation, certain mutations (MDM2/4) family amplification or EFGR) aberrations[65]*
Dissociated response/Mixed response	Growth of certain lesions accompanied by the paradoxic shrinkage in baseline lesions. *Potential association with favorable prognosis in comparison with patients with homogeneous progression. Therefore, patients might get a better benefit by not discontinuing initial immunotherapy treatment. In addition, it can identify oligometastatic patients who may benefit from local therapies.*
Sustained response	Enduring responses post-treatment with immunotherapy. *Observed in 10%–25% of metastatic patients.*

3 and 6 months after initiation of treatment. Retrospective cohort trials using FDG-PET showed TLG as the best predictive biomarker in melanoma-specific survival, with a statistically significant relationship between TLG and overall survival when treated with immunotherapy.[88]

Further studies are required to define the utility of non-FDG PET tracers, novel technologies and

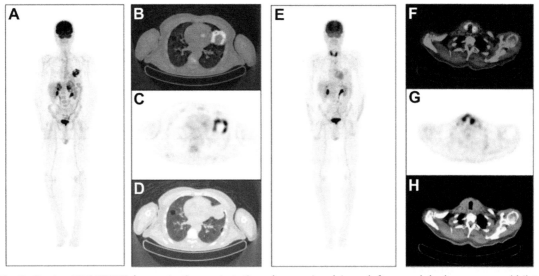

Fig. 9. Staging FDG-PET/CT demonstrating metastatic melanoma involving a left upper lobe lung mass and bilateral adrenal metastases (*A–D*). Restaging PET/CT demonstrating near complete response of metastatic disease to Ipilimumab/Nivolumab immunotherapy with evidence of thyroiditis (*E–H*).

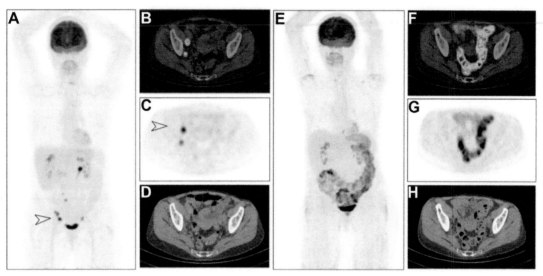

Fig. 10. FDG-PET/CT scan demonstrating biopsy confirmed nodal metastatic melanoma within the retroperitoneal, right common and external iliac nodal stations (*white arrows*) (*A–D*). Restaging FDG-PET/CT scan post cycle 2 Ipilimumab-Nivolumab demonstrated complete metabolic response with evidence of immune mediated colitis (*E–H*).

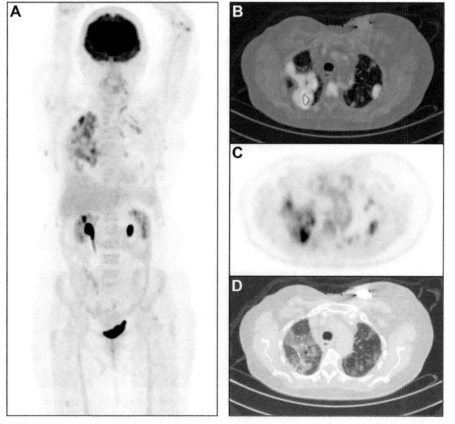

Fig. 11. FDG-PET/CT in a patient with immunotherapy associated pneumonitis on Ipilimumab and Nivolumab therapy for melanoma. Maximum intensity projection (*A*), axial CT (*B*), axial PET (*C*), axial fused PET/CT (*D*).

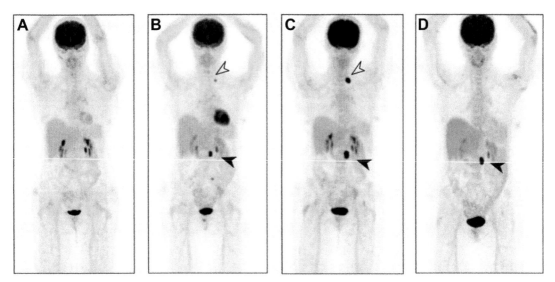

Fig. 12. FDG-PET demonstrating complete metabolic response to Ipilimumab/Nivolumab immunotherapy, which was ceased due to clinical toxicity. Maximum intensity projection images at cessation (*A*), 3-month (*B*) and 6-month restaging (*C*) demonstrate progressive disease within the left supraclavicular (*white arrows*) and para-aortic (*black arrows*) lymph nodes while off therapy, with partial response to carboplatin and paclitaxel chemotherapy (*D*).

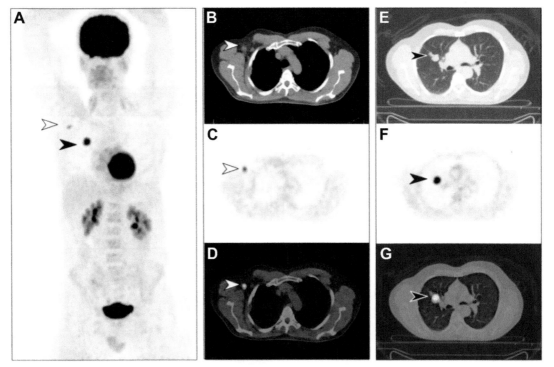

Fig. 13. FDG-PET/CT of patient with basal cell carcinoma resected from the right neck. Staging scan showed right axillary node (*white arrow*) seen on MIP (*A*) and corresponding axial CT (*B*), axial PET (*C*), axial fused PET/CT (*D*); and an intensely FDG-avid biopsy proven right lung metastasis (*black arrows*) on axial CT (*E*), axial PET (*F*), axial fused PET/CT (*G*).

radiomics in melanoma and other high risk cutaneous malignancies.

SUMMARY

PET imaging has an important role in the management of the most common cutaneous malignancies. FDG PET is not typically used in the characterization of the primary lesion, but for assessing for distant metastatic disease, particularly those with late stage or advanced disease. In the era of increasing immunotherapies and small molecule inhibitors in the treatment of metastatic melanoma, FDG-PET/CT has increasing use in assessment of treatment response over conventional imaging, and prognostication. A good understanding of immune modulation effects on FDG-PET is important to accurately interpret PET scans in these setting. In restaging, PET may be indicated where there are suspicious clinical symptoms, in-transit disease or palpable lymphadenopathy, or other suggestions of possible locoregional or metastatic disease. PET clearly impacts on patient management and can guide treatment decisions. Although there is controversy over the role of PET in surveillance, the sensitivity of FDG PET/CT makes it valuable in patients with high-risk disease. The use of new PET tracers and advanced PET technology may assist in more accurate staging of disease in the future and assist in developing biologic therapies targeted to specific oncogenic pathways in melanomas.

CLINICS CARE POINTS

- FDG PET is recommended in AJCC Stage III (regional nodal) and Stage IV (systemic) disease for staging, restaging, treatment monitoring with significant management impact.
- FDG PET can detect clinically relevant immune-related adverse effect prior to clinical diagnoses, including endocrinopathies and enterocolitis.
- The distinction between pseudoprogression, hyperprogression, dissociated/mixed response and sustained response categories in interpretation of FDG PET is important to understand.

DISCLOSURE

The authors have no relevant disclosures to report.

FUNDING

Sze-Ting Lee is supported by a Victorian Cancer Agency Early Career Research Fellowship, and Andrew M. Scott is supported by an NHMRC Investigator Fellowship No. 1177837.

REFERENCES

1. American Cancer Society, Key Statistics for Melanoma Skin Cancer, Available at: https://www.cancer.org/cancer/types/melanoma-skin-cancer/about/key-statistics.html. Accessed October 31, 2023.
2. Arnold M, Singh D, Laversanne M, et al. Global burden of cutaneous melanoma in 2020 and Projections to 2040. JAMA Dermatol 2022;158(5):495–503.
3. Gandini S, Sera F, Cattaruzza M, et al. Meta-analysis of risk factors for cutaneous melanoma: III. Family history, actinic damage and phenotypic features. Eur J Cancer 2005;41(14):2040–59.
4. Pampena R, Kyrgidis A, Lallas A, et al. A meta-analysis of nevus-associated melanoma: prevalence and practical implications. J Am Acad Dermatol 2017;77(5):938.
5. Lazovich D, Isaksson VR, Weinstock M, et al. Association between indoor tanning and melanoma in younger men and women. JAMA Dermatol 2016;152(3):268.
6. Kubica AW, Brewer JD. Melanoma in immunosuppressed patients. Mayo Clin Proc 2012;87(10):991–1003.
7. Brewer JD, Christenson LJ, Weaver AL, et al. Malignant melanoma in solid transplant recipients: collection of database cases and comparison with surveillance, epidemiology, and end results data for outcome analysis. Arch Dermatol 2011;147(7):790.
8. Leachman SA, Lucero OM, Sampson JE, et al. Identification, genetic testing, and management of hereditary melanoma. Cancer Metastasis Rev 2017;36(1):77.
9. Long GV, Menzies AM, Nagrial AM, et al. Prognostic and clinicopathologic associations of oncogenic BRAF in metastatic melanoma. J Clin Oncol 2011;29(10):1239.
10. Thoelke A, Willrodt S, Hauschild A, et al. Primary Extracutaneous malignant melanoma: a comprehensive review with emphasis on treatment. Onkologie 2004;27(5):492–9.
11. Keung EZ, Balch CM, Gershenwald JE, et al. Key changes in the AJCC eight edition melanoma staging system. The Melanoma Letter 2018;36(1).
12. Leiter U, Meier F, Schittek B, et al. The natural course of cutaneous melanoma. J Surg Oncol 2004;86:172–8.
13. Thomas NE, Edmiston SN, Alexander A, et al. Association between NRAS and BRAF mutational status

and melanoma-specific survival among patients with higher-risk primary melanoma. JAMA Oncol 2015; 1(3):359.

14. Morton DL, Thompson JF, Cochran AJ, et al. Final trial report of sentinel-node biopsy versus nodal observation in melanoma. N Engl J Med 2014; 370(7):599.

15. Faries MB, Thompson JF, Cochran AJ, et al. Completion dissection or observation for sentinel-node metastasis in melanoma. N Engl J Med 2017; 376(23):2211.

16. Robert C, Long GV, Brady B, et al. Nivolumab in previously untreated nivolumab without BRAF mutation. N Engl J Med 2015;372(4):320–30.

17. Robert C, Schachter J, Long GV, et al. Pembrolizumab versus ipilimumab in advanced melanoma. N Engl J Med 2015;372(36):2521–32.

18. Larkin J, Chiarion-Sileni V, Gonzalez R, et al. Five-year survival with combined nivolumab and ipilimumab in advanced melanoma. N Engl J Med 2019; 381:1535–46.

19. Robert C, Grob J, Stroyakovskiy D, et al. Five-year outcomes with dabrafenib plus trametinib in metastatic melanoma. N Engl J Med 2019;381:626–36.

20. Luke JJ, Rutkowski P, Queirolo P, et al. Pembrolizumab versus placebo as adjuvant therapy in completely resected stage IIB or IIC melanoma (KEYNOTE-716): a randomised,m double-blind, phase 3 trial. Lancet 2022;399(10336):1718–29.

21. Kirkwood JM, Del Vecchio M, Weber J, et al. Adjuvant nivolumab in resected stage IIB/C melanoma: primary results from the randomized, phase 3 CheckMate 76K trial. Nat Med 2023. https://doi.org/10.1038/s41591-023-02583-2.

22. Menzies AM, Amaria RN, Rozeman EA, et al. Pathological response and survival with neoadjuvant therapy in melanoma: a pooled analysis from the International Neoadjuvant Melanoma Consortium (INMC). Nat Med 2021;27:301–9.

23. Larkin J, Ascierto PA, et al. Combined vemurafenib and cobimetinib in BRAF-mutated melanoma. N Engl J Med 2014;371(20):1867–76.

24. Dummer R, Ascierto PA, et al. Encorafenib plus binimetinib versus vemurafenib or encorafenib in patients with BRAF-mutant melanoma (COLUMBUS): a multicenter, open-label, randomised phase 3 trial. Lancet Oncol 2018;19(5):603–15.

25. McArthur G, Puzanov I, Amaravadi R, et al. Marked, Homogenous, and early 18F-fluorodeoxyglucose positron emission tomography responses to vemurafenib in BRAF-mutant advanced melanoma. J Clin Oncol 2012;30:1628–34.

26. Schadendorf D, Hodi FS, Robert C, et al. Pooled analysis of long-term survival data from phase II and phase III trials of ipilimumab in unresectable or metastatic melanoma. J Clin Oncol 2015;33(17): 1889–94.

27. Robert C, Carlino MS, McNeil C, et al. Seven-year follow-up of the phase III KEYNOTE-006 study: pembrolizumab versus ipilimumab in advanced melanoma. J Clin Oncol 2023;41(24):3998–4003.

28. Wolchok JD, Chiarion-Sileni V, Gonzalez R, et al. Long-term outcomes with nivolumab plus ipilimumab or nivolumab alone versus ipilimumab in patients with advanced melanoma. J Clin Oncol 2022;40(2):127–37.

29. Wolchok JD, Chiarion-Sileni V, Gonzalez R, et al. Overall survival with combined nivolumab and ipilimumab in advanced melanoma. N Engl J Med 2017;377:1345–56.

30. Morton DL, Thompson JF, Cochran AJ, et al. Sentinel-node biopsy or nodal observation in melanoma. N Engl J Med 2006;355:1307–17.

31. Gershenwald JE, Scolyer RA, Hess KR, et al. Melanoma staging: evidence-based changes in the American joint Committee on Cancer eighth edition cancer staging manual. CA Cancer J Clin 2017; 67(6):472.

32. Belhocine TZ, Scott AM, Even-Sapir E, et al. The role of nuclear medicine in the management of cutaneous malignant melanoma. J Nucl Med 2006;47: 957–67.

33. Schafer A, Herbst RA, Beiteke U, et al. Sentinel lymph node excision (SLNE) and positron emission tomography in the staging of stage I–II melanoma patients. Hautarzt 2003;54:440–7.

34. Fink AM, Holle-Robatsch S, Herzog N, et al. Positron emission tomography is not useful in detecting metastasis in the sentinel lymph node in patients with primary malignant melanoma stage I and II. Melanoma Res 2004;14:141–5.

35. Crippa F, Leutner M, Belli F, et al. Which kinds of lymph node metastases can FDG PET detect? A clinical study in melanoma. J Nucl Med 2000;41: 1491–4.

36. Xing Y, Bronstein Y, Ross MI, et al. Contemporary diagnostic imaging modalities for the staging and surveillance of melanoma patients: a meta-analysis. J Natl Cancer Inst 2011;103:129–42.

37. Fletcher JW, Djulbegovic B, Soares HP, et al. Recommendations on the use of 18F-FDG PET in oncology. J Nucl Med 2008;49:480–508.

38. Harris MT, Berlangieri SU, Cebon JS, et al. Impact of 2-deoxy-2[F-18]fluoro-d-glucose positron emission tomography on the management of patients with advanced melanoma. Mol Imaging Biol 2005;7: 304–8.

39. Bastiaannet E, Wobbes T, Hoekstra OS, et al. Prospective comparison of [(18)F] fluorodeoxyglucose positron emission tomography and computed tomography in patients with melanoma with palpable lymph node metastases: diagnostic accuracy and impact on treatment. J Clin Oncol 2009;27: 4774–80.

40. Perng P, Marcus C, Subramaniam RM. 18F-FDG PET/CT and melanoma: staging, immune modulation and mutation-targeted therapy assessment and prognosis. Am J Roentgenol 2015;205:259–70.

41. Garbe C, Amaral T, Peris K, et al. European consensus-based interdisciplinary guideline for melanoma. Part 1: Diagnostics - Update 2019. Eur J Cancer 2020;126:141–58.

42. Strobel K, Bode B, Dummer R, et al. Limited value of 18F-FDG PET/CT and S-100B tumour marker in the detection of liver metastases from uveal melanoma compared to liver metastases from cutaneous melanoma. Eur J Nucl Med Mol Imag 2009; 36:1774–82.

43. Schröer-Günther MA, Wolff RF, Westwood ME, et al. F-18-fluoro-2-deoxyglucose positron emission tomography (PET) and PET/computed tomography imaging in primary staging of patients with malignant melanoma: a systematic review. Syst Rev 2012;1:62.

44. Loffler M, Weckesser M, Franzius Ch, et al. Malignant melanoma and (18)F-FDG-PET: should the whole body scan include the legs? Nuklearmedizin 2003;42:167–72.

45. Coleman RE, Delbeke D, Guiberteau MJ, et al. Concurrent PET/CT with an integrated imaging system: intersociety dialogue from the joint Working Group of the American College of Radiology, the Society of nuclear medicine, and the Society of computed body tomography and magnetic resonance. J Nucl Med 2005;46:1225–39.

46. Balch CM, Soong SJ, Gershenwald JE, et al. Prognostic factors analysis of 17,600 melanoma patients: validation of the American Joint Committee on Cancer melanoma staging system. J Clin Oncol 2001; 19:3622–34.

47. Stas M, Stroobants S, Dupont P, et al. 18F-FDG PET scan in the staging of recurrent melanoma: additional value and therapeutic impact. Melanoma Res 2002;12:479–90.

48. Jiménez-Requena F, Delgado-Bolton RC, Fernandez-Perez C, et al. Meta-analysis of the performance of (18)F-FDG PET in cutaneous melanoma. Eur J Nucl Med Mol Imag 2010;37:284–300.

49. Brady MS, Akhurst T, Spanknebel K, et al. Utility of preoperative [(18)]F fluorodeoxyglucose-positron emission tomography scanning in high-risk melanoma patients. Ann Surg Oncol 2006;13:525–32.

50. Fulham MJ, Kelley B, Ramshaw J, et al. Impact of FDG PET on the management of patients with suspected or proven metastatic melanoma prior to surgery: a prospective, multi-centre study as part of the Australian PET Data Collection Project. J Nucl Med 2007;48(Suppl 2):191P.

51. Macapinlac HA. The utility of 2-deoxy-2-[18F]fluoro-d-glucose-positron emission tomography and combined positron emission tomography and computed tomography in lymphoma and melanoma. Mol Imaging Biol 2004;6:200–7.

52. Veit-Haibach P, Vogt FM, Jablonka R, et al. Diagnostic accuracy of contrast enhanced FDG-PET/CT in primary staging of cutaneous malignant melanoma. Eur J Nucl Med Mol Imag 2009;36:910–8.

53. Pfannenberg C, Aschoff P, Schanz S, et al. Prospective comparison of 18F-fluorodeoxyglocose positron emission tomography/computed tomography and whole-body magnetic resonance imaging in staging of advanced melanoma. Eur J Cancer 2007;43:557–64.

54. Strobel K, Dummer R, Steinert HC, et al. Chemotherapy response assessment in stage IV melanoma patients-comparison of 18F-FDG-PET/CT, CT, brain MRI, and tumormarker S-100B. Eur J Nucl Med Mol Imag 2008;35:1786–95.

55. Hofman MS, Constantinidou A, Acland K, et al. Assessing response to chemotherapy in metastatic melanoma with FDG PET: early experience. Nucl Med Commun 2007;28:902–6.

56. Filippi L, Bianconi F, Schillaci O, et al. The role and potential of 18F-FDG PET/CT in malignant melanoma:prognostication, monitoring response to targeted and immunotherapy, and radiomics. Diagnostics 2022;12(4):929.

57. Tan AC, Emmett L, Lo S, et al. FDG-PET response and outcome from anti-PD-1 therapy in metastatic melanoma. Ann Oncol 2018;29(10):2115–20.

58. Iravani A, Osman MM, Weppler AM, et al. FDG PET/CT for tumoral and systemic immune response monitoring of advanced melanoma during first-line combination ipilimumab and nivolumab treatment. Eur J Nucl Med Mol Imaging 2020;47:2776–86.

59. Kong BY, Menzies AM, Saunders CA, et al. Residual FDG-PET metabolic activity in metastatic melanoma patients with prolonged response to anti-PD-1 therapy. Pigment Cell & Melanoma Research 2016;29: 572–7.

60. Ayati N, Sadeghi R, Kiamanesh Z, et al. The value of 18F-FDG PET/CT for predicting or monitoring immunotherapy response in patients with metastatic melanoma: a systematic review and meta-analysis. Eur J Nucl Med Mol Imaging 2021;48:428–48.

61. Lopci E. Immunotherapy monitoring with immune checkpoint inhibitors based on [18F]FDG PET/CT in metastatic melanomas and lung cancer. J Clin Med 2021;10:5160.

62. Anwar H, Sachpekidis C, Winkler J, et al. Absolute number of new lesions on 18F-FDG PET/CT is more predictive of clinical response than SUV changes in metastatic melanoma patients receiving ipilimumab. Eur J Nucl Med Mol Imaging 2018;45:376–83.

63. Losada MM, Robles LR, Melero AM, et al. [18F]FDG PET/CT in the evaluation of melanoma patients treated with immunotherapy. Diagnostics 2023;13:978.

64. Leon-Mateos L, Garcia-Velloso MJ, García-Figueiras R, et al. A multidisciplinary consensus on

the morphological and functional responses to immunotherapy treatment. Clin Transl Oncol 2021; 23:434–49.

65. Lin M, Vanneste BGL, Yu Q, et al. Hyperprogression under immunotherapy: a new form of immunotherapy response? A narrative literature review. Transl Lung Cancer Res 2021;10:3276–91.

66. Wolchok JD, Hoos A, O'Day S, et al. Guidelines for the evaluation of immune therapy activity in solid tumors: immune-related response criteria. Clin Cancer Res 2009;15:7412–20.

67. Hofman MS, Hicks RJ. How we read oncologic FDG PET/CT. Cancer Imag 2016;16:35–48.

68. Gulec SA, Faries MB, Lee CC, et al. The role of fluorine-18 deoxyglucose positron emission tomography in the management of patients with metastatic melanoma: impact on surgical decision making. Clin Nucl Med 2003;28:961–5.

69. Niebling MG, Bastiaannet E, Hoekstra OS, et al. Outcome of clinical stage III melanoma patients with FDG-PET and whole-body CT added to the diagnostic workup. Ann Surg Oncol 2013;20:3098–105.

70. Kaleem A, Patel N, Chandra SR, et al. Imaging and laboratory workup for melanoma. Oral Maxillofac Surg Clin North Am 2022 May;34(2):235–50.

71. Eigtved A, Andersson AP, Dahlstrom K, et al. Use of fluorine-18 fluorodeoxyglucose positron emission tomography in the detection of silent metastases from malignant melanoma. Eur J Nucl Med 2000;27:70–5.

72. Krug B, Crott R, Roch I, et al. Cost-effectiveness analysis of FDG PET-CT in the management of pulmonary metastases from malignant melanoma. Acta Oncol 2010;49(2):192–200.

73. Johnston L, Starkey S, Mukovozov I, et al. Surveillance after a previous cutaneous melanoma diagnosis: a scoping review of melanoma follow-up guidelines. J Cutan Med Surg 2023. https://doi.org/10.1177/12034754231188434.

74. Fujiwara M, Suzuki T, Takiguchi T, et al. Evaluation of positron emission tomography imaging to detect lymph node metastases in patients with high-risk cutaneous squamous cell carcinoma. J Fermatol 2016;43:1314–20.

75. Mahajan S, Barker CA, Singh B, et al. Clinical value of FDG-PET/CT in staging cutaneous squamous cell carcinoma. Nucl Med Commun 2019;40(7):744–51.

76. McLean LS, Cavanagh K, Hicks RJ, et al. FDG-PET/CT imaging for evaluating durable responses to immune checkpoint inhibitors in patients with advanced cutaneous squamous cell carcinoma. Cancer Imag 2021; 21:57.

77. Poulsen M, MacFarlane D, Veness M, et al. Prospective analysis of the utility of 18-FDG-PET in Merkel cell carcinoma of the skin: a Trans Tasman radiation oncology Group study, TROG 09:03. J Med Imag Radiat Oncol 2018;62:412–9.

78. Sachpekidis C, Sidiropoulou P, Hassel JC, et al. Positron emission tomography in Merkel cell carcinoma. Cancers 2020;12:2897.

79. Zijlker LP, Bakker M, van der Hiel B, et al. Baseline ultrasound and FDG-PET/CT in Merkel cell carcinoma. J Surg Oncol 2023;127:841–7.

80. Juan YH, Saboo SS, Tirumani SH, et al. Malignant skin and subcutaneous neoplasms in adults: multimodality imaging with CT, MRI, and 18F-FDG PET/CT. Am J Roentdenol 2014;202(5):W422–38.

81. Thacker CA, Weiss GJ, Tibes R, et al. 18-FDG PET/CT assessment of basal cell carcinoma with vismodegib. Cancer Med 2012;1(2):230–6.

82. Prendergast CM, Capaccione KM, Lopci E, et al. More than Just skin-Deep: a review of Imaging's role in guiding CAR T-cell therapy for advanced melanoma. Diagnostics 2023;13:992.

83. Cobben DCP, Jager PL, Elsinga PH, et al. '3-^{18}F-fluoro-3'-deoxy-$_L$-thymidine: a new tracer for staging of metastatic melanoma? J Nucl Med 2003;44: 1927–32.

84. Ishiwata K, Kubota K, Kubota R, et al. Selective 2-[18F]fluorodopa uptake for melanogenesis in murine metastatic melanomas. J Nucl Med 1991;32:95–101.

85. Dimitrakopoulou-Strauss A, Strauss LG, Burger C. Quantitative PET studies in pretreated melanoma patients: a comparison of 6-[18F]fluoro-L-dopa with 18F-FDG and 15O-water using compartment and non-compartment analysis. J Nucl Med 2001;42: 248–56.

86. Zhang C, Zhang Z, Lin K-S, et al. Melanoma imaging using 18F-labeled α-melanocyte-stimulating hormone derivatives with positron emission tomography. Mol Pharm 2018;15:2116–22.

87. Greguric I, Taylor SR, Denoyer D, et al. Discovery of [18F]N-(2-(diethylamino)ethyl)-6-fluoronicotinamide: a melanoma positron emission tomography imaging radiotracer with high tumor to body contrast ratio and rapid renal clearance. J Med Chem 2009;52: 5299–302.

88. Sanli Y, Leake J, Odu A, et al. Tumor Heterogeneity on FDG PET/CT and immunotherapy: an imaging biomarker for predicting treatment response in patients with metastatic melanoma. Am J Roentgenol 2019;212:1318–26.

Positron Emission Tomography/Computed Tomography Transformation of Oncology: Multiple Myeloma

Salikh Murtazaliev, MD[a], Steven P. Rowe, MD, PhD[a],
Sara Sheikhbahaei, MD, MPH[a], Rudolf A. Werner, MD[a,b],
Lilja B. Sólnes, MD, MBA[a,*]

KEYWORDS

- Multiple myeloma • FDG PET CT • CXCR4 • Overall survival • Whole body MRI

KEY POINTS

- Imaging plays a crucial role in the evaluation of patients with suspected multiple myeloma (MM).
- International Myeloma Working Group updated the diagnostic criteria for MM to include additional biomarkers to identify patients with the near-inevitable risk of progressing to MM but who have not yet developed end-organ damage and CRAB features
- Patients with 3 or greater focal lesions or extramedullary disease on 2-deoxy-2-[18F]fluoro-D-glucose (^{18}F FDG) positron emission tomography/computed tomography had significantly shorter progression-free survival and overall survival
- Solitary bone plasmacytoma (SBP) is more prevalent than solitary extramedullary plasmacytoma
- A promising new approach for imaging and treatment of MM is C-X-C motif chemokine receptor 4-directed theranostics

INTRODUCTION

Multiple myeloma (MM) is a hematologic malignancy caused by the neoplastic proliferation of plasma cells that produce monoclonal immunoglobulin and free light chains (FLCs). MM is consistently preceded by the precursor states of monoclonal gammopathy of undetermined significance (MGUS) and smoldering myeloma and is part of a broader spectrum of clonal plasma cell disorders.[1] In the United States, MM accounts for almost 2% of all cancers and is the second most common hematological malignancy after lymphoma. Each year, 7 out of 100,000 people with a median age of 70 will be diagnosed with MM, and 3 out of 100,000 will die from the disease or treatment-related complications.[2] Despite the introduction of new targeted therapies and transplant techniques that have resulted in an increase in median survival from 3 to up to 10 years during the last 2 decades, MM remains an incurable disease.[3]

2-deoxy-2-[18F]fluoro-D-glucose (^{18}F FDG) positron emission tomography/computed tomography (PET/CT) has emerged as a valuable imaging modality for diagnosis, therapy assessment,

The first author of this article (S. Murtazaliev) is a nonnative English speaker who used ChatGPT as a language editor for this text.*
* All rights are reserved, including those for text and data mining, artificial intelligence training, and similar technologies.
[a] Division of Nuclear Medicine and Molecular Imaging, The Russell H. Morgan Department of Radiology and Radiological Science at Johns Hopkins Hospital, 601 North Caroline St., JHOC 3, Baltimore, MD 21287, USA;
[b] Department of Nuclear Medicine, University Hospital Würzburg, Würzburg, Germany
* Corresponding author.
E-mail address: lsolnes1@jh.edu

PET Clin 19 (2024) 249–260
https://doi.org/10.1016/j.cpet.2023.12.010
1556-8598/24/© 2024 Elsevier Inc. All rights reserved.

and prognostication in the setting of MM. [18]F FDG PET/CT integrates the metabolic findings from the FDG component with the anatomic information provided by the CT component, allowing for accurate localization of abnormal hypermetabolism/active disease. This article provides an in-depth review of the role of ^{18}F FDG PET/CT in MM and related clonal plasma cell disorders. We will address the role of ^{18}F FDG PET/CT in relation to other imaging techniques and explore new diagnostic and therapeutic directions for novel PET radiotracers.

INITIAL DIAGNOSIS

Diagnosis of active MM is based on a combination of factors. Earlier, the diagnosis primarily relied on identifying MM-induced end-organ damage using the CRAB criteria: "C" hypercalcemia (>11 mg/dL), "R" renal insufficiency (creatinine clearance <40 mL/min or serum creatinine >2 mg/dL), "A" anemia (hemoglobin <10 g/dL), and "B" the presence of lytic bone lesions.[4] However, in 2014, the International Myeloma Working Group (IMWG) updated the diagnostic criteria for MM to include additional biomarkers to identify patients with the near-inevitable risk of progressing to MM but who have not yet developed end-organ damage and CRAB features.

The new biomarkers can be remembered using the acronym "SLiM," which is short for "Sixty," "Light chain ratio," and "MRI." The first is the presence of at least 60% clonal plasma cells in the bone marrow (BM). The second is an involved/uninvolved free light chain (FLC) ratio of 100 or more (provided that the involved FLC level is at least 100 mg/L). The third is an MRI scan that shows 2 or more focal lesions.[5] Furthermore, the criteria were revised to allow CT, PET-CT, and MRI to diagnose MM bone disease.

In approximately one-third (26%–34%) of patients, the first presentation of MM is a pathologic fracture resulting from osteolytic lesions.[6] They originate from plasma cells infiltrating the BM and secreting cytokines, leading to an imbalance in bone resorption by increasing osteoclast activity, decreasing osteoblast activity, and generally producing purely osteolytic lesions.[7] Weakened bones with multiple punched-out lesions may lead to complications, such as pathologic fractures, vertebral collapse, and spinal cord compression, significantly affecting the patient's quality of life and functional status.[8]

Imaging plays a crucial role in the evaluation of patients with suspected MM. According to the latest guidelines from IMWG, advanced imaging techniques such as MRI, PET/CT, and CT should be used for the evaluation of suspected MM because they can detect up to 80% more lesions than conventional skeletal radiography, which has been the primary imaging modality for nearly 4 decades.[9]

MRI and ^{18}F FDG PET/CT are complementary imaging. MRI analyzes the tissue composition of water and fat, whereas ^{18}F FDG PET/CT uses anatomic and metabolic data within the region of interest.[5] In initial studies, the comparative performance between whole-body ^{18}F FDG PET/CT and spine MRI showed similar results in detecting single lesions, and superior performance of MRI in detecting diffuse BM infiltration, whereas ^{18}F FDG PET/CT had the advantage of detecting extramedullary disease (EMD), which was outside of the routine spine MRI field of view.[10–13] Consequently, there has been increased usage of whole-body MRI. A recent meta-analysis by Rama and colleagues compared the performance of both whole-body ^{18}F FDG PET/CT and whole-body MRI, revealing that the specificity of PET/CT was higher than that of MRI at 82% (95% CI, 75%–88%) compared with 57% (95% CI, 37%–76%), with a statistically significant difference ($P = .01$). In contrast, the sensitivity of MRI was higher than that of PET/CT at 87% (95% CI, 75%–93%) compared with 64% (95% CI, 45%–79%) but the difference was not statistically significant ($P = .29$). Overall, these data suggest that whole-body MRI and ^{18}F FDG PET/CT provide complementary information for the assessment of disease, with each modality having its strengths and weaknesses.[14]

According to the most recent consensus by IMWG on first-diagnosis imaging in MM, the recommended starting point is whole-body CT (WBCT) to determine the presence and extent of osteolytic lesions. However, when available, ^{18}F FDG PET/CT is the preferred imaging modality, offering a comprehensive evaluation of the total metabolically active disease burden, detection of EMD, and identification of clinically relevant damage to affected skeletal structures or organs. Alternatively, if the ^{18}F FDG PET/CT is not feasible, whole-body magnetic resonance imaging (WBMRI) can be performed instead.[15]

INITIAL STAGING

MM is a heterogeneous disease that can progress rapidly in some patients, whereas others may have a more indolent disease course. Several staging systems have been developed to better risk stratify patients, predict survival, and help interpret data from clinical trials. These systems include the Durie-Salmon staging system from 1975,[16] the International Staging System (ISS) from 2005,[17] and the most recent Revised International Staging

System (R-ISS), introduced in 2015. The R-ISS 3-stage risk classification system uses a combination of blood and genetic parameters, namely the serum levels of albumin, LDH, and β2 microglobulin, as well as genetic risk assessment using fluorescence in situ hybridization. Palumbo and colleagues demonstrated the validity of this system in a study of 3060 newly diagnosed MM patients who were stratified into 3 categories based on the abovementioned parameters. The observed 5-year overall survival (OS) rates for the R-ISS I, R-ISS II, and R-ISS III groups were 82%, 62%, and 40%, respectively.[18]

The Durie-Salmon staging system was the last to incorporate imaging findings as a part of the evaluation criteria for MM. However, a recent study emphasized the potential advantages of using ^{18}F FDG PET/CT for initial staging to stratify patients and their prognoses further. In a retrospective analysis of 167 newly diagnosed patients with MM who were stratified according to the R-ISS, those in the R-ISS II group with positive PET/CT findings, as indicated by the presence of 3 or more focal lesions or EMD, had significantly shorter progression-free survival (PFS) and OS than those who were PET/CT negative (PFS: 15.4 vs 29.7 months, $P = .001$; OS: 43.3 months vs not reached, $P = .020$). Similarly, PET/CT-positive patients with R-ISS III had significantly shorter PFS and OS compared with those who were not PET/CT-positive (PFS: 4.9 vs 22.7 months, $P < .001$; OS: 21.0 months vs not reached, $P = .008$).[19] This study emphasizes the complementary prognostic value of PET/CT in addition to IMWG R-ISS criteria alone. Perhaps, with the recent introduction of advanced imaging in the initial diagnosis of MM, it may also be included in the initial staging of the disease.

[18]F FDG PET/CT PROGNOSTIC VALUE

Pretreatment PET/CT scan at the initial diagnosis is a valuable tool for prognostication in MM. A meta-analysis of 1670 patients demonstrated that the presence of 3 or more focal lesions, EMD, and high ^{18}F FDG uptake on PET/CT scans was strongly associated with shorter PFS and OS.[20] Hazard ratios for PFS for 3 or more focal lesions, EMD, and high ^{18}F FDG uptake were 2.38 (95% CI, 1.84–3.07), 2.12 (95% CI, 1.52–2.96), and 2.02 (95% CI, 1.51–2.68), respectively. The hazard ratios for OS for these 3 parameters were 3.29 (95% CI, 2.38–4.56), 2.37 (95% CI, 1.77–3.16), and 2.28 (95% CI, 1.67–3.13), respectively (**Fig. 1**).

Those markers accurately reflect the underlying disease biology and significantly affect patient outcomes through established mechanisms. Specifically, the number of focal lesions reflects the

degree of tumor burden, whereas the presence of EMD indicates a propensity for disease formation in an unusual site, and ^{18}F FDG uptake intensity indicates tumor aggressiveness.[21] Despite their prognostic value, guidelines for escalating or deescalating therapy based on those results are yet to be developed. Therefore, with further research on disease prognostication, more tailored guidelines can come forth, leading to personalized treatment management for patients.

The Italian myeloma criteria for PET use (IMPeTUs) were proposed with the aim of streamlining and standardizing the interpretation of ^{18}F FDG PET/CT scans in patients with MM.[22] The significance of these criteria has been supported by several studies, validating their prognostic value.[23,24] The details of IMPeTUs are summarized in **Box 1**. In essence, IMPeTUs criteria provide a visual interpretation framework that encompasses 2 key aspects. First, it outlines the distribution of FDG-avid disease, including BM, focal bone (FL), paramedullary (PM), or extramedullary (EM) lesions. Second, IMPeTUs uses the 5-point scale of the Deauville score (DS) to assess the relative metabolic activity of lesions. Notably, patients displaying FDG uptake above the liver (DS $\geq$ 4) in either the BM or at least 1 focal lesion tend to have significantly shorter PFS and OS. Despite its advantages, these criteria come with their own set of limitations. The subjective nature of IMPeTUs introduces the risk of interrater variability and the time-consuming analysis of scans with numerous lesions, posing challenges for their implementation in clinical settings.

ASSESSMENT OF TREATMENT RESPONSE

[18]F FDG PET/CT is a valuable tool for assessing treatment response in patients with MM. One of the main advantages of ^{18}F FDG PET/CT is its ability to detect changes in tumor metabolism, which tends to precede any morphologic changes observed in other modalities.

In 2018, Davies and colleagues further investigated the prognostic value of ^{18}F FDG activity resolution in focal lesions at various posttreatment time points, including day 7, postinduction, posttransplant, and during maintenance therapy. Consistent with earlier findings, patients with 3 or more focal lesions at the initial imaging had a higher risk of shorter PFS and OS. Interestingly, patients with focal lesions at the initial imaging that resolved on subsequent scans had a similar prognosis to those without lesions at the initial imaging. Furthermore, this study found that ongoing ^{18}F FDG activity in focal lesions maintained its negative prognostic significance at all testable time points. These findings

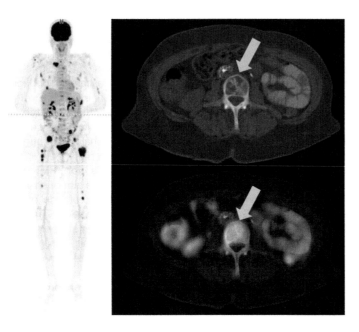

Fig. 1. [18]F FDG PET/CT image of a 50-year-old female patient with MM. The image reveals multiple lytic bone lesions, indicated by the yellow arrows, which exhibit high ^{18}F FDG uptake. The presence of more than 3 intensely avid lytic lesions is indicative of a potentially unfavorable prognosis, suggesting a decreased PFS and OS for the patient.

support serial PET/CT scanning at distinct time points to accurately decipher the true prognostic significance of these lesions for individual patients, to aid in determining the effectiveness of therapy, and to help tailor individualized treatment plans for patients with MM[25] (**Fig. 2**).

[18]F FDG PET/CT AND STEM CELL TRANSPLANTATION

Both autologous and allogeneic stem cell transplantation have been used in the treatment of MM since the 1980s.[26,27] Auto-SCT has been found to significantly prolong OS and PFS, have manageable short-term toxicities, and low treatment-related mortality rates but it is not considered a curative treatment.[28] Allo-SCT, however, offers potential curative benefits, including a tumor-free graft and graft-versus-myeloma effect, frequently leading to sustained remission. However, allo-SCT remains controversial due to significant toxicity related to immunosuppression and subsequent infections, the risk of graft-versus-host disease, and potentially high nonrelapse mortality.[29] As a result, allo-SCT is not routinely performed in patients with MM, although the number of transplantations has been steadily increasing in recent decades.[30] Earlier studies have shown that complete ^{18}F FDG suppression in focal lesions and EMD before the first transplantation was associated with better survival outcomes, including longer OS and event-free survival. Specifically, 30 months after the first auto-SCT, the rates of being alive and event-free were 92% and 89%,

respectively, compared with only 71% and 63% among those with less than 100% suppression of ^{18}F FDG uptake in focal lesions and EMD.[21]

Several studies have investigated the role of ^{18}F FDG PET/CT in monitoring the response to allo-SCT in patients with MM. Patriarca and colleagues evaluated the significance of PET positivity before and 6 months after allo-SCT. They found that patients who achieved or maintained complete PET remission had significantly higher PFS and OS than those with persistent PET findings. Reportedly, the 2-year PFS and OS rates for patients with complete PET remission versus those with persistent PET findings were 51% and 81% versus 25% and 47%, respectively.[31]

These findings were supported by Stolzenburg and colleagues, who analyzed heavily pretreated patients with MM before allo-SCT and ~100 days after allo-SCT. Their study also concluded that the persistence of metabolically active disease after allo-SCT is an unfavorable prognostic factor. Specifically, patients with a negative PET had significantly longer PFS (26.9 ± 2.0 m vs 3.5 ± 0.8 m, $P < .001$) and OS (10.3 ± 2.4 m vs not reached with longest OS 92.5 m, $P = .012$), compared with those with positive PET.[32]

MINIMAL RESIDUAL DISEASE

As MM treatment advances, the need for more precise treatment response criteria has become apparent. In the past 15 years, new therapies, including multidrug combinations, posttransplant consolidation, and prolonged maintenance

Box 1
IMPeTUs criteria description

IMPeTUs Criteria

Diffuse BM uptake + DS

Deauville criteria:

(1) : No uptake at all

(2) : $\leq$ mediastinal blood pool uptake

(3) : >mediastinal blood pool uptake, $\leq$ liver uptake (4): > liver uptake +10%

(5) : >> liver uptake (twice or more)

A appended if there is hypermetabolism in limbs and ribs

Focal bone lesions (F)

Lesion location and number group (x)

S: skull Sp: spine Extra Sp: all the rest

x = (1): no lesions (2): 1 to 3 lesions (3): 4 to 10 lesions (4): greater than 10 lesions

DS of target focal bone lesion (target lesion is the hottest area)

Lytic lesions (L) at CT associated to PET

Lesion number group (x)

x = (1): no lesions (2): 1 to 3 lesions (3): 4 to 10 lesions (4): greater than 10 lesions

Presence of at least one fracture on CT images (Fr)

Presence of PM disease:

A bone lesion involving surrounding soft tissues with bone cortical interruption

Presence of EM disease

Nodal disease (N) plus site:

LC: laterocervical SC: supraclavicular M: mediastinal Ax: axillary Rp: retroperitoneal Mes: mesentery In: inguinal

Extranodal disease (EN) plus site

Li: liver Mus: muscle Spl: spleen Sk: skin Oth: other

DS of target extramedullary lesion (hottest lesion)

M-protein, less than 5% plasma cells in the BM, and disappearance of soft tissue plasmacytomas, plus more stringent requirements, including a normal FLC ratio and absence of clonal plasma cells on the trephine biopsy. Notably, radiographic findings were not part of the complete response criteria.[38] However, clinical criteria alone may not accurately identify the presence of minimal residual disease, as demonstrated in a Mayo Clinic study of 195 newly diagnosed patients with MM. The study found that despite achieving the clinical criteria for complete remission, 21% of patients had persistently positive ^{18}F FDG PET/CT after treatment. Those patients demonstrated a shorter time to next treatment (TTNT) and significantly shorter OS than those with negative ^{18}F FDG PET/CT (TTNT: 39.2 vs 58.9 months, $P = .27$; OS: 72 months vs unreached, $P = .01$). Importantly, ^{18}F FDG PET/CT retained prognostic significance even after adjusting for multiple other variables, such as ISS score, high-risk genetic profile, and presence of EMD.[39]

In a study conducted by Derlin and colleagues, they evaluated the effectiveness of ^{18}F FDG PET/CT in detecting and localizing residual or recurrent disease in 99 patients with MM following stem cell transplantation. The results were compared with the IMWG Uniform Response Criteria for MM, which uses clinical and biochemical information to assess response. The study found that ^{18}F FDG PET/CT had a remarkable specificity of 82.1% and positive predictive value of 82.3%. However, they found an underwhelming sensitivity of 54.6%, negative predictive value of 54.2%, and overall accuracy of 65.5%. Interestingly, further analysis revealed that sensitivity varied widely depending on the patient's clinical remission status per IMWG Response Criteria, with the better treatment response having lower PET sensitivity. The sensitivity rates were 80.0%, 63.6%, 55.9%, and 34.1% for patients with recurrent disease, stable disease, partial response (PR), and very good PR, respectively.[40]

That variability in sensitivity is not surprising and can be attributed to several factors. For example, patients who achieve a very good PR have a serum paraprotein reduction of 90% or greater, which is dictated by a significant myeloma volume reduction. That may lead to disease manifestations that are too small to be depicted by PET due to the limited resolution of the imaging modality and partial volume effects. Additionally, extensive prior high-dose chemotherapy may lead to the selection of slow-growing cell colonies that are less metabolically active and do not accumulate a notable amount of ^{18}F FDG, evading detection on imaging.

Rama and colleagues performed a meta-analysis that aimed to compare the diagnostic performance

therapy, have resulted in more than 50% of patients achieving complete response.[33–37] Despite this significant improvement, many patients still experience relapse, highlighting the need for more sensitive methods to detect and quantify minimal residual disease levels.

In 2011, a complete response was defined as negative serum and urine immunofixation for an

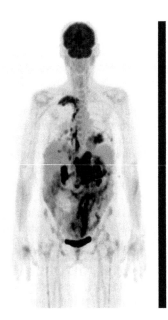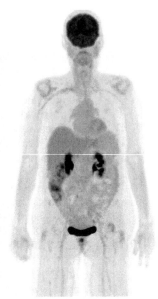

Fig. 2. A 59-year-old woman with MM, with large soft tissue mass with vascular encasement and extension to the pelvis, lytic bone lesions, and pleural involvement exhibited a remarkable response following chimeric antigen receptor (CAR) T-cell therapy.

of WBMRI versus ^{18}F FDG PET/CT in patients with MM. The study included 373 patients, and the results showed that MRI was able to detect more lesions than PET/CT, with a detection rate of 87% versus 64%, respectively. However, MRI was found to be less specific, with a specificity of 57%, compared with PET/CT, which had a specificity of 82%.[14] The lower specificity of MRI is likely due to residual anatomic changes in otherwise treated and inactive lesions. In addition to accurately identifying residual or recurrent disease, ^{18}F FDG PET/CT also offers the advantage of prompt abnormal uptake resolution. Resolution of PET uptake can occur quickly, whereas normalization of MRI signal in focal lesions can take weeks to years, depending on the size of the lesion.[41] Because of these advantages, the updated IMWG consensus published in 2016 concluded that the present data favor the use of ^{18}F FDG PET. They defined MRD negativity as the resolution of increased tracer uptake in lesions seen at baseline or a preceding PET/CT, or a decrease to a level less than the mediastinal blood pool or less than that of surrounding normal background tissue[42] (**Fig. 3**).

MONOCLONAL GAMMOPATHY OF UNDETERMINED SIGNIFICANCE

MGUS is a common asymptomatic condition that carries the risk of progression to MM. The incidence of MGUS is 3.2% in individuals aged older than 50 years and increases to 5.3% in those aged older than 70 years.[43] The risk factors for non-IgM MGUS progression to active MM include an M-protein level of 1.5 g/dL or higher and an

abnormal serum FLC ratio. IgM MGUS does not progress to MM. According to the Southeastern Minnesota cohort analysis, patients with neither risk factor had a 7% progression rate, those with one risk factor had a 20% progression rate, and those with both risk factors had a 30% progression rate during a 20-year period.[44] Given these risks, the IMWG recommends whole-body CT only for patients with high-risk MGUS. In negative cases, follow-up bone imaging is not recommended unless there are signs of disease progression,

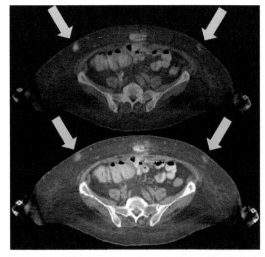

Fig. 3. A 73-year-old female with MM in complete response found to have increasing FLCs. [18]F FDG PET/CT demonstrates multiple new subcutaneous lesions, indicated by the yellow arrows, confirmed to be an extraosseous MM relapse.

such as new bone pain or an increase in serologic markers. [15] ^{18}F FDG PET/CT is the preferred next-step imaging method for investigating equivocal findings.[15]

SMOLDERING MYELOMA

Smoldering multiple myeloma (SMM) is a condition that falls between MGUS and MM. Compared with the active form of MM, SMM has a lower disease burden, with plasma cells occupying 10% to 60% of BM. SMM is highly likely to progress to MM early in the disease course at a rate of 10% per year during the first 5 years, 3% per year during the next 5 years, and 1.5% per year thereafter. Therefore, early detection of bone disease is critical.[45] IMWG recommends starting with WBCT to evaluate for osteolytic lesions or WBMRI, where identifying 2 or more focal lesions should be considered diagnostic of MM.

However, if available, ^{18}F FDG PET/CT is a viable alternative to WBCT and WBMRI. Several studies have investigated the potential value of ^{18}F FDG PET/CT in predicting disease progression in SMM with promising results. For instance, in a prospective study of 120 patients with SMM, Zamagni and colleagues found that patients with FL lesions without an osteolytic component, and thus did not meet the criteria for a CRAB feature, had a higher risk of progressing to symptomatic MM within 2 years compared with those with a negative scan (58% vs 33%). Furthermore, the risk of progression increased with the number of focal lesions identified on the scan.[46] Those findings were consistent with the findings of Siontis and colleagues, who studied a larger cohort of 188 patients with SMM and found that those with positive ^{18}F FDG PET/CT had a 75% probability of progressing to MM within 2 years, compared with 30% in patients with negative ^{18}F FDG PET/CT. The median time to progression was also significantly shorter in the ^{18}F FDG PET/CT positive group (21 months vs 60 months, respectively; $P = .0008$).[47]

SOLITARY PLASMACYTOMA

Solitary plasmacytoma (SPC) is characterized by biopsy-proven localized clonal plasma cell proliferation in bone (solitary bone plasmacytoma, SBP) or soft tissue (extramedullary plasmacytoma, EMP). SBP is more prevalent than solitary EMP, with a 40% higher incidence.[48] Additionally, SBP had a higher progression rate to MM, 35% for SBP, and 7% for EMP at 2 years. In SPC, imaging plays a crucial role in excluding additional osteolytic lesions or further soft tissue masses, which would define the progression of the disease.[49] Depending on the type of SPC, different imaging modalities are recommended. Although WBMRI or ^{18}F FDG PET/CT can be used for SBP, ^{18}F FDG PET/CT is the imaging modality of choice for EMP[15] (**Fig. 4**).

Several studies have investigated the role of ^{18}F FDG PET/CT in determining PFS in patients with SPC. The results indicate that patients with negative ^{18}F FDG PET/CT have a significantly longer PFS, whereas having 2 or more hypermetabolic lesions on ^{18}F FDG PET/CT is a documented risk factor for a significantly shorter time to transformation to MM.[50,51] In a study by Paiva and colleagues, 64 patients with SPC were followed until progression to MM, death, or the last follow-up, with a median follow-up of 3 years. The results showed that 38% of patients with SBP and 14% of EMP cases evolved into treatment-requiring MM, with 82% of total progressions observed during the first 3 years.[52]

Given these findings, the IMWG recommends yearly imaging of patients with SPC for at least 5 years using the same imaging modality (WBCT, WBMRI, or PET/CT). After 5 years, further imaging is only necessary if there is a clinical or biochemical concern for disease progression. Such an approach can help monitor patients with SPC accurately, detect disease progression early, and guide effective treatment strategies.[15]

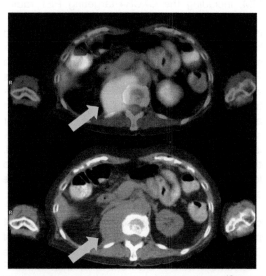

Fig. 4. A 68-year-old woman with back pain. ^{18}F FDG PET CT demonstrated a single paraspinal lesion, indicated by the yellow arrow. CT-guided lesional biopsy revealed infiltration of monoclonal cells, and after the systemic disease was excluded by BM biopsy and blood test, the patient was diagnosed with extramedullary plasmacytoma.

NOVEL IMAGING TARGETS

In the realm of management of MM, a promising new approach has gained traction involving the chemokine receptor C-X-C motif 4 (CXCR4). That receptor is found in a variety of hematopoietic cells and can bind to a protein present in the BM called CXCL12, also known as stromal cell-derived factor 1α. The CXCR4-CXCL12 interaction is critical for directing hematopoietic cells to their correct location in the BM niche; however, blocking this interaction can cause these cells to be released into the circulation.[53]

A study conducted by Bao and colleagues investigated 227 patients with MM and showed that CXCR4 upregulation in the BM was associated with prolonged survival compared with those without CXCR4 expression.[54] This finding emphasizes the importance of further research on CXCR4. Schottelius and colleagues have proposed a general direction for possible future radiotracer targeting of CXCR4. To address the marked interindividual and intraindividual differences in CXCR4 receptor expression and clonal heterogeneity, they suggest conducting further studies, preferably in vivo and with whole-body image acquisitions.[55] This approach could provide valuable insights into the potential use of CXCR4 as a target for radiotracer imaging in various malignancies, including MM.

Recent advancements in nuclear medicine have led to the development of several radiotracers for MM, including the CXCR4-targeting PET radiotracer [68]Ga PentixaFor.[55,56] This diagnostic radiopharmaceutical has been extensively tested and has a therapeutic counterpart (^{177}Lu/^{90}Y-PentixaTher). High CXCR4 expression reflected by [68]Ga PentixaFor may enable the treatment of patients with its beta-emitting equivalent, offering the potential for anti-MM activity and BM eradication. Such an approach could potentially prepare patients for stem cell transplantation and provide a longlasting effect within the stem cell niche.[57] Overall, the approach offers the potential for improved lesion identification and effective myeloablative strategies in the management of MM.

A prospective study performed a head-to-head comparison of [68]Ga PentixaFor and ^{18}F FDG in 34 patients with MM. The study found that 23 out of 34 patients (68%) showed more extensive disease involvement with [68]Ga PentixaFor than with ^{18}F FDG. Moreover, the CXCR4-directed radiopharmaceutical produced images with a higher target-to-background ratio, indicating a better image contrast. Furthermore, [68]Ga PentixaFor led to upstaging in more individuals, whereas a higher rate of downstaging was observed with ^{18}F FDG.[58] These results

suggest that CXCR4-targeted imaging with [68]Ga PentixaFor may have a potential advantage over the standard ^{18}F FDG radiotracer in identifying more extensive disease involvement and improved image contrast. Finally, as mentioned earlier, whole-body PET imaging in patients with MM should also preferably reveal intralesional and interlesional heterogeneities.[55] Additionally, the authors reported BM lesions observed with CXCR4-directed PET in 5 patients, whereas ^{18}F FDG identified such disease involvement in only 3 subjects. These findings suggest that a dual-tracer approach may provide more comprehensive information on heterogeneity at the lesion-by-lesion level in patients with MM.[58] However, despite the promising results, the wide range (21%–68%) of positive findings in patients with MM after injection of [68]Ga PentixaFor should be investigated in future studies.[59]

The potential use of CXCR4-directed PET extends beyond its ability to detect MM lesions and disease activity. A recent study explored the utility of this imaging modality in monitoring adverse events in Idecabtagen Vicleucel, a CAR T-cell therapy targeted against MM. In this study, [68]Ga PentixaFor helped differentiate between true disease progression and treatment-related adverse events, such as sarcoid-like lesions in the lung, which may seem identical on ^{18}F FDG PET.[60] Considered together, these findings highlight the diverse potential applications of CXCR4-directed PET in the management of MM, ranging from improved lesion detection in treatment-naïve patients to monitoring treatment response and adverse events in patients undergoing novel treatment regimens.

Recent studies have not only investigated the use of CXCR4 in imaging in various clinical scenarios but also explored its potential as a theranostic agent in MM. Pretherapeutic dosimetry studies have shown that after a low amount of PentixaTher injection, stable radiotracer retention in the BM can be observed. This accounts for the high doses to that organ, which can lead to high myeloablative efficacy and play a significant role in the treatment plan (**Fig. 5**).[61]

Herrmann and colleagues were among the first who conducted radioligand therapy using ^{177}Lu/^{90}Y-PentixaTher after identifying intense in vivo CXCR4 expression on [68]Ga PentixaFor PET in 3 patients with MM. Of those patients, 2 showed a significant decline in ^{18}F FDG uptake, indicating a positive treatment response.[62] In another study, 8 heavily pretreated patients with MM were scheduled for 10 RLT cycles using PentixaTher. Doses of up to 70 Gy were recorded in both intramedullary and extramedullary lesions. Complete remission was observed in 1 patient, PR in 5 patients, and 2 patients died due to complications. One patient

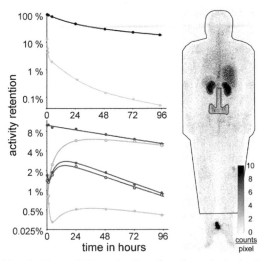

Fig. 5. The activity retention for the whole body (black), per liter of whole blood (gray), red bone marrow (BM, red), liver (green), kidneys (purple), and spleen (blue). The stable activity retention in the BM over many hours after injection of the radiotracer explains the high doses to this organ, which is a desirable phenomenon to achieve myeloablation and prepare for a subsequent conditioning regimen, followed by stem cell transplantation. (This research was originally published in JNM. Hänscheid et al, Biokinetics and Dosimetry of 177 Lu-Pentixather. Journal of Nuclear Medicine 2022;63(5):754-60. © SNMMI.)

died of sepsis during the aplastic phase, and the second patient died of tumor lysis syndrome, emphasizing the importance of implementing prophylaxis protocols to avoid such major complications.[57,63] Those cases demonstrate that PentixaTher has the potential to exert significant anti-MM activity in selected patients.

Although CXCR4 is the most widely used target for diagnostic and therapeutic applications in patients with MM, another promising approach is to leverage the widespread expression of CD38 on plasma cells. In a study by Ulaner and colleagues, the therapeutic monoclonal antibody daratumumab (anti-CD38) was labeled with zirconium-89, which allowed for the successful imaging of MM cells in both mouse models and humans.[64] In the future, comparison to ^{18}F FDG for the sensitive detection of lesions from MM should be pursued.

SUMMARY

[18]F FDG PET/CT has established itself as a valuable imaging modality in the management of MM. It plays a crucial role in the initial diagnosis, staging, prognostication, assessment of treatment response, and monitoring of minimal residual disease. [18]F FDG PET/CT allows for accurate localization of active disease, which was consistently associated with shorter PFS and OS. Looking ahead, the future of molecular imaging holds great potential in further improving the management of MM. Emerging radiotracers and novel imaging techniques may offer enhanced sensitivity and specificity, enabling more precise disease characterization and personalized treatment strategies.

CLINICS CARE POINTS

- Role of ^{18}F FDG PET/CT in initial diagnosis: [18]F FDG PET/CT is recommended as a valuable imaging modality for the evaluation of suspected MM. It provides accurate localization of abnormal hypermetabolism and active disease, detects more lesions than conventional skeletal radiography, and helps in the detection of EMD.

- Prognostic value of ^{18}F FDG PET/CT: Pretreatment ^{18}F FDG PET/CT scans at the initial diagnosis of MM can provide valuable prognostic information. The presence of 3 or more focal lesions, EMD, and high ^{18}F FDG uptake on PET/CT scans is associated with shorter PFS and OS.

- Assessment of treatment response: [18]F FDG PET/CT is a valuable tool for assessing treatment response in patients with MM. It can detect changes in tumor metabolism, which may precede morphologic changes observed in other imaging modalities. Serial PET/CT scanning at distinct time points, such as postinduction, posttransplant, and during maintenance therapy, can help determine the effectiveness of therapy and aid in tailoring individualized treatment plans for patients.

DISCLOSURE

L.B. Sólnes receives research funding from Novartis AG Pharmaceutical Company, Cellectar, Inc, and Precision Molecular, Inc. Consultant for Progenics Pharmaceuticals, Inc, R.A. Werner has received speaker honoraria from Novartis/AAA and PentixaPharm, and reports advisory board work for Novartis/AAA and Bayer. S.P. Rowe is a consultant for Progenics Pharmaceuticals, Inc and owns equity in and is a consultant for Precision Molecular, Inc

REFERENCES

1. Landgren O, Kyle RA, Pfeiffer RM, et al. Monoclonal gammopathy of undetermined significance (MGUS)

consistently precedes multiple myeloma: a prospective study. Blood 2009;113(22):5412–7.

2. Padala SA, Barsouk A, Barsouk A, et al. Epidemiology, staging, and management of multiple myeloma. Med Sci 2021;9(1):3.

3. Gulla' A, Anderson KC. Multiple myeloma: the (r) evolution of current therapy and a glance into the future. Haematologica 2020;105(10):2358–67.

4. Group TIMW. Criteria for the classification of monoclonal gammopathies, multiple myeloma and related disorders: a report of the International Myeloma Working Group. Br J Haematol 2003;121(5):749–57.

5. Rajkumar SV, Dimopoulos MA, Palumbo A, et al. International Myeloma Working Group updated criteria for the diagnosis of multiple myeloma. Lancet Oncol 2014;15(12):e538–48.

6. Kyle RA, Gertz MA, Witzig TE, et al. Review of 1027 patients with newly diagnosed multiple myeloma. Mayo Clin Proc 2003;78(1):21–33.

7. Kuroda J, Chinen Y. Multiple myeloma: pathophysiology and progress in management. Jpn J Clin Hematol 2017;58(5):487–97.

8. Mukkamalla SKR, Malipeddi D. Myeloma bone disease: a comprehensive review. Int J Mol Sci 2021;22(12):6208.

9. Regelink JC, Minnema MC, Terpos E, et al. Comparison of modern and conventional imaging techniques in establishing multiple myeloma-related bone disease: a systematic review. Br J Haematol 2013;162(1):50–61.

10. Hur J, Yoon CS, Ryu YH, et al. Efficacy of multidetector row computed tomography of the spine in patients with multiple myeloma: comparison with magnetic resonance imaging and fluorodeoxyglucose-positron emission tomography. J Comput Assist Tomogr 2007;31(3):342–7.

11. Zamagni E, Nanni C, Patriarca F, et al. A prospective comparison of 18F-fluorodeoxyglucose positron emission tomography-computed tomography, magnetic resonance imaging and whole-body planar radiographs in the assessment of bone disease in newly diagnosed multiple myeloma. Haematologica 2007;92(1):50–5.

12. Hur J, Yoon CS, Ryu YH, et al. Comparative study of fluorodeoxyglucose positron emission tomography and magnetic resonance imaging for the detection of spinal bone marrow infiltration in untreated patients with multiple myeloma. Acta Radiol Stockh Swed 1987 2008;49(4):427–35.

13. Fonti R, Salvatore B, Quarantelli M, et al. 18F-FDG PET/CT, 99mTc-MIBI, and MRI in evaluation of patients with multiple myeloma. J Nucl Med Off Publ Soc Nucl Med 2008;49(2):195–200.

14. Rama S, Suh CH, Kim KW, et al. Comparative performance of whole-body MRI and FDG PET/CT in evaluation of multiple myeloma treatment response: systematic review and meta-analysis. Am J Roentgenol 2022;218(4):602–13.

15. Hillengass J, Usmani S, Rajkumar SV, et al. International myeloma working group consensus recommendations on imaging in monoclonal plasma cell disorders. Lancet Oncol 2019;20(6):e302–12.

16. Durie BG, Salmon SE. A clinical staging system for multiple myeloma. Correlation of measured myeloma cell mass with presenting clinical features, response to treatment, and survival. Cancer 1975;36(3):842–54.

17. Greipp PR, Miguel JS, Durie BGM, et al. International staging system for multiple myeloma. J Clin Oncol 2005;23(15):3412–20.

18. Palumbo A, Avet-Loiseau H, Oliva S, et al. Revised international staging system for multiple myeloma: a report from international myeloma working group. J Clin Oncol 2015;33(26):2863–9.

19. Jung SH, Kwon SY, Min JJ, et al. 18F-FDG PET/CT is useful for determining survival outcomes of patients with multiple myeloma classified as stage II and III with the Revised International Staging System. Eur J Nucl Med Mol Imag 2019;46(1):107–15.

20. Han S, Woo S, Kim Y il, et al. Prognostic value of 18F-fluorodeoxyglucose positron emission tomography/computed tomography in newly diagnosed multiple myeloma: a systematic review and meta-analysis. Eur Radiol 2021;31(1):152–62.

21. Bartel TB, Haessler J, Brown TLY, et al. F18-fluorodeoxyglucose positron emission tomography in the context of other imaging techniques and prognostic factors in multiple myeloma. Blood 2009;114(10):2068–76.

22. Nanni C, Zamagni E, Versari A, et al. Image interpretation criteria for FDG PET/CT in multiple myeloma: a new proposal from an Italian expert panel. IMPeTUs (Italian Myeloma criteria for PET USe). Eur J Nucl Med Mol Imag 2016;43(3):414–21.

23. Sachpekidis C, Merz M, Raab MS, et al. The prognostic significance of [18F]FDG PET/CT in multiple myeloma according to novel interpretation criteria (IMPeTUs). EJNMMI Res 2021;11(1):100.

24. Nanni C, Versari A, Chauvie S, et al. Interpretation criteria for FDG PET/CT in multiple myeloma (IMPeTUs): final results. IMPeTUs (Italian myeloma criteria for PET USe). Eur J Nucl Med Mol Imag 2018;45(5):712–9.

25. Davies FE, Rosenthal A, Rasche L, et al. Treatment to suppression of focal lesions on positron emission tomography-computed tomography is a therapeutic goal in newly diagnosed multiple myeloma. Haematologica 2018;103(6):1047–53.

26. Fermand JP, Levy Y, Gerota J, et al. Treatment of aggressive multiple myeloma by high-dose chemotherapy and total body irradiation followed by blood stem cells autologous graft. Blood 1989;73(1):20–3.

27. Yee GC, McGuire TR. Allogeneic bone marrow transplantation in the treatment of hematologic diseases. Clin Pharm 1985;4(2):149–60.

28. Al Hamed R, Bazarbachi AH, Malard F, et al. Current status of autologous stem cell transplantation for multiple myeloma. Blood Cancer J 2019;9(4):44.

29. Dhakal B, Vesole DH, Hari PN. Allogeneic stem cell transplantation for multiple myeloma: is there a future? Bone Marrow Transplant 2016;51(4):492–500.

30. Sobh M, Michallet M, Gahrton G, et al. Allogeneic hematopoietic cell transplantation for multiple myeloma in Europe: trends and outcomes over 25 years. A study by the EBMT Chronic Malignancies Working Party. Leukemia 2016;30(10):2047–54.

31. Patriarca F, Carobolante F, Zamagni E, et al. The role of positron emission tomography with 18F-fluoro-deoxyglucose integrated with computed tomography in the evaluation of patients with multiple myeloma undergoing allogeneic stem cell transplantation. Biol Blood Marrow Transplant J Am Soc Blood Marrow Transplant 2015;21(6):1068–73.

32. Stolzenburg A, Lückerath K, Samnick S, et al. Prognostic value of [18F]FDG-PET/CT in multiple myeloma patients before and after allogeneic hematopoietic cell transplantation. Eur J Nucl Med Mol Imag 2018;45(10):1694–704.

33. Kumar S, Flinn I, Richardson PG, et al. Randomized, multicenter, phase 2 study (EVOLUTION) of combinations of bortezomib, dexamethasone, cyclophosphamide, and lenalidomide in previously untreated multiple myeloma. Blood 2012;119(19):4375–82.

34. Attal M, Lauwers-Cances V, Marit G, et al. Lenalidomide maintenance after stem-cell transplantation for multiple myeloma. N Engl J Med 2012;366(19):1782–91.

35. McCarthy PL, Owzar K, Hofmeister CC, et al. Lenalidomide after stem-cell transplantation for multiple myeloma. N Engl J Med 2012;366(19):1770–81.

36. Jakubowiak AJ, Dytfeld D, Griffith KA, et al. A phase 1/2 study of carfilzomib in combination with lenalidomide and low-dose dexamethasone as a frontline treatment for multiple myeloma. Blood 2012;120(9):1801–9.

37. Cavo M, Terpos E, Nanni C, et al. Role of 18F-FDG PET/CT in the diagnosis and management of multiple myeloma and other plasma cell disorders: a consensus statement by the International Myeloma Working Group. Lancet Oncol 2017;18(4):e206–17.

38. Rajkumar SV, Harousseau JL, Durie B, et al. Consensus recommendations for the uniform reporting of clinical trials: report of the International Myeloma Workshop Consensus Panel 1. Blood 2011;117(18):4691–5.

39. Charalampous C, Goel U, Broski SM, et al. Utility of PET/CT in assessing early treatment response in patients with newly diagnosed multiple myeloma. Blood Adv 2022;6(9):2763–72.

40. Derlin T, Weber C, Habermann CR, et al. 18F-FDG PET/CT for detection and localization of residual or recurrent disease in patients with multiple myeloma after stem cell transplantation. Eur J Nucl Med Mol Imag 2012;39(3):493–500.

41. Walker RC, Brown TL, Jones-Jackson LB, et al. Imaging of multiple myeloma and related plasma cell dyscrasias. J Nucl Med 2012;53(7):1091–101.

42. Kumar S, Paiva B, Anderson KC, et al. International Myeloma Working Group consensus criteria for response and minimal residual disease assessment in multiple myeloma. Lancet Oncol 2016;17(8):e328–46.

43. Kyle RA, Therneau TM, Rajkumar SV, et al. Prevalence of monoclonal gammopathy of undetermined significance. N Engl J Med 2006;354(13):1362–9.

44. Kyle RA, Larson DR, Therneau TM, et al. Long-term follow-up of monoclonal gammopathy of undetermined significance. N Engl J Med 2018;378(3):241–9.

45. Rajkumar SV, Landgren O, Mateos MV. Smoldering multiple myeloma. Blood 2015;125(20):3069–75.

46. Zamagni E, Nanni C, Gay F, et al. 18F-FDG PET/CT focal, but not osteolytic, lesions predict the progression of smoldering myeloma to active disease. Leukemia 2016;30(2):417–22.

47. Siontis B, Kumar S, Dispenzieri A, et al. Positron emission tomography-computed tomography in the diagnostic evaluation of smoldering multiple myeloma: identification of patients needing therapy. Blood Cancer J 2015;5(10):e364.

48. Dores GM, Landgren O, McGlynn KA, et al. Plasmacytoma of bone, extramedullary plasmacytoma, and multiple myeloma: incidence and survival in the United States, 1992-2004. Br J Haematol 2009;144(1):86–94.

49. Nahi H, Genell A, Wålinder G, et al. Incidence, characteristics, and outcome of solitary plasmacytoma and plasma cell leukemia. Population-based data from the Swedish Myeloma Register. Eur J Haematol 2017;99(3):216–22.

50. Warsame R, Gertz MA, Lacy MQ, et al. Trends and outcomes of modern staging of solitary plasmacytoma of bone. Am J Hematol 2012;87(7):647–51.

51. Fouquet G, Guidez S, Herbaux C, et al. Impact of initial FDG-PET/CT and serum-free light chain on transformation of conventionally defined solitary plasmacytoma to multiple myeloma. Clin Cancer Res Off J Am Assoc Cancer Res 2014;20(12):3254–60.

52. Paiva B, Chandia M, Vidriales MB, et al. Multiparameter flow cytometry for staging of solitary bone plasmacytoma: new criteria for risk of progression to myeloma. Blood 2014;124(8):1300–3.

53. Bao L, Lai Y, Liu Y, et al. CXCR4 is a good survival prognostic indicator in multiple myeloma patients. Leuk Res 2013;37(9):1083–8.

54. Chatterjee S, Behnam Azad B, Nimmagadda S. The intricate role of CXCR4 in cancer. Adv Cancer Res 2014;124:31–82.

55. Schottelius M, Herrmann K, Lapa C. In Vivo targeting of CXCR4-new horizons. Cancers 2021;13(23):5920.

56. Poty S, Désogère P, Nicholson K, et al. New imaging agents targeting chemokine receptor CXCR4 for PET/SPECT and MRI. EJNMMI Phys 2014;1(Suppl 1):A81.

57. Buck AK, Serfling SE, Lindner T, et al. CXCR4-targeted theranostics in oncology. Eur J Nucl Med Mol Imag 2022;49(12):4133–44.

58. Shekhawat AS, Singh B, Malhotra P, et al. Imaging CXCR4 receptors expression for staging multiple myeloma by using 68Ga-Pentixafor PET/CT: comparison with 18F-FDG PET/CT. Br J Radiol 2022;95(1136):20211272.

59. Lapa C, Schreder M, Schirbel A, et al. [68Ga]Pentixafor-PET/CT for imaging of chemokine receptor CXCR4 expression in multiple myeloma - comparison to [18F]FDG and laboratory values. Theranostics 2017;7(1):205–12.

60. Leipold AM, Werner RA, Düll J, et al. Th17.1 cell driven sarcoidosis-like inflammation after anti-BCMA CAR T cells in multiple myeloma. Leukemia 2023;37(3):650–8.

61. Hänscheid H, Schirbel A, Hartrampf P, et al. Biokinetics and dosimetry of 177Lu-pentixather. J Nucl Med Off Publ Soc Nucl Med 2022;63(5):754–60.

62. Herrmann K, Schottelius M, Lapa C, et al. First-in-Human experience of CXCR4-directed endoradiotherapy with 177Lu- and 90Y-labeled pentixather in advanced-stage multiple myeloma with extensive intra- and extramedullary disease. J Nucl Med Off Publ Soc Nucl Med 2016;57(2):248–51.

63. Lapa C, Herrmann K, Schirbel A, et al. CXCR4-directed endoradiotherapy induces high response rates in extramedullary relapsed Multiple Myeloma. Theranostics 2017;7(6):1589–97.

64. Cartia GL. [Evaluation of the effects of thymopentin on the incidence of leucopenia in patients treated with chemotherapy for breast carcinoma]. Minerva Med 1990;81(11):815–7.

Clinical Positron Emission Tomography/Computed Tomography
Quarter-Century Transformation of Prostate Cancer Molecular Imaging

David C. Chen, BMedSc[a,b], Siyu Huang, MD[c], James P. Buteau, MD[a,b],
Raghava Kashyap, MD[a,b], Michael S. Hofman, MBBS[a,b],*

KEYWORDS

- Radiopharmaceuticals • Radiotracers • Prostate-specific membrane antigen • PSMA • PET
- PET/CT

INTRODUCTION

Prostate cancer (CaP) is the second most common cancer diagnosis and fifth most common cause of death in men worldwide.[1,2] The disease course can vary from indolent to highly aggressive metastatic cancer that may develop resistance to hormonal or other systemic therapies.[3] Around 5% to 10% of patients in the United States are diagnosed with de novo metastatic cancer at first presentation, with bone and distant lymph nodes being the most common sites of metastasis.[4,5]

Positron emission tomography (PET) imaging represents a paradigm shift in CaP compared with conventional computed tomography (CT), magnetic resonance imaging (MRI) and bone scintigraphy modalities, and now plays a fundamental role in clinical decision-making.[6,7] In the last quarter of a century, PET imaging has advanced dramatically to become a pillar of cancer imaging. Implementation in CaP, however, has come relatively late compared with many other tumor types (**Table 1**). Radiolabeled peptide-like small molecules that bind prostate-specific membrane antigen (PSMA) have now transitioned into clinical practice and the role of PET imaging in CaP cannot be understated. The current renaissance of PET in CaP is principally driven by the exponential growth in PSMA ligand research. However, the role of other tracers is still of great interest.

The aim of this review is to highlight the milestone events of the past quarter century and the development of tracers in the imaging of CaP with PET/CT technology.

BEFORE THE ERA OF PROSTATE-SPECIFIC MEMBRANE ANTIGEN
Fluorine-18-Sodium-Fluoride

Fluorine-18-sodium-fluoride (^{18}F-NaF) was first described by Blau and colleagues in 1962 to be a bone-seeking agent with 10 times higher uptake in areas of increased bone formation compared with normal bone.[8] Fluoride ions are deposited in the bone matrix and enable imaging of osteoblastic activity.[9] Given significant burden of bone involvement in metastatic prostate cancer (mCaP), ^{18}F-NaF offered a molecular basis for identifying advanced disease.[5,10] However, as gamma cameras became ubiquitous in the 1970s, Technetium-99m (^{99m}Tc)-

[a] Prostate Cancer Theranostics and Imaging Centre of Excellence, Molecular Imaging and Therapeutic Nuclear Medicine, Cancer Imaging, Peter MacCallum Cancer Centre, Melbourne, Victoria, Australia; [b] Sir Peter MacCallum Department of Oncology, University of Melbourne, Melbourne, Victoria, Australia; [c] Department of Surgery, The University of Melbourne
* Corresponding author. Department of Cancer Imaging, Peter MacCallum Cancer Centre, 305 Grattan Street, Melbourne, Victoria 3052, Australia.
E-mail address: michael.hofman@petermac.org

PET Clin 19 (2024) 261–279
https://doi.org/10.1016/j.cpet.2023.12.011
1556-8598/24/© 2023 Elsevier Inc. All rights reserved.

Table 1
Timeline of landmark events in the development of prostate cancer molecular imaging tracers

Year	Significant Event in CaP Molecular Imaging Tracer Development
1962	Blau et al. first described the use of ^{18}F-NaF
1973	Advent of PET/CT saw a re-emerging interest in ^{18}F-NaF
1987	Horoszewicz et al. discovers specific prostate antigenic marker
1993	The PSMA gene is cloned for the first time at MSKCC
1996	^{111}In-Capromab is the first FDA-approved CaP molecular imaging agent
1997	J591 antibody is identified by Bander et al. to target extracellular epitopes
1998	Hara et al. demonstrate first application of ^{11}C-choline
	Heston and O'Keefe identify the molecular structure of PSMA
2004	Urea-based PSMA inhibitors under investigation
2011	^{11}C-choline demonstrated to assess ADT treatment response
2013	First reports of ^{68}Ga-PSMA-11 from Heidelberg, Germany
2019	Fendler et al. trial results on the role of ^{68}Ga-PSMA-11 in BCR published
2020	Hofman et al. trial (proPSMA) results published, ^{68}Ga-PSMA-11 PET/CT superior to conventional imaging (bone scan, CT)
	^{68}Ga-PSMA-11 as a tracer is FDA approved
2021	^{18}F-DCFPyL is FDA approved
	Hope et al. trial results on the role of ^{68}Ga-PSMA-11 in primary staging published
	Morris et al. trial (CONDOR) results on the role of ^{18}F-DCFPyL in BCR published
	Pienta et al. trial (OSPREY) results on the role of ^{18}F-DCFPyL in primary staging published
2023	^{18}F-rhPSMA-7.3 is FDA approved

labeled bisphosphonates including methylene diphosphonate (MDP) and hydroxy diphosphonate largely replaced the use of ^{18}F-NaF.[11]

The increasing availability of hybrid PET/CT from the late 1970s onwards saw a resurgence of interest in ^{18}F-NaF for functional skeletal imaging.[12]

[18]F-NaF PET/CT proved to be more sensitive and specific than planar or single photon emission computed tomography (SPECT)/CT bone scanning in differentiating between benign and malignant bone metastasis (**Fig. 1**).[13,14] Sheikhbahaei and colleagues highlighted in a 6 study meta-analysis the superior sensitivity and specificity of ^{18}F-NaF compared with ^{99m}Tc bone scintigraphy both on a per-patient (AUC 0.990 vs 0.842, $P < .001$, n = 148), and per-lesion level analysis (AUC 0.998 vs 0.771, $P < .001$, n = 744).[15] Radiotracer uptake alone, however, is insufficient to delineate benign disease and malignant metastasis, thus consequent anatomic correlation is necessary.[16]

In the setting of biochemical recurrence (BCR), ^{18}F-NaF may localize occult bone metastases. Within a limited prospective study of 37 patients, Jadvar and colleagues found 6 patients with bone metastases and biochemical failure. Additionally, detection rates increased with increasing prostate-specific antigen (PSA) levels.[17] ^{18}F-NaF PET/CT also can assess suitability and therapeutic efficacy of Radium-223 dichloride ([223]Ra) alpha particle therapy for metastatic castration-resistant prostate cancer (mCRPC) in the treatment of bone metastasis.[18-20]

Fluorine-18 or Carbon-11 Choline Derivatives

Fluorine-18 (^{18}F) or Carbon-11 (^{11}C)-labeled choline-derived tracers for PET imaging have been used for investigation of primary or recurrent CaP.[21-23] In 1998, Hara and colleagues highlighted the first application of ^{11}C-choline PET, harnessing the increased expression of choline kinase and phospholipase enzymes in CaP comparative to normal tissue.[22] Increased activity of phospholipid biosynthesis and degradation pathways leads to an elevated turnover of phosphatidylcholine. Given that choline is a precursor to phosphatidylcholine, this heightened flux of radiolabeled choline accumulates in CaP cells and thus suitable for PET imaging.[24]

[11]C-choline exhibits rapid and selective uptake in CaP cells. In a systematic review of ^{18}F or ^{11}C-choline PET, Evangelista and colleagues highlighted the detection rate of CaP across 9 studies in initial staging ranged between 11% and 100%, with high variability between intraprostatic primary cancer, lymph node metastases or occult bone metastasis. It should be noted that the difference in detection rate is not related to serum PSA before radical prostatectomy but most likely linked to baseline characteristics including disease staging and International Society of Urological Pathology (ISUP) grade group.[25] Compared with conventional imaging with bone scan and contrast-enhanced CT

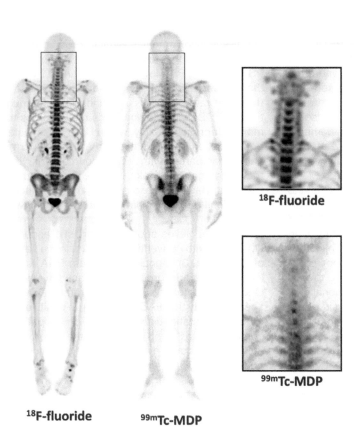

Fig. 1. Superior resolution of ^{18}F-NaF PET/CT for imaging bone compared with ^{99m}Tc-MDP.

[18]F-fluoride

^{99m}Tc-MDP

[18]F-fluoride   ^{99m}Tc-MDP

in bone metastases, ^{18}F-choline PET/CT was more sensitive (Choline PET: 100% vs CT: 46.2%, BS: 90%) and specific (Choline PET: 92.3% vs CT: 92.3%, BS: 77.2%). Similar results were found comparing MRI to ^{18}F or ^{11}C-choline PET/CT (Sensitivity of Choline PET or PET/CT: 9.4%–78% vs 18.8%–57.1%, specificity of Choline PET or PET/CT: 86.4%–92.3% vs DWI-MRI: 77.2%–92.3%) in nodal staging.[26–29]

At restaging, the detection rate for choline PET varies depending on sites of recurrence and serum PSA levels. However, in a retrospective study by Michaud and colleagues, they suggested that even at low serum PSA levels of less than 0.5 ng/mL, choline PET is effective in detecting CaP recurrence with a detection rate of 28%.[30–32] Detection rate for skeletal metastases and metastatic lymph nodes are reported to be approximately 20% to 50%, and 30%, respectively.[33–35] Choline PET is more specific than conventional imaging when assessing bone metastases.[36] However, depending on the per-lesion characteristics, the uptake of choline may be variable. Van den Berg and colleagues reported that the sensitivity of detecting intraprostatic lesions is reported to be superior in choline PET compared with MRI (Choline PET: 77% [at

maximum standardized uptake value (SUVmax) cut off 2.7] vs MRI: 34%) in local recurrences.[37]

Beyond initial and secondary staging, choline PET can contribute to salvage radiation planning and treatment response assessment. Given the increased sensitivity of identifying lymph node metastasis on choline PET, radiation therapy planning changes 10% to 15% across various studies and may be useful in dose escalation.[38,39] In 2011, Fuccio and colleagues first reported the role of ^{11}C-choline PET assessing response to androgen deprivation therapy (ADT) in 14 patients with BCR.[40] Fuccio's findings and consequent studies highlighted the relationship between metabolic choline pathways and a biochemical serum PSA response with systemic treatments in patients with hormone-sensitive or castration-resistant CaP.[25,41,42]

2-Fluorine-18-Fluoro-2-Deoxy-D-Glucose

First described by Warburg, cancer cells are known to have a greater glucose uptake due to increased glycolysis.[43] Applying this concept, 2-fluorine-18-fluoro-2-deoxy-D-glucose (^{18}F-FDG), a radiolabeled glucose derivative, became the most commonly used radiotracer in cancer detection. However, the role of ^{18}F-FDG PET/CT is perceived to be limited in CaP due to the lower rate of glucose metabolism compared with other tumor types, especially in hormone-sensitive CaP.[44] With higher ISUP grade group, castration resistance or metastasis, ^{18}F-FDG uptake also increases because of higher metabolic demand. Beauregard and colleagues demonstrate a prognostic role for ^{18}F-FDG PET/CT in staging in high-risk CaP.[45]

Beyond the limitations of CaP in diagnosis and restaging, ^{18}F-FDG PET/CT can assess for discordant metastases compared with PSMA PET/CT (FDG positive/PSMA negative) before radioligand therapy (RLT) in patients with mCRPC. This strategy identifies ineligible patients with poor prognosis, avoiding futile RLT and redirecting toward more appropriate management.[46] Additionally, in a prespecified imaging biomarker analysis of the prospective TheraP trial, a metabolic tumor volume of 200 mL or greater on ^{18}F-FDG PET/CT was prognostic for worse outcomes regardless if patients received cabazitaxel or Lutetium-177 (^{177}Lu)-PSMA-617.[47] This readily available prognostic biomarker identifies a group of patients who may benefit most from treatment intensification, such as combination treatments.

Anti-1-Amino-3-Fluorine-18-Fluorocyclobutane-1-Carboxylic Acid or ^{18}F-Fluciclovine

In 2016, the Food and Drug Administration (FDA) approved ^{18}F-fluciclovine (FACBC) for the detection of CaP recurrence. FACBC is a leucine amino acid analog, which is overexpressed in CaP and absorbed via amino acid transporters (Fig. 2). Comparative to conventional bone scans, FACBC has the ability to detect bone metastasis and also soft tissue involvement.[48] Similar to other tracers, FACBC detection rate improves with higher serum PSA levels. At PSA levels of less than 1, 1 to less than 2, and 2 ng/mL or greater, FACBC had a detection rate of 72%, 83%, and 100%, respectively.[48-50] Because amino acids move across tumor membranes rapidly within 4 to 10 minutes post-injection, images can be obtained within 5 minutes compared with FDG counterparts that require images to be taken 45 to 90 minutes post-injection. A fasting state of at least 4 hours is necessary to limit free serum amino acid competing with FACBC.

FACBC achieves superior diagnostic accuracy compared with conventional imaging in the setting of BCR (Fig. 3). Agnostic to serum PSA levels, initial ISUP grade group or PSA doubling times, Odewole and colleagues demonstrated in a retrospective study that FACBC had a true positive rate for extraprostatic disease in 12 of 53 patients compared with 3 of 53 patients for the CT group.[51] Further prospective evidence from the multicenter, phase III FALCON trial highlighted that 52 of 85 patients had revised treatment plans secondary to FACBC findings for salvage radiotherapy.[52] In patients who underwent significant management changes, 60% shifted from radiotherapy to systemic treatment or watchful waiting. The remaining 40% of changed management involved modifying initial radiotherapy plans including boosts to prostate beds. Such accuracy in a salvage setting lends the tracer to significantly change radiotherapy management decision post-RP with BCR.

FACBC seems to be a better correlate with PSA response than conventional imaging in CT or bone scan. In the context of mCRPC under treatment with docetaxel, FACBC uptake correlated with PSA change after 1 and 6 cycles of docetaxel

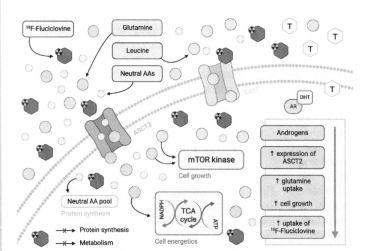

Fig. 2. FACBC uptake with illustrated changes of associated metabolic and androgenic pathways. AA, amino acids; AR, androgen receptor; ASCT2, alanine, serine, cysteine transporter 2; ATP, adenosine triphosphate; DHT, dihydrogentestosterone; LAT1, L-type amino acid transporter 1; mTOR kinase, mammalian target of rapamycin kinase; NADPH, nicotinamide adenine dinucleotide phosphate; T, testosterone; TCA cycle, tricarboxylic acid cycle.

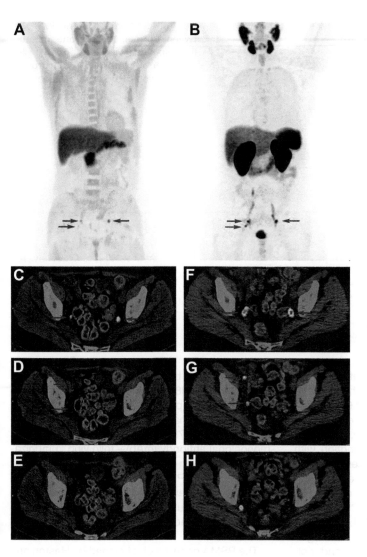

Fig. 3. Comparative FACBC and ^{68}Ga-PSMA-11 PET/CT of a patient with BCR (PSA 12 ng/mL) with 1-week interval between scans. FACBC PET maximum intensity projection (MIP) (*A*) and PET/CT (*C–E*) images show physiologic distribution of this tracer and increased uptake in bilateral subcentimeter pelvic LNs (*arrows*). ^{68}Ga-PSMA-11 PET MIP (*B*) and PET/CT (*F–H*) images demonstrate bilateral pelvic LNs (*arrows*) with 2- to 3-fold higher tumor-to-background contrast and maximum standardized uptake value range of 7 to 19 compared with 3 to 9 in FACBC. (Reproduced with permission.[149])

in an exploratory analysis.[48] SUVmax, mean standardized uptake value (SUVmean), and peak standardized uptake value (SUVpeak) were higher in patients who experienced disease progression than those who had a favorable response after 6 cycles of docetaxel, with a 75% correlation of PET with PSA response in these patients with mCRPC.

[18]F-Fluoro-5α-Dihydrotestosterone

Since Huggins' first discovery of CaP and its hormone-dependent nature, ADT and more recently androgen-receptor (AR) pathway inhibitors have been widely used to target the AR signaling axis.[53] Contemporary understanding of castration resistance is thought to be a result of amplified AR gene mutations or ligand-independent AR activation through cytokines and extraneous growth factors rather than a loss of AR expression. AR

continues to be expressed in virtually all mCRPC.[54,55] Clearly, in vivo AR signaling pathways studies are needed to better understand the development of CaP at its various disease stages and for the assessment of treatment response.

The initial assessment of ^{18}F-fluoro-5α-dihydrotestosterone (^{18}F-FDHT) reported by Scher and colleagues in 2004 with a prospective cohort of 7 men with mCaP provided feasibility into a new AR ligand tracer.[56] Consequently, in 2005, a larger prospective cohort of 20 men was reported by Dehdashti and colleagues to further validate binding selectivity.[57] The team identified ^{18}F-FDHT to be of high affinity for ARs, in line with the tracer's chemical similarity to DHT (**Fig. 4**). Biodistribution and degrees of estimated radiation exposure were first measured on baboon prostates. Although ^{18}F-FDG is more sensitive for CaP detection, ^{18}F-FDHT has superior clinical relevance for measuring

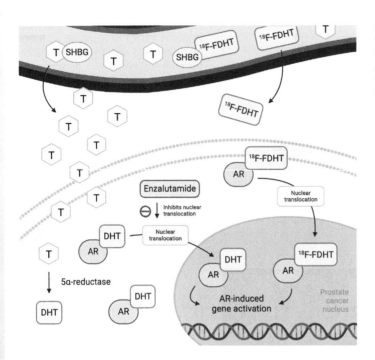

Fig. 4. Identifying interactions between normal testosterone metabolisms in CaP cells and ^{18}F-FDHT. AR, androgen receptor; DHT, dihydrogentestosterone; SHBG, sex hormone binding globulin; T, testosterone.

treatment response (^{18}F-FDG sensitivity: 96% vs ^{18}F-FDHT sensitivity: 86%).[56] Dehdashti and colleagues reported a lower sensitivity of 63%; however, positive PET findings were correlated with increased PSA levels.[57] More recently, ^{18}F-FDHT PET/CT has also been used in conjunction with ^{18}F-FDG PET/CT to assess for the presence of concurrent AR and glycolytic lesions as an imaging phenotype and their negative impact on survival with AR pathway inhibitors resistance.[58]

A great potential of ^{18}F-FDHT PET/CT lies in assessing treatment response to antiandrogen therapy. Published in 2010 by Scher and colleagues, the initial phase I/II study assessed the antitumor effect of enzalutamide or MDV3100 in men with mCRPC regardless of chemotherapy resistance or sensitivity. ^{18}F-FDHT PET/CT was fundamental in measuring pre-enzalutamide and post-enzalutamide AR saturation, ultimately providing insight to drug dosing.[59] In the recent years, Hoving and colleagues demonstrated in a pilot study of 18 men with chemotherapy-naive mCRPC, that baseline ^{18}F-FDHT PET/CT using SUVpeak of all metastatic sites predicts enzalutamide treatment response.[60]

DEVELOPMENT OF PROSTATE-SPECIFIC MEMBRANE ANTIGEN
Prostate-Specific Membrane Antigen Discovery and Development of Antibodies

The current success of theranostics and oncologic PSMA imaging would not be a reality without high-quality, rigorous basic science research from the late 1980s. In 1987, Horoszewicz and colleagues established the potential of a specific antigenic marker to CaP that may have clinical impact. The team isolated 7E11-C5—a immunoglobulin G monoclonal antibody (mAb)—following immunization of mice with CaP lymph node cells isolated from human CaP.[61] Through immunoperoxidase staining, Horoszewicz and colleagues recognized that 7E11-C5 could identify an antigen expressed at highly elevated levels in neoplastic cells and metastases.

The PSMA gene was first cloned by Heston and Fair's group at Memorial Sloan Kettering (MSKCC) in 1993 using 7E11-C5 (Capromab).[62,63] Consequently in 1996, Capromab was used in the form of ^{111}In-capromab as the first US FDA approved molecular imaging agent targeting PSMA with a sensitivity of a sensitivity and specificity of 62% and 72%, respectively, in the setting of primary staging.[64–69] However, Capromab is limited to targeting intracellular PSMA epitopes, binding only to dying or dead cells. Given that mCaP bone metastases are often highly vascular, 7E11-C5 has relatively poor performance as an imaging agent.[61,70] This is further exacerbated in the context of stand-alone SPECT imaging if lacking transmission attenuation correction or precise anatomic correlation without CT.

In attempts to combat limitations of Capromab, Bander and colleagues in 1997 developed an antibody, J591, to target extracellular epitopes of PSMA (**Fig. 5**). Liu and Bander's team reported

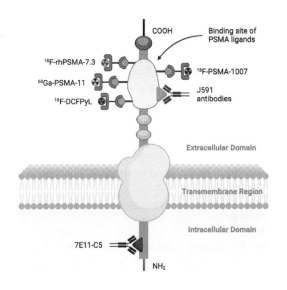

Fig. 5. PSMA representation at a molecular level. COOH, carboxylic acid; NH₂, amino group.

that viable CaP lymph node cells can internalize J591.[71] Ahead of their time, the authors remarked that this characteristic enables for "novel therapeutic methods to target the delivery of toxins, drugs, or short-range isotopes into the interior of CaP cells" heralding the next era of PSMA-based therapies.

In an attempt to further understanding of the extracellular epitope, Heston and O'Keefe in 1998 identified PSMA as a 100-kDA type II transmembrane protein with folate and N-acetyl-alpha-linked-acidic-dipeptidase (NAALADase) activity (see **Fig. 6**).[72] Although both PSMA and NAADLADase describe the same glycoprotein, the former is used in CaP oncology with the latter used primarily in neuroscience.

PSMA expression is elevated in benign prostatic hyperplasia, however, increasingly upregulated with malignant changes. With increasing ISUP grade group, CaP can increase in PSMA expression to upwards of a 1000 times.[73–76] PSMA is physiologically distributed in other areas including the jejunal brush border, nervous system astrocytes and schwann cells, proximal renal tubules, salivary glands, and neovasculature of epithelial malignancies.[73,75–77] Despite characterizing PSMA function in the brain and jejunal brush border, the functional role of PSMA in the prostatic epithelium and renal proximal tubules has still not been well defined.

Prostate-Specific Membrane Antigen-Based Tracers for Imaging

Contemporary CaP imaging uses small molecules over antibodies given superior qualities as an

imaging tracer (**Table 2** and **Fig. 6**). Antibodies have a long circulating half-life to clear from nontarget tissues, thus creating low signal/noise ratios, needing around 3 days between antibody injection and imaging.[78] Peptides and small molecules (**Fig. 7**) greatly reduce this clinical delay, overall costs involved and are less likely to undergo cross-reactivity leading to increased false-positive rates.[79]

Gallium-68-Prostate Specific Membrane Antigen-11

Although urea-based PSMA inhibitors were first reported in 2001, preclinical and clinical development occurred in the later parts of the 2000s and early 2010s. The initial experience and preclinical assessment of gallium-68-PSMA-11 (^{68}Ga-PSMA-11), also known as [[68] Ga]Glu-Urea-Lys(Ahx)-HBED-CC, were first reported clinically in 2013.[80–83] Two pivotal studies validated the approval of ^{68}Ga-PSMA-11 in the staging and BCR setting. In a staging setting, Hope and colleagues prospectively recruited 277 patients in a single-arm trial who underwent radical prostatectomy.[84] Additionally, Hope and colleagues reported sensitivity and specificity for pelvic nodal metastases to be 40% and 95%, respectively. Fendler and colleagues, prospectively recruited 635 patients with BCR after definitive treatment in a single-arm trial. The team found a sensitivity of 90% to 92% and a 92% positive predictive value (PPV) by composite reference standard.[85]

In 2020, Hofman and colleagues published results to the proPSMA trial—a multicenter, two-arm, randomized study investigating whether novel imaging using ^{68}Ga-PSMA-11 PET/CT for staging may improve accuracy and affect management compared with CT and bone scan in men with biopsy-proven CaP and high-risk features.[86] The study found that ^{68}Ga-PSMA-11 PET had a 27% greater accuracy. ^{68}Ga-PSMA-11 PET/CT superiority in detecting lymph node metastases was demonstrated when compared with conventional imaging at 97% to 65%, respectively.

In December 2020, ^{68}Ga-PSMA-11 was the first FDA-approved PSMA-targeted tracer for men with CaP. From 2012, in the lead up to FDA approval, more than 1700 studies were published on PSMA PET.[78] As the most extensively studied and ubiquitous tracer, ^{68}Ga-PSMA-11 was proven in a high-volume meta-analysis to have a high sensitivity (80%) and specificity (97%) in detecting CaP in a BCR setting.[87]

As robust clinical trials and results are published, PSMA PET for initial staging with suspected metastasis has been widely accepted both clinically and

Table 2
Appropriate use criteria for prostate-specific membrane antigen PET imaging[99]

Scenario	Description	Appropriateness	Score
1	Patients with suspected CaP (eg, high/increasing PSA levels, abnormal digital rectal examination results) evaluated for targeted biopsy, and detection of intraprostatic tumor	Rarely appropriate	3
2	Patients with very-low risk, low-risk, and favorable intermediate-risk CaP	Rarely appropriate	2
3	Newly diagnosed unfavorable intermediate-risk, high-risk, or very-high-risk CaP	Appropriate	8
4	Newly diagnosed unfavorable intermediate-risk, high-risk, or very-high-risk CaP with negative/equivocal or oligometastatic disease on conventional imaging	Appropriate	8
5	Newly diagnosed CaP with widespread metastatic disease on conventional imaging	May be appropriate	4
6	PSA persistence or PSA rise from undetectable level after radical prostatectomy	Appropriate	9
7	PSA rise above nadir after definitive radiotherapy	Appropriate	9
8	PSA rise after focal therapy of the primary tumor	May be appropriate	5
9	nmCRPC (M0) on conventional imaging	Appropriate	7
10	Posttreatment PSA increase in the mCRPC setting	May be appropriate	6
11	Evaluation of response to therapy	May be appropriate	5

Abbreviations: mCRPC, metastatic castration resistant prostate cancer; nmCRPC, nonmetastatic castration-resistant prostate cancer; PSA, prostate-specific antigen.

This research was originally published in JNM. Hossein Jadvar et al., Appropriate Use Criteria for Prostate-Specific Membrane Antigen PET Imaging. Journal of Nuclear Medicine January 2022, 63 (1) 59-68. © SNMMI.

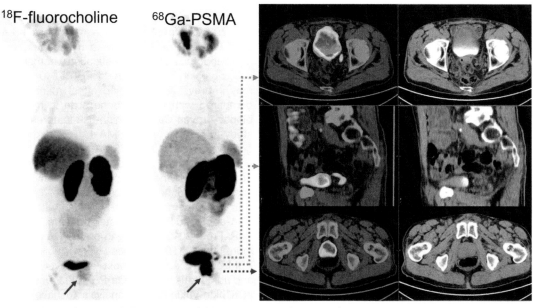

Fig. 6. Left Panel. Fluorocholine PET MIP (oblique projection) image of a 70-year-old man with Gleason 9 (ISUP grade group 5) CaP and PSA of 100 demonstrates mildly avid primary CaP. Right panel. PSMA PET MIP image and corresponding PET/CT images show intensely PSMA expressing locally advanced CaP with extension of tumor along the seminal vesicle and vas deferens (curvilinear uptake). *Dotted red arrow* demonstrates high PSMA avidity in the prostate. *Solid red arrow* highlights the location of the prostate. (Reproduced with permission.[148])

Fig. 7. Chemical structure of PSMA.

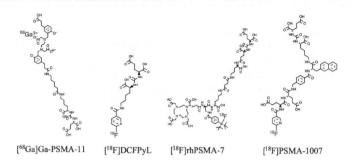

[^{68}Ga]Ga-PSMA-11   [^{18}F]DCFPyL   [^{18}F]rhPSMA-7   [^{18}F]PSMA-1007

by regulatory bodies. The current NCCN guideline recommends PSMA PET/CT for staging of newly diagnosed CaP with unfavorable intermediate or high-grade disease.[88]

In recent years, PSMA PET/CT has been combined with other imaging modalities with the aim to determine whether a combination of imaging can be superior to a single imaging technique alone for detecting clinically significant CaP. Of note, the PRIMARY study by Emmett and colleagues investigated the additive diagnostic value of ^{68}Ga-PSMA-11 PET/CT in men with suspected CaP before biopsy.[89] They demonstrated a combination of MRI and PSMA PET significantly improved the negative predictive value (91% in combined imaging modalities vs 72% MRI alone) and sensitivity (97% vs 83%).[89]

Fluoride-18-DCFPyL

Before fluoride-18-DCFPyL (^{18}F-DCFPyL), ^{18}F-DCFBC was assessed as a fluorinated alternative to ^{68}Ga tracers.[90,91] However, ^{18}F-DCFBC faced significant limitations with high blood pool activity interfering with the detection of lymph node metastases proximal to large blood vessels in the retroperitoneum and pelvis. In turn, ^{18}F-DCFPyL superseded ^{18}F-DCFBC and was proven to have a 5-fold binding affinity increase in initial evaluations.[92]

Trials of ^{18}F-DCFPyL demonstrated results that were comparable to earlier studies of ^{68}Ga-PSMA-11, although almost no high-quality head-to-head studies have been performed. The phase II/III, prospective, multicenter, open label, OSPREY imaging study assessed two cohorts of men. Cohort A included men with high-risk CaP planned for radical prostatectomy and lymph node dissection, and Cohort B assessed men with suspected recurrent metastatic CaP on conventional imaging.[93] Cohort A consisted of 252 patients, and

sensitivity for pelvic lymph node detection was 40% and specificity was 98%. Cohort B, with biopsy as comparison, had a 96% detection rate and PPV of 82%. The phase III, prospective, multicenter, CONDOR study consisting of 208 patients with BCR after definitive therapy found the detection rate and PPV to be 59% to 66% and 78% to 93%, respectively.[94] Both of these studies made significant contributions to the FDA approval for ^{18}F-DCFPyL in May 2021 with the same indications as ^{68}Ga-PSMA-11.

Although slight differences are observed between ^{18}F-DCFPyL and ^{68}Ga-PSMA-11, they are all comparable and vastly superior to conventional imaging with CT or bone scanning.[95,96,97] In particular, in intra-individual comparison demonstrated normal tissue biodistribution was similar between these 2 radiotracers.[98] Use of either aligns with the Society of Nuclear Medicine and Molecular Imaging (SNMMI) appropriate use criteria for PSMA PET.[99] However, there is increasing interest to use fluorinated tracers as ^{68}Ga generators are limited by a maximum activity of up to 1.85 GBq ^{68}Ga per elution in most generators, which ultimately limits mean batch production to 2 to 4 patient doses. Additionally, given the longer half-life of fluorinated tracers, satellite site tracer production may be feasible improving supply chain sustainability.[100]

Fluoride-18-rhPSMA-7.3

FDA recently approved fluoride-18-rhPSMA-7.3 (^{18}F-rhPSMA-7.3) in May 2023 for CaP initial staging and recurrence.[101] As a hybrid tracer, denoted by the "rh" prefix, ^{18}F-rhPSMA-7.3 incorporates a silicon-fluoride-acceptor building block to allow for efficient labeling of ^{18}F to the PSMA binding molecule. In addition, the hybrid molecule contains a metal-chelator in its structure, decreasing its lipophilicity. Such a property allows it to bind to alpha or beta emitters for therapeutic purposes.

Two industry-sponsored prospective phase III trials, namely LIGHTHOUSE and SPOTLIGHT, were designed to establish the safety and diagnostic accuracy of ^{18}F-rhPSMA-7.3 in initial CaP staging and BCR. LIGHTHOUSE evaluated 352 patients with high-risk disease planned to undergo radical prostatectomy.[102] Sensitivity and specificity of pelvic lymph node detection ranged between 23% to 30% and 93% to 97% across 3 readers, respectively. No adverse effects related to the imaging tracer were noted. In the BCR setting, SPOTLIGHT demonstrated ^{18}F-rhPSMA-7.3 detection rates with histopathology as reference, ranging from 51% to 54%, and a combined region-level PPV of 46% to 60%.[103,104]

Fluoride-18-PSMA-1007

Fluoride-18-PSMA-1007 (^{18}F-PSMA-1007) is not currently FDA approved. ^{18}F-PSMA-1007 is excreted through the hepatobiliary route. Limited studies report its detection rate in comparison to ^{68}Ga-PSMA-11 for primary staging. Head-to-head comparison indicates ^{18}F-PSMA-1007 to have a similar lesion-detection rate for local CaP lesions in primary staging at approximately 92%.[96,105] Detection rates of 94% 90.9%, 74.5%, and 61.5% were achieved for PSA levels greater than or equal to 2, 1 to less than 2, 0.5 to less than 1, and 0.2 to less than 0.5 ng/mL, respectively.[106] Higher detection rates of 86% were reported at a PSA level of less or equal to 0.5 ng/mL in another retrospective series of 100 patients by Rahbar and colleagues.[107]

Despite the apparent noninferiority of ^{18}F-PSMA-1007 PET/CT to ^{68}Ga-PSMA-11 PET/CT, with high PET positivity rates and sensitivity on a per region basis, the tracer is limited by a lower PPV (86%).[108] Specific bone lesion PPV is reported to be around 79%, due to nonspecific uptake in bones.[108,109] Given the prevalence of bone metastasis in advanced mCaP, this is a significant diagnostic limitation.

PROSTATE SPECIFIC MEMBRANE ANTIGEN PET-GUIDED TREATMENTS
Prostate Specific Membrane Antigen PET-Guided Treatment of Oligometastatic Disease

Oligometastatic CaP is considered to be a transitional stage between local and metastatic disease. Given the limited metastatic sites, it is proposed to be potentially curable.[110] Definitions vary for what constitutes oligometastatic disease, from 1 to less than or equal to 5 bony or visceral metastases.[111-113] In turn, metastasis-directed therapy (MDT) is of high interest using PSMA PET as a more sensitive imaging modality with the goal of prolonging time to systemic treatment.[114]

MDT heavily relies on highly accurate imaging to guide therapy, in contrast to conventional imaging with CT and bone scan, which has low sensitivity for oligometastases.[115] The prospective, randomized phase II STOMP trial validated that MDT using stereotactic ablative body radiotherapy (SABR) delayed time-to-initiation of ADT in men with metastatic hormone sensitive CaP with 3 or lesser metastasis on ^{18}F-choline PET/CT. The MDT arm experienced an increased ADT-free survival time of 21 months compared with the control group that received surveillance alone, which only achieved an ADT-free time of 13 months.[116] It should be noted that at the last follow-up, 30% of patients treated with ADT continued to progress with oligo-recurrence potentially suggesting the presence of micrometastatic disease not visualized on ^{18}F-choline PET/CT and may be improved with the higher sensitivity of PSMA PET/CT.[117]

In the prospective POPSTAR trial, 33 patients underwent ^{18}F-NaF PET/CT and received SABR to sites of oligometastases. The study demonstrated safety and efficacy in patients with low volume advanced CaP.[118] Importantly, ADT-free survival time was evident in almost half of the participants at 2 years. Multiple retrospective studies have highlighted the potential for PSMA PET/CT in identifying true oligometastatic CaP for further treatment.[119] Several studies currently underway will define whether MDT using PSMA PET/CT can improve patient outcomes.

Prostate specific membrane antigen PET/Computed Tomography Enables Prostate Specific Membrane Antigen Radioligand Therapy

At the heart of theranostics is "seeing what you treat." The visualization of striking tumor-to-background contrast combined with ability to label to ^{177}Lu spearheaded early translation from PET/CT imaging to RLT (**Fig. 8**).[120,121] In the post-docetaxel treatment landscape for mCRPC, the TheraP trial established Lutetium-177-PSMA-617 (^{177}Lu-PSMA-617) as an effective alternative to cabazitaxel, whereas VISION demonstrated that ^{177}Lu-PSMA-617 improves survival compared with trial-defined standard care.[122,123] The TheraP trial included patients with PSMA PET/CT avid lesions and excluded based on FDG PET/CT positive, PSMA PET/CT negative sites of disease ("discordant disease") (**Fig. 9**). In VISION, PSMA-positive uptake on metastasis was defined by SUV greater than liver.[124] Both trials indicate that higher uptake is associated with higher rates of PSA response of greater or equal to 50%.[125] Moreover, data from the TheraP trial demonstrated that PSMA and FDG PET/CT are predictive and prognostic

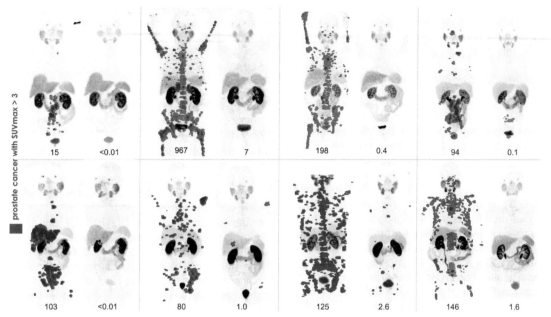

Fig. 8. SNMMI Image of the Year 2018. 68Ga-PSMA-11 visualizing response to up to 4 cycles of 177Lu-PSMA-617. (This research was originally published in JNM. Violet J, Sandhu S, Iravani A, et al. Long-Term Follow-up and Outcomes of Retreatment in an Expanded 50-Patient Single-Center Phase II Prospective Trial of Lu-PSMA-617 Theranostics in Metastatic Castration-Resistant Prostate Cancer. J Nucl Med. 2020;61(6):857-865. © SNMMI.)

biomarkers for response. A SUVmean of greater or equal to 10 on baseline PSMA PET/CT before the first dose of 177Lu-PSMA-617 predicted higher likelihood of favorable response to RLT than cabazitaxel.[47] Further biomarker research from prospective cohorts will allow for improved precision in treatment sequence decision-making.

THE NEXT QUARTER-CENTURY IN CLINICAL PET/COMPUTED TOMOGRAPHY FOR PROSTATE CANCER
Cost Effectiveness of Prostate Specific Membrane Antigen PET/Computed Tomography

Within an Australian context, PSMA PET/CT has already become a new standard-of-care with reimbursement for initial staging and BCR of CaP. A cost–benefit subanalysis of the proPSMA trial estimated PSMA PET cost of 1203 Australian dollars (AUD) compared with conventional imaging at 1412 AUD.[126] Furthermore, 959 AUD was saved per additional accurate detection of nodal disease. After introduction of PSMA PET/CT, a marked decline in the use of bone scan has occurred.[127] Given PSMA PET/CT is vital for patient selection, patients who are better directed to appropriate care due to advanced imaging can potentially save on treatment associated costs.

However, the cost of PSMA PET scans and accessibility remain a barrier of entry globally.[128] In particular, access to PET/CT remains limited in rural settings.[129] Further infrastructure and supply issues may develop in providing high-quality care

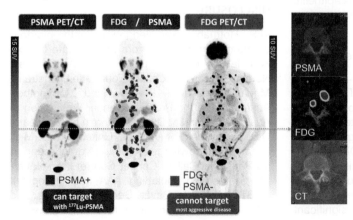

Fig. 9. 68Ga-PSMA-11 and 18F-FDG PET/CT performed on the same day in a patient with metastatic castration-resistant CaP being evaluated for 177Lu-PSMA-617 treatment. On 68Ga-PSMA-11 and CT alone the patient seems suitable for 177Lu therapy. 18F-FDG PET/CT identifies a large burden of PSMA-negative disease, which is also invisible on CT. Treatment options other than 177Lu-PSMA such as cabazitaxel should be considered in this patient. (Reproduced with permission.[150])

regardless of geography. Satellite production of tracers that can be feasibly transported will play a crucial role in the future.[96]

Prostate-Specific Membrane Antigen Biologic-Guided Radiotherapy

PET/CT technology continues to evolve. Biology-guided radiotherapy allows for the delivery of external beam radiotherapy by combining PET/CT and a linear accelerator. This technology allows for real-time delivery of radiotherapy at latency of less than a second to PET emissions.[130] In the setting of BCR and biochemical persistence, PSMA-guided radiotherapy (PSMAgRT) may allow for an improved PSA response and duration of ADT-free survival. PSMAgRT allows for increased dosage to areas that have increased molecular activity and spare healthy tissue. However, there are significant costs and data for PSMAgRT data are currently limited largely to feasibility assessments.[131–133]

Targets Beyond Prostate-Specific Membrane Antigen

Around 5% to 10% of patients will have low PSMA expression, and the clinical utility of PSMA PET/CT is therefore limited.[134,135] Up to 30% of patients referred for RNT who have either low PSMA expression or discordant PSMA-negatives sites with increased glycolytic activity.[122] Further research needs to occur in identifying theranostic targets in PSMA negative and FDG positive CaP.[56,136,137]

In vitro studies demonstrate that in patients who have neuroendocrine prostate cancer (NEPC) are positive for delta-like ligand 3 (DLL3) and negative for AR, PSA, and PSMA at a transcriptional and translational level.[138] SC16 is a humanized mAb selectively binding to human and murine DLL3. Consequently, the development of zirconium-98 labeled DLL3 targeting SC16 provides a suitable PET radiopharmaceutical imaging agent in identifying the presence of DLL3 positive NEPC.[139] Other markers include 6-transmembrane epithelial antigen of the prostate, glypican 3, and somatostatin receptors.[140–142]

Implementation of Artificial Intelligence into Clinical Workflows

With the rapid adoption of PSMA PET/CT in the clinic, there are new patterns of physiologic uptake and pitfalls to learn.[143] Reproducible interpretation of PSMA PET can be enhanced by using standardized criteria such as E-PSMA, PROMISE2, or RECIP.[144–146] To further enhance clinician identification and safety net for possible undetected lesions, radiomics and artificial intelligence incorporated with machine learning have a significant

role in the future to standardize diagnostic performance across sites.[147]

SUMMARY

The rapid growth and utility of PSMA PET/CT in recent years was not an overnight success. The development of the earlier tracers including NaF, choline, and fluciclovine PET/CT for staging, assessing recurrence and treatment response paved the way for PSMA PET today. The superiority of PET/CT over conventional imaging is striking across various indications and has revolutionized how we manage men diagnosed with localized or advanced disease. FDG PET/CT still has a complementary role especially as a prognostic biomarker and evaluation of suitability for RLT. The future of PSMA PET research continues to refine our clinical practice and more prospective trials are necessary to validate further clinical experience.

CLINICS CARE POINTS

- PSMA PET/CT has become a new standard-of-care for imaging patients with CaP with improved accuracy
- PSMA PET/CT is currently indicated for staging of newly diagnosed patients with intermediate-to-high risk CaP, BCR, and assessment of suitability for RLT
- NaF, choline, and fluciclovine PET/CT have also represented significant advances in the last quarter-century but their role is now limited in the PSMA PET/CT era
- FDG PET/CT is a powerful prognostic tool for patients with CaP and is currently underutilized

DISCLOSURE

M.S. Hofman acknowledged philanthropic/government grant support from the Prostate Cancer Foundation, Australia funded by CANICA Oslo Norway, Peter MacCallum Foundation, Australia, Medical Research Future Fund, Movember, Australia, and the Prostate Cancer Foundation of Australia, Australia. Other funding in last 10 years: U.S. Department of Defense, United States. M.S. Hofman acknowledges research grant support (to Peter MacCallum Cancer Centre) from Novartis, Switzerland (including AAA and Endocyte), ANSTO, Australia, Bayer, Germany, Isotopia, and MIM, Australia. Consulting fees for lectures or advisory boards from Astellas and AstraZeneca in the last 2 years, and Janssen, Merck/MSD and Mundipharma in the last 5 years. J.P. Buteau receives PhD support through an Australian Government Research Training Program Scholarship. All other authors declare no relevant disclosures.

REFERENCES

1. Rawla P. Epidemiology of prostate cancer. World J Oncol 2019;10(2):63–89.

2. Sung H, Ferlay J, Siegel RL, et al. Global cancer Statistics 2020: GLOBOCAN Estimates of Incidence and Mortality worldwide for 36 cancers in 185 Countries. CA Cancer J Clin 2021;71(3):209–49.

3. Dong L, Zieren RC, Xue W, et al. Metastatic prostate cancer remains incurable, why? Asian J Urol 2019;6(1):26–41.

4. Borno HT, Cowan JE, Zhao S, et al. Examining initial treatment and survival among men with metastatic prostate cancer: an analysis from the CaP-SURE registry. Urol Oncol 2020;38(10):793.e1-11.

5. Gandaglia G, Abdollah F, Schiffmann J, et al. Distribution of metastatic sites in patients with prostate cancer: a population-based analysis. Prostate 2014;74(2):210–6.

6. Gillessen S, Bossi A, Davis ID, et al. Management of patients with advanced prostate cancer. Part I: intermediate-/high-risk and locally advanced disease, biochemical Relapse, and side effects of hormonal treatment: report of the advanced prostate cancer consensus Conference 2022. Eur Urol 2023;83(3):267–93.

7. Gillessen S, Bossi A, Davis ID, et al. Management of patients with advanced prostate cancer-metastatic and/or castration-resistant prostate cancer: report of the Advanced Prostate Cancer Consensus Conference (APCCC) 2022. Eur J Cancer 2023;185:178–215.

8. Blau M, Nagler W, Bender MA. Fluorine-18: a new isotope for bone scanning. J Nucl Med 1962;3:332–4. Available at: https://www.ncbi.nlm.nih.gov/pubmed/13869926.

9. Park PSU, Raynor WY, Sun Y, et al. 18F-Sodium fluoride PET as a diagnostic modality for metabolic, Autoimmune, and Osteogenic bone Disorders: Cellular Mechanisms and clinical applications. Int J Mol Sci 2021;22(12). https://doi.org/10.3390/ijms22126504.

10. Wong SK, Mohamad NV, Giaze TR, et al. Prostate cancer and bone metastases: the Underlying Mechanisms. Int J Mol Sci 2019;20(10). https://doi.org/10.3390/ijms20102587.

11. Tapscott E. Nuclear medicine pioneer, Hal O. Anger, 1920-2005. J Nucl Med Technol 2005;33(4):250–3. Available at: https://www.ncbi.nlm.nih.gov/pubmed/16397975.

12. Hicks RJ, Hofman MS. Is there still a role for SPECT-CT in oncology in the PET-CT era? Nat Rev Clin Oncol 2012;9(12):712–20.

13. Kulshrestha RK, Vinjamuri S, England A, et al. The role of 18F-Sodium fluoride PET/CT bone scans in the diagnosis of metastatic bone disease from Breast and prostate cancer. J Nucl Med Technol 2016;44(4):217–22.

14. Beheshti M, Rezaee A, Geinitz H, et al. Evaluation of prostate cancer bone metastases with 18F-NaF and 18F-fluorocholine PET/CT. J Nucl Med 2016;57(Suppl 3):55S–60S.

15. Sheikhbahaei S, Jones KM, Werner RA, et al. 18F-NaF-PET/CT for the detection of bone metastasis in prostate cancer: a meta-analysis of diagnostic accuracy studies. Ann Nucl Med 2019;33(5):351–61.

16. Bastawrous S, Bhargava P, Behnia F, et al. Newer PET application with an old tracer: role of 18F-NaF skeletal PET/CT in oncologic practice. Radiographics 2014;34(5):1295–316.

17. Jadvar H, Desai B, Ji L, et al. Prospective evaluation of 18F-NaF and 18F-FDG PET/CT in detection of occult metastatic disease in biochemical recurrence of prostate cancer. Clin Nucl Med 2012;37(7):637–43.

18. Medina-Ornelas S, Garcia-Perez FO. Clinical utility of 18F-NaF and 68Ga-PSMA PET/CT as prognostic marker in patients with metastatic prostate cancer treated with Radium-223. J Nucl Med 2020;61(supplement 1):1283. Available at: https://jnm.snmjournals.org/content/61/supplement_1/1283. Accessed August 14, 2023.

19. Cook G Jr, Parker C, Chua S, et al. 18F-fluoride PET: changes in uptake as a method to assess response in bone metastases from castrate-resistant prostate cancer patients treated with 223Ra-chloride (Alpharadin). EJNMMI Res 2011;1(1):4.

20. Jadvar H, Colletti PM. 18F-NaF/223RaCl2 theranostics in metastatic prostate cancer: treatment response assessment and prediction of outcome. Br J Radiol 2018;91(1091):20170948.

21. Reske SN, Blumstein NM, Neumaier B, et al. Imaging prostate cancer with 11C-choline PET/CT. J Nucl Med 2006;47(8):1249–54. https://www.ncbi.nlm.nih.gov/pubmed/16883001.

22. Hara T, Kosaka N, Kishi H. PET imaging of prostate cancer using carbon-11-choline. J Nucl Med 1998;39(6):990–5. https://www.ncbi.nlm.nih.gov/pubmed/9627331.

23. Hara T, Kosaka N, Kishi H. Development of (18)F-fluoroethylcholine for cancer imaging with PET: synthesis, biochemistry, and prostate cancer imaging. J Nucl Med 2002;43(2):187–99. https://www.ncbi.nlm.nih.gov/pubmed/11850483.

24. Rodríguez-González A, Ramírez de Molina A, Benítez-Rajal J, et al. Phospholipase D and choline kinase: their role in cancer development and their

potential as drug targets. Prog Cell Cycle Res 2003; 5:191–201. https://www.ncbi.nlm.nih.gov/pubmed/14593713.

25. Evangelista L, Briganti A, Fanti S, et al. New clinical indications for (18)F/(11)C-choline, new tracers for positron emission tomography and a Promising hybrid Device for prostate cancer staging: a systematic review of the Literature. Eur Urol 2016; 70(1):161–75.

26. Budiharto T, Joniau S, Lerut E, et al. Prospective evaluation of 11C-choline positron emission tomography/computed tomography and diffusion-weighted magnetic resonance imaging for the nodal staging of prostate cancer with a high risk of lymph node metastases. Eur Urol 2011;60(1):125–30.

27. Heck MM, Souvatzoglou M, Retz M, et al. Prospective comparison of computed tomography, diffusion-weighted magnetic resonance imaging and [11C] choline positron emission tomography/computed tomography for preoperative lymph node staging in prostate cancer patients. Eur J Nucl Med Mol Imaging 2014;41(4):694–701.

28. Pinaquy JB, De Clermont-Galleran H, Pasticier G, et al. Comparative effectiveness of [(18) F]-fluorocholine PET-CT and pelvic MRI with diffusion-weighted imaging for staging in patients with high-risk prostate cancer. Prostate 2015;75(3):323–31.

29. Evangelista L, Cimitan M, Zattoni F, et al. Comparison between conventional imaging (abdominal-pelvic computed tomography and bone scan) and [(18)F]choline positron emission tomography/computed tomography imaging for the initial staging of patients with intermediate- tohigh-risk prostate cancer: a retrospective analysis. Scand J Urol 2015;49(5):345–53.

30. Mamede M, Ceci F, Castellucci P, et al. The role of 11C-choline PET imaging in the early detection of recurrence in surgically treated prostate cancer patients with very low PSA level <0.5 ng/mL. Clin Nucl Med 2013;38(9):e342–5.

31. Welle CL, Cullen EL, Peller PJ, et al. ^{11}C-Choline PET/CT in recurrent prostate cancer and Nonprostatic neoplastic Processes. Radiographics 2016; 36(1):279–92.

32. Michaud L, Touijer KA, Mauguen A, et al. 11C-Choline PET/CT in recurrent prostate cancer: retrospective analysis in a large U.S. Patient series. J Nucl Med 2020;61(6):827–33.

33. Mitchell CR, Lowe VJ, Rangel LJ, et al. Operational characteristics of (11)c-choline positron emission tomography/computerized tomography for prostate cancer with biochemical recurrence after initial treatment. J Urol 2013;189(4):1308–13.

34. Ceci F, Castellucci P, Graziani T, et al. 11C-choline PET/CT identifies osteoblastic and osteolytic lesions in patients with metastatic prostate cancer. Clin Nucl Med 2015;40(5):e265–70.

35. Soyka JD, Muster MA, Schmid DT, et al. Clinical impact of 18F-choline PET/CT in patients with recurrent prostate cancer. Eur J Nucl Med Mol Imaging 2012;39(6):936–43.

36. Picchio M, Spinapolice EG, Fallanca F, et al. [11C] Choline PET/CT detection of bone metastases in patients with PSA progression after primary treatment for prostate cancer: comparison with bone scintigraphy. Eur J Nucl Med Mol Imaging 2012; 39(1):13–26.

37. Van den Bergh L, Koole M, Isebaert S, et al. Is there an additional value of 11C-choline PET-CT to T2-weighted MRI images in the localization of intraprostatic tumor nodules? Int J Radiat Oncol Biol Phys 2012;83(5):1486–92.

38. Souvatzoglou M, Krause BJ, Pürschel A, et al. Influence of (11)C-choline PET/CT on the treatment planning for salvage radiation therapy in patients with biochemical recurrence of prostate cancer. Radiother Oncol 2011;99(2):193–200.

39. Alongi F, Comito T, Villa E, et al. What is the role of [11C]choline PET/CT in decision making strategy before post-operative salvage radiation therapy in prostate cancer patients? Acta Oncol 2014;53(7):990–2.

40. Fuccio C, Schiavina R, Castellucci P, et al. Androgen deprivation therapy influences the uptake of 11C-choline in patients with recurrent prostate cancer: the preliminary results of a sequential PET/CT study. Eur J Nucl Med Mol Imaging 2011; 38(11):1985–9.

41. De Giorgi U, Caroli P, Burgio SL, et al. Early outcome prediction on 18F-fluorocholine PET/CT in metastatic castration-resistant prostate cancer patients treated with abiraterone. Oncotarget 2014;5(23):12448–58.

42. Ceci F, Castellucci P, Graziani T, et al. 11)C-Choline PET/CT in castration-resistant prostate cancer patients treated with docetaxel. Eur J Nucl Med Mol Imaging 2016;43(1):84–91.

43. Liberti MV, Locasale JW. The Warburg effect: How Does it benefit cancer cells? Trends Biochem Sci 2016;41(3):211–8.

44. Gonzalez-Menendez P, Hevia D, Mayo JC, et al. The dark side of glucose transporters in prostate cancer: are they a new feature to characterize carcinomas? Int J Cancer 2018;142(12):2414–24.

45. Beauregard JM, Blouin AC, Fradet V, et al. FDG-PET/CT for pre-operative staging and prognostic stratification of patients with high-grade prostate cancer at biopsy. Cancer Imag 2015;15(1):2.

46. Thang SP, Violet J, Sandhu S, et al. Poor Outcomes for Patients with Metastatic Castration-resistant Prostate Cancer with Low Prostate-specific Membrane Antigen (PSMA) Expression Deemed

Ineligible for ^{177}Lu-labelled PSMA Radioligand Therapy. Eur Urol Oncol 2019;2(6):670–6.

47. Buteau JP, Martin AJ, Emmett L, et al. PSMA and FDG-PET as predictive and prognostic biomarkers in patients given [^{177}Lu]Lu-PSMA-617 versus cabazitaxel for metastatic castration-resistant prostate cancer (TheraP): a biomarker analysis from a randomised, open-label, phase 2 trial. Lancet Oncol 2022;23(11):1389–97.

48. Akin-Akintayo OO, Jani AB, Odewole O, et al. Change in salvage radiotherapy management based on guidance with FACBC (fluciclovine) PET/CT in Postprostatectomy recurrent prostate cancer. Clin Nucl Med 2017;42(1):e22–8.

49. Marzola MC, Chondrogiannis S, Ferretti A, et al. Role of 18F-choline PET/CT in biochemically relapsed prostate cancer after radical prostatectomy: correlation with trigger PSA, PSA velocity, PSA doubling time, and metastatic distribution. Clin Nucl Med 2013;38(1):e26–32.

50. Bluemel C, Krebs M, Polat B, et al. 68Ga-PSMA-PET/CT in patients with biochemical prostate cancer recurrence and negative 18F-Choline-PET/CT. Clin Nucl Med 2016;41(7):515–21.

51. Odewole OA, Tade FI, Nieh PT, et al. Recurrent prostate cancer detection with anti-3-[(18)F]FACBC PET/CT: comparison with CT. Eur J Nucl Med Mol Imaging 2016;43(10):1773–83.

52. Teoh E, Bottomley D, Scarsbrook A, et al. Impact of 18F-fluciclovine PET/CT on clinical management of patients with recurrent prostate cancer: results from the phase 3 FALCON trial. Int J Radiat Oncol Biol Phys 2017;99(5):1316–7.

53. Huggins C, Stevens RE, Hodges CV. Studies ON prostatic cancer: II. The effects OF CASTRATION ON advanced CARCINOMA OF the prostate GLAND. Arch Surg 1941;43(2):209–23.

54. Wong CI, Zhou ZX, Sar M, et al. Steroid requirement for androgen receptor dimerization and DNA binding. Modulation by intramolecular interactions between the NH2-terminal and steroid-binding domains. J Biol Chem 1993;268(25):19004–12. Available at: https://www.ncbi.nlm.nih.gov/pubmed/8360187.

55. Culig Z, Hobisch A, Hittmair A, et al. Expression, structure, and function of androgen receptor in advanced prostatic carcinoma. Prostate 1998;35(1):63–70.

56. Larson SM, Morris M, Gunther I, et al. Tumor localization of 16beta-18F-fluoro-5alpha-dihydrotestosterone versus 18F-FDG in patients with progressive, metastatic prostate cancer. J Nucl Med 2004;45(3):366–73. Available at: https://www.ncbi.nlm.nih.gov/pubmed/15001675.

57. Dehdashti F, Picus J, Michalski JM, et al. Positron tomographic assessment of androgen receptors in prostatic carcinoma. Eur J Nucl Med Mol Imaging 2005;32(3):344–50.

58. Fox JJ, Gavane SC, Blanc-Autran E, et al. Positron emission tomography/computed tomography-based assessments of androgen receptor expression and glycolytic activity as a prognostic biomarker for metastatic castration-resistant prostate cancer. JAMA Oncol 2018;4(2):217–24.

59. Scher HI, Beer TM, Higano CS, et al. Antitumour activity of MDV3100 in castration-resistant prostate cancer: a phase 1-2 study. Lancet 2010;375(9724):1437–46.

60. Hoving H, Palthe S, Vallinga M, et al. Early 18F-FDHT PET/CT as a predictor of treatment response in mCRPC treated with enzalutamide. J Clin Orthod 2019;37(7_suppl):232.

61. Horoszewicz JS, Kawinski E, Murphy GP. Monoclonal antibodies to a new antigenic marker in epithelial prostatic cells and serum of prostatic cancer patients. Anticancer Res 1987;7(5B):927–35. Available at: https://www.ncbi.nlm.nih.gov/pubmed/2449118.

62. Israeli RS, Powell CT, Fair WR, et al. Molecular cloning of a complementary DNA encoding a prostate-specific membrane antigen. Cancer Res 1993;53(2):227–30. Available at: https://www.ncbi.nlm.nih.gov/pubmed/8417812.

63. O'Keefe DS, Su SL, Bacich DJ, et al. Mapping, genomic organization and promoter analysis of the human prostate-specific membrane antigen gene. Biochim Biophys Acta 1998;1443(1–2):113–27.

64. Miyahira AK, Soule HR. The history of prostate-specific membrane antigen as a theranostic target in prostate cancer: the Cornerstone role of the prostate cancer Foundation. J Nucl Med 2022;63(3):331–8.

65. Lopes AD, Davis WL, Rosenstraus MJ, et al. Immunohistochemical and Pharmacokinetic characterization of the site-specific Immunoconjugate CYT-356 derived from Antiprostate monoclonal antibody 7E11-C5. Cancer Res 1990;50(19):6423–9. Available at: https://aacrjournals.org/cancerres/article-pdf/50/19/6423/2441053/cr0500196423.pdf. Accessed March 13, 2023.

66. Kahn D, Williams RD, Seldin DW, et al. Radioimmunoscintigraphy with 111indium labeled CYT-356 for the detection of occult prostate cancer recurrence. J Urol 1994;152(5 Pt 1):1490–5.

67. Wynant GE, Murphy GP, Horoszewicz JS, et al. Immunoscintigraphy of prostatic cancer: preliminary results with 111In-labeled monoclonal antibody 7E11-C5.3 (CYT-356). Prostate 1991;18(3):229–41.

68. Rosenthal SA, Haseman MK, Polascik TJ. Utility of capromab pendetide (ProstaScint) imaging in the management of prostate cancer. Tech Urol 2001;7(1):27–37. Available at: https://www.ncbi.nlm.nih.gov/pubmed/11272670.

69. Murphy GP, Maguire RT, Rogers B, et al. Comparison of serum PSMA, PSA levels with results of Cytogen-356 ProstaScint scanning in prostatic cancer patients. Prostate 1997;33(4):281–5.

70. Troyer JK, Feng Q, Beckett ML, et al. Biochemical characterization and mapping of the 7E11-C5.3 epitope of the prostate-specific membrane antigen. Urol Oncol 1995;1(1):29–37.

71. Liu H, Moy P, Kim S, et al. Monoclonal antibodies to the extracellular domain of prostate-specific membrane antigen also react with tumor vascular endothelium. Cancer Res 1997;57(17):3629–34. Available at: https://www.ncbi.nlm.nih.gov/pubmed/9288760.

72. Carter RE, Feldman AR, Coyle JT. Prostate-specific membrane antigen is a hydrolase with substrate and pharmacologic characteristics of a neuropeptidase. Proc Natl Acad Sci U S A 1996;93(2):749–53.

73. Silver DA, Pellicer I, Fair WR, et al. Prostate-specific membrane antigen expression in normal and malignant human tissues. Clin Cancer Res 1997;3(1):81–5. Available at: https://www.ncbi.nlm.nih.gov/pubmed/9815541.

74. Woythal N, Arsenic R, Kempkensteffen C, et al. Immunohistochemical validation of PSMA expression measured by 68Ga-PSMA PET/CT in primary prostate cancer. J Nucl Med 2018;59(2):238–43.

75. Sweat SD, Pacelli A, Murphy GP, et al. Prostate-specific membrane antigen expression is greatest in prostate adenocarcinoma and lymph node metastases. Urology 1998;52(4):637–40.

76. Bostwick DG, Pacelli A, Blute M, et al. Prostate specific membrane antigen expression in prostatic intraepithelial neoplasia and adenocarcinoma: a study of 184 cases. Cancer 1998;82(11):2256–61.

77. Ghosh A, Heston WDW. Tumor target prostate specific membrane antigen (PSMA) and its regulation in prostate cancer. J Cell Biochem 2004;91(3):528–39.

78. Kuppermann D. Calais J, Marks LS. Imaging prostate cancer: clinical utility of prostate-specific membrane antigen. J Urol 2022;207(4):769–78.

79. Ristau BT, O'Keefe DS, Bacich DJ. The prostate-specific membrane antigen: lessons and current clinical implications from 20 years of research. Urol Oncol 2014;32(3):272–9.

80. Kozikowski AP, Nan F, Conti P, et al. Design of remarkably simple, yet potent urea-based inhibitors of glutamate carboxypeptidase II (NAALADase). J Med Chem 2001;44(3):298–301.

81. Eder M, Schäfer M, Bauder-Wüst U, et al. 68Ga-complex lipophilicity and the targeting property of a urea-based PSMA inhibitor for PET imaging. Bioconjug Chem 2012;23(4):688–97.

82. Afshar-Oromieh A, Haberkorn U, Eder M, et al. [68Ga]Gallium-labelled PSMA ligand as superior PET tracer for the diagnosis of prostate cancer: comparison with 18F-FECH. Eur J Nucl Med Mol Imaging 2012;39(6):1085–6.

83. Afshar-Oromieh A, Haberkorn U, Hadaschik B, et al. PET/MRI with a 68Ga-PSMA ligand for the detection of prostate cancer. Eur J Nucl Med Mol Imaging 2013;40(10):1629–30.

84. Hope TA, Eiber M, Armstrong WR, et al. Diagnostic accuracy of 68Ga-PSMA-11 PET for pelvic nodal metastasis detection prior to radical prostatectomy and pelvic lymph node dissection: a multicenter prospective phase 3 imaging trial. JAMA Oncol 2021;7(11):1635–42.

85. Fendler WP, Calais J, Eiber M, et al. Assessment of 68Ga-PSMA-11 PET accuracy in localizing recurrent prostate cancer: a prospective single-arm clinical trial. JAMA Oncol 2019;5(6):856–63.

86. Hofman MS, Lawrentschuk N, Francis RJ, et al. Prostate-specific membrane antigen PET-CT in patients with high-risk prostate cancer before curative-intent surgery or radiotherapy (proPSMA): a prospective, randomised, multicentre study. Lancet 2020;395(10231):1208–16.

87. Perera M, Papa N, Roberts M, et al. Gallium-68 prostate-specific membrane antigen positron emission tomography in advanced prostate cancer-Updated diagnostic utility, sensitivity, specificity, and distribution of prostate-specific membrane antigen-avid lesions: a systematic review and meta-analysis. Eur Urol 2020;77(4):403–17.

88. National Comprehensive Cancer Network. NCCN Prostate Cancer Guidelines. 2023. Available at: https://www.nccn.org/login?ReturnURL=https://www.nccn.org/professionals/physician_gls/pdf/prostate.pdf. Accessed June 1, 2023.

89. Emmett L, Buteau J, Papa N, et al. The additive diagnostic value of prostate-specific membrane antigen positron emission tomography computed tomography to Multiparametric magnetic resonance imaging triage in the diagnosis of prostate cancer (PRIMARY): a prospective multicentre study. Eur Urol 2021;80(6):682–9.

90. Cho SY, Gage KL, Mease RC, et al. Biodistribution, tumor detection, and radiation dosimetry of 18F-DCFBC, a low-molecular-weight inhibitor of prostate-specific membrane antigen, in patients with metastatic prostate cancer. J Nucl Med 2012;53(12):1883–91.

91. Mease RC, Dusich CL, Foss CA, et al. N-[N-[(S)-1,3-Dicarboxypropyl]Carbamoyl]-4-[18F]Fluorobenzyl-l-Cysteine, [18F]DCFBC: a new imaging Probe for prostate cancer. Clin Cancer Res 2008;14(10):3036–43.

92. Szabo Z, Mena E, Rowe SP, et al. Initial evaluation of [(18)F]DCFPyL for prostate-specific membrane antigen (PSMA)-Targeted PET imaging of prostate cancer. Mol Imaging Biol 2015;17(4):565–74.

93. Pienta KJ, Gorin MA, Rowe SP, et al. A phase 2/3 prospective multicenter study of the diagnostic

accuracy of prostate specific membrane antigen PET/CT with 18F-DCFPyL in prostate cancer patients (OSPREY). J Urol 2021;206(1):52–61.

94. Morris MJ, Rowe SP, Gorin MA, et al. Diagnostic performance of 18F-DCFPyL-PET/CT in men with biochemically recurrent prostate cancer: results from the CONDOR phase III, multicenter study. Clin Cancer Res 2021;27(13):3674–82.

95. Dietlein F, Kobe C, Neubauer S, et al. PSA-stratified performance of 18F- and 68Ga-PSMA PET in patients with biochemical recurrence of prostate cancer. J Nucl Med 2017;58(6):947–52.

96. Kuten J, Fahoum I, Savin Z, et al. Head-to-Head comparison of 68Ga-PSMA-11 with 18F-PSMA-1007 PET/CT in staging prostate cancer using histopathology and Immunohistochemical analysis as a reference standard. J Nucl Med 2020;61(4):527–32.

97. Huang S, Ong S, McKenzie D, et al. Comparison of ^{18}F-based PSMA radiotracers with [68Ga]Ga-PSMA-11 in PET/CT imaging of prostate cancer-a systematic review and meta-analysis. Prostate Cancer Prostatic Dis 2023. https://doi.org/10.1038/s41391-023-00755-2.

98. Ferreira G, Iravani A, Hofman MS, et al. Intra-individual comparison of Ga-PSMA-11 and F-DCFPyL normal-organ biodistribution. Cancer Imag 2019; 19(1):23.

99. H Jadvar, J Calais, S Fanti, et al. Appropriate use criteria for prostate-Specific Membrane Antigen (PSMA) PET imaging. Society of Nuclear Medicine and Molecular Imaging. Published 03/2022. Available at: https://www.snmmi.org/ClinicalPractice/content.aspx?ItemNumber=38657. Accessed March 13, 2023.

100. Cardinale J, Roscher M, Schäfer M, et al. Development of PSMA-1007-related series of 18F-labeled Glu-Ureido-type PSMA inhibitors. J Med Chem 2020;63(19):10897–907.

101. FDA Approves Flotufolastat Fluorine-18 injection, first Radiohybrid PSMA-targeted PET imaging agent for prostate cancer. Available at: https://ascopost.com/news/may-2023/fda-approves-flotufolastat-fluorine-18-injection-first-radiohybrid-psma-targeted-pet-imaging-agent-for-prostate-cancer/. Accessed August 15, 2023.

102. Surasi DS, Eiber M, Maurer T, et al. Diagnostic performance and safety of positron emission tomography with 18F-rhPSMA-7.3 in patients with newly diagnosed Unfavourable intermediate- to very-high-risk prostate cancer: results from a phase 3, prospective, multicentre study (LIGHTHOUSE). Eur Urol 2023. https://doi.org/10.1016/j.eururo.2023.06.018.

103. Jani AB, Ravizzini GC, Gartrell BA, et al. Diagnostic performance and safety of 18F-rhPSMA-7.3 positron emission tomography in men with suspected prostate cancer recurrence: results from a phase

3, prospective, multicenter study (SPOTLIGHT). J Urol 2023;210(2):299–311.

104. Kroenke M, Mirzoyan L, Horn T, et al. Matched-pair comparison of 68Ga-PSMA-11 and 18F-rhPSMA-7 PET/CT in patients with primary and biochemical recurrence of prostate cancer: frequency of non-tumor-related uptake and tumor positivity. J Nucl Med 2021;62(8):1082–8.

105. Pattison DA, Debowski M, Gulhane B, et al. Prospective intra-individual blinded comparison of [18F]PSMA-1007 and [68 Ga]Ga-PSMA-11 PET/CT imaging in patients with confirmed prostate cancer. Eur J Nucl Med Mol Imaging 2022;49(2):763–76.

106. Giesel FL, Knorr K, Spohn F, et al. Detection efficacy of 18F-PSMA-1007 PET/CT in 251 patients with biochemical recurrence of prostate cancer after radical prostatectomy. J Nucl Med 2019;60(3):362–8.

107. Rahbar K, Afshar-Oromieh A, Seifert R, et al. Diagnostic performance of 18F-PSMA-1007 PET/CT in patients with biochemical recurrent prostate cancer. Eur J Nucl Med Mol Imaging 2018;45(12):2055–61.

108. Mingels C, Bohn KP, Rominger A, et al. Diagnostic accuracy of [18F]PSMA-1007 PET/CT in biochemical recurrence of prostate cancer. Eur J Nucl Med Mol Imaging 2022;49(7):2436.

109. Grünig H, Maurer A, Thali Y, et al. Focal unspecific bone uptake on [18F]-PSMA-1007 PET: a multicenter retrospective evaluation of the distribution, frequency, and quantitative parameters of a potential pitfall in prostate cancer imaging. Eur J Nucl Med Mol Imaging 2021;48(13):4483–94.

110. Hellman S, Weichselbaum RR. Oligometastases. J Clin Oncol 1995;13(1):8–10.

111. Guckenberger M, Lievens Y, Bouma AB, et al. Characterisation and classification of oligometastatic disease: a European Society for radiotherapy and oncology and European Organisation for research and treatment of cancer consensus recommendation. Lancet Oncol 2020;21(1):e18–28.

112. Ahmed KA, Barney BM, Davis BJ, et al. Stereotactic body radiation therapy in the treatment of oligometastatic prostate cancer. Front Oncol 2012;2:215.

113. Decaestecker K, De Meerleer G, Lambert B, et al. Repeated stereotactic body radiotherapy for oligometastatic prostate cancer recurrence. Radiat Oncol 2014;9:135.

114. Alberto M, Yim A, Papa N, et al. Role of PSMA PET-guided metastases-directed therapy in oligometastatic recurrent prostate cancer. Front Oncol 2022;12:929444.

115. Crawford ED, Stone NN, Yu EY, et al. Challenges and recommendations for early identification of

metastatic disease in prostate cancer. Urology 2014;83(3):664–9.

116. Ost P, Reynders D, Decaestecker K, et al. Surveillance or metastasis-directed therapy for oligometastatic prostate cancer recurrence: a prospective, randomized, multicenter phase II trial. J Clin Oncol 2018;36(5):446–53.

117. Ost P, Reynders D, Decaestecker K, et al. Surveillance or metastasis-directed therapy for oligometastatic prostate cancer recurrence (STOMP): five-year results of a randomized phase II trial. J Clin Orthod 2020;38(6_suppl):10.

118. Siva S, Bressel M, Murphy DG, et al. Stereotactic Abative body radiotherapy (SABR) for oligometastatic prostate cancer: a prospective clinical trial. Eur Urol 2018;74(4):455–62.

119. Deijen CL, Vrijenhoek GL, Schaake EE, et al. PSMA-11-PET/CT versus choline-PET/CT to guide stereotactic ablative radiotherapy for androgen deprivation therapy deferral in patients with oligometastatic prostate cancer. Clin Transl Radiat Oncol 2021;30:1–6.

120. Afshar-Oromieh A, Hetzheim H, Kratochwil C, et al. The theranostic PSMA ligand PSMA-617 in the diagnosis of prostate cancer by PET/CT: biodistribution in humans, radiation dosimetry, and first evaluation of tumor lesions. J Nucl Med 2015; 56(11):1697–705.

121. Hofman MS, Violet J, Hicks RJ, et al. [177Lu]-PSMA-617 radionuclide treatment in patients with metastatic castration-resistant prostate cancer (LuPSMA trial): a single-centre, single-arm, phase 2 study. Lancet Oncol 2018;19(6):825–33.

122. Hofman MS, Emmett L, Sandhu S, et al. [^{177}Lu]Lu-PSMA-617 versus cabazitaxel in patients with metastatic castration-resistant prostate cancer (TheraP): a randomised, open-label, phase 2 trial. Lancet 2021;397(10276):797–804.

123. Sartor O, de Bono J, Chi KN, et al. Lutetium-177-PSMA-617 for metastatic castration-resistant prostate cancer. N Engl J Med 2021;385(12):1091–103.

124. Kuo PH, Yoo DC, Avery R, et al. A VISION Substudy of reader Agreement on Ga-PSMA-11 PET/CT scan interpretation to determine patient Eligibility for Lu-PSMA-617 radioligand therapy. J Nucl Med 2023; 64(8):1259–65.

125. Gafita A, Marcus C, Kostos L, et al. Predictors and real-World Use of prostate-specific radioligand therapy: PSMA and beyond. Am Soc Clin Oncol Educ Book 2022;42:1–17.

126. de Feria Cardet RE, Hofman MS, Segard T, et al. Is prostate-specific membrane antigen positron emission tomography/computed tomography imaging cost-effective in prostate cancer: an analysis Informed by the proPSMA trial. Eur Urol 2021; 79(3):413–8.

127. Haran C, McBean R, Parsons R, et al. Five-year trends of bone scan and prostate-specific membrane antigen positron emission tomography utilization in prostate cancer: a retrospective review in a private centre. J Med Imaging Radiat Oncol 2019;63(4):495–9.

128. Hricak H, Abdel-Wahab M, Atun R, et al. Medical imaging and nuclear medicine: a Lancet oncology Commission. Lancet Oncol 2021;22(4):e136–72.

129. Australian Government Department of Health, Care A. PET units in Australia. Australian Government Department of Health and Aged Care. Published August 15, 2023. Available at: https://www.health.gov.au/topics/diagnostic-imaging/mri-and-pet-locations/PET-Australia. Accessed August 15, 2023.

130. Shirvani SM, Huntzinger CJ, Melcher T, et al. Biology-guided radiotherapy: redefining the role of radiotherapy in metastatic cancer. Br J Radiol 2021;94(1117):20200873.

131. Gaudreault M, Chang D, Hardcastle N, et al. Feasibility of biology-guided radiotherapy using PSMA-PET to boost to dominant intraprostatic tumour. Clin Transl Radiat Oncol 2022;35:84–9.

132. Gaudreault M, Chang D, Hardcastle N, et al. Utility of biology-guided radiotherapy to metastases diagnosed during staging of high-risk biopsy-proven prostate cancer. Front Oncol 2022;12:854589.

133. Gaudreault M, Chang D, Hardcastle N, et al. Combined biology-guided radiotherapy and Lutetium PSMA theranostics treatment in metastatic castrate-resistant prostate cancer. Front Oncol 2023;13: 1134884.

134. Violet J, Jackson P, Ferdinandus J, et al. Dosimetry of 177Lu-PSMA-617 in metastatic castration-resistant prostate cancer: Correlations between Pretherapeutic imaging and Whole-body tumor dosimetry with treatment outcomes. J Nucl Med 2019;60(4):517–23.

135. Current K, Meyer C, Magyar CE, et al. Investigating PSMA-targeted radioligand therapy efficacy as a function of Cellular PSMA levels and Intratumoral PSMA Heterogeneity. Clin Cancer Res 2020; 26(12):2946–55.

136. Jadvar H. Is there Use for FDG-PET in prostate cancer? Semin Nucl Med 2016;46(6):502–6.

137. Gomes Marin JF, Nunes RF, Coutinho AM, et al. Theranostics in nuclear medicine: Emerging and Re-emerging Integrated imaging and therapies in the era of precision oncology. Radiographics 2020;40(6):1715–40.

138. Korsen JA, Kalidindi TM, Khitrov S, et al. Molecular imaging of neuroendocrine prostate cancer by targeting delta-like ligand 3. J Nucl Med 2022;63(9): 1401–7.

139. Sharma SK, Pourat J, Abdel-Atti D, et al. Noninvasive Interrogation of DLL3 expression in metastatic

small cell Lung cancer. Cancer Res 2017;77(14): 3931–41.

140. Hubert RS, Vivanco I, Chen E, et al. STEAP: a prostate-specific cell-surface antigen highly expressed in human prostate tumors. Proc Natl Acad Sci U S A 1999;96(25):14523–8.

141. Shimizu Y, Suzuki T, Yoshikawa T, et al. Next-generation cancer Immunotherapy targeting glypican-3. Front Oncol 2019;9:248.

142. Savelli G, Muni A, Falchi R, et al. Somatostatin receptors over-expression in castration resistant prostate cancer detected by PET/CT: preliminary report of in six patients. Ann Transl Med 2015; 3(10):145.

143. Hofman MS, Hicks RJ, Maurer T, et al. Prostate-specific membrane antigen PET: clinical utility in prostate cancer, normal patterns, Pearls, and pitfalls. Radiographics 2018;38(1):200–17.

144. Gafita A, Djaileb L, Rauscher I, et al. Response evaluation criteria in PSMA PET/CT (RECIP 1.0) in metastatic castration-resistant prostate cancer. Radiology 2023;308(1):e222148.

145. Seifert R, Emmett L, Rowe SP, et al. Second version of the prostate cancer molecular imaging standardized evaluation Framework including response evaluation for clinical trials (PROMISE V2). Eur Urol 2023;83(5):405–12.

146. Ceci F, Oprea-Lager DE, Emmett L, et al. E-PSMA: The EANM standardized reporting guidelines v1.0 for PSMA-PET. Eur J Nucl Med Mol Imaging 2021;48(5):1626–38.

147. Zang S, Ai S, Yang R, et al. Development and validation of 68Ga-PSMA-11 PET/CT-based radiomics model to detect primary prostate cancer. EJNMMI Res 2022;12(1):63.

148. Hofman MS, Iravani A. Gallium-68 prostate-specific membrane antigen PET imaging. Pet Clin 2017; 12(2):219–34.

149. Hofman MS, Iravani A, Nzenza T, et al. Advances in Urologic imaging: prostate-specific membrane antigen ligand PET imaging. Urol Clin North Am 2018; 45(3):503–24.

150. Sutherland DEK, Azad AA, Murphy DG, et al. Role of FDG PET/CT in management of patients with prostate cancer. Semin Nucl Med 2023. https://doi.org/10.1053/j.semnuclmed.2023.06.005.

Quarter-Century PET/CT Transformation of Oncology: Lymphoma

Ashwin Singh Parihar, MBBS, MD[a,b,*,1], Niharika Pant, MBBS, MD[a,1],
Rathan M. Subramaniam, MD, PhD, MPH, MBA[c,d,e]

KEYWORDS

- Lymphoma • FDG PET/CT • Response assessment • Fluorodeoxyglucose • Deauville • Hodgkin
- Non-Hodgkin

KEY POINTS

- FDG PET/CT is central to initial staging and response assessment for the majority of lymphomas.
- The 5-point scale is a visual scoring system used to determine treatment response in the FDG-avid lymphomas using the Lugano criteria.
- FDG PET/CT is superior to conventional imaging in differentiating metabolically active residual malignancy from metabolically inactive residual fibrosis.

INTRODUCTION

The clinical landscape of lymphomas has changed dramatically over the last 2 decades, including significant progress made in the understanding and utilization of imaging modalities and the available treatment options for both indolent and aggressive lymphomas. Since the introduction of hybrid PET/CT scanners in 2001, the indications of [18F]fluorodeoxyglucose (FDG) PET/CT in the management of lymphomas have grown rapidly. In today's clinical practice, FDG PET/CT is used in successful management of the vast majority patients with lymphomas.

In this review, the authors start with providing a historical overview of management of lymphomas from a diagnostic imaging perspective, describing how FDG-PET/CT was integrated in the management algorithm. The subsequent sections elaborate on the clinical indications of performing FDG-PET/CT in patients with lymphoma, describing the currently followed Lugano system for initial staging

and response assessment. Special emphasis is given to the interim response assessment and its value in disease prognostication. The authors conclude with discussing the areas of current research and future advances.

CLASSIFICATION OF LYMPHOID NEOPLASMS

Lymphoid neoplasms are broadly categorized as those originating from B-cell, T-cell, or natural killer (NK)-cell lineage. Further subcategories are based on whether they derive from precursor cells or mature lymphocytes and plasma cells.[1] hodgkin lymphoma (HL) arises from precursor B cells with characteristic malignant Reed–Sternberg cells. Despite being the hallmark of HL, the Reed–Sternberg cells composed of less than 1% of the tumor microenvironment, with the majority being comprised by the inflammatory cells (such as macrophages, eosinophils, T cells, B cells, and plasma cells).[2] Thus, from an imaging perspective, it is important to recognize that the bulk of a "malignant

[a] Mallinckrodt Institute of Radiology; [b] Siteman Cancer Center, Washington University School of Medicine, St Louis, MO, USA; [c] Faculty of Medicine, Nursing, Midwifery & Health Sciences, The University of Notre Dame Australia, Sydney, Australia; [d] Department of Radiology, Duke University, Durham, NC, USA; [e] Department of Medicine, University of Otago Medical School, Dunedin, New Zealand
[1] Contributed equally.
* Corresponding author. Mallinckrodt Institute of Radiology, Washington University School of Medicine, 4525 Scott Avenue, #3433, St Louis, MO 63110.
E-mail address: ashwinp@wustl.edu

PET Clin 19 (2024) 281–290
https://doi.org/10.1016/j.cpet.2023.12.014
1556-8598/24/© 2023 Elsevier Inc. All rights reserved.

pet.theclinics.com

lesion" seen on structural imaging in patients with HL represents the inflammatory cell population. NHLs arise from malignant, monoclonal proliferations of B cells or T cells. Definitive distinction between HL and non-Hodgkin lymphoma (NHL) requires a pathologic examination; however, there are pertinent differences in the imaging characteristics of these lymphomas. Most patients with HL have localized, predominantly nodal disease that spreads in a contiguous manner with infrequent extranodal involvement. Conversely, most patients with NHL have a disseminated disease involving several nodal groups, with frequent involvement of extranodal sites.

HISTORICAL OVERVIEW

Imaging in lymphoma has advanced from the use of plain films (commonly chest x-rays) to FDG-PET/CT, the latter of which is now the standard of care for the majority of lymphomas. The staging of lymphomas was commonly done using a combination of invasive (nodal biopsies, laparotomy, splenectomy) and relatively noninvasive techniques (lymphangiography, fluoroscopy in the 1960s).[3] The advent of CT and subsequent technological improvements enabled noninvasive staging of lymphomas. Even though imaging was mainstream in the staging and response assessment of lymphomas, there were obvious limitations to the available techniques. The most common problems were low inter-reader, and even intra-reader reproducibility of measurements on anatomic imaging, discordance between tumor size and survival outcomes following treatment,

and difficulties in measuring certain patterns of disease involvement, such as malignant effusions and sclerotic osseous lesions.[4]

The international workshop criteria (IWC) first incorporated the FDG-PET findings in the traditional response assessment criteria of NHL.[5] Further modifications to the IWC + PET criteria, including descriptions for assessment of FDG uptake based on the lesion size led to the International Harmonization Project (IHP).[6,7] The IHP recommended the use of mediastinal blood-pool activity as a reference for comparing the FDG uptake in lesions with size greater than 2 cm in their largest transaxial diameter. For smaller lesions, the background activity was recommended as the reference standard. Additional guidance was also provided for the timing of PET following treatment to avoid false positives due to therapy-related inflammation. PET was recommended to be performed at least 3 weeks, and preferably 6 to 8 weeks following chemotherapy, and at 8 to 12 weeks following radiation therapy.[6] These distinctions led to the elimination of "Complete response unconfirmed (CRu)" from the categorical response assessment framework. The IHP also provided standardized definitions for relevant end points of therapeutic efficacy in the lymphoma clinical trials. The Deauville criteria, initially proposed in 2009 and subsequently modified, were a major landmark in simplifying the interpretation of FDG-PET with robust patient-specific internal comparators and high inter-reader reproducibility.[8] The Deauville criteria provided for a five-point scale, comparing the FDG uptake at disease sites to that of the blood pool and the liver (**Fig. 1**).

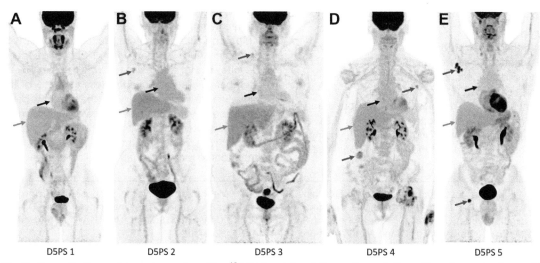

D5PS 1 D5PS 2 D5PS 3 D5PS 4 D5PS 5

Fig. 1. Deauville five-point scoring system. The ^{18}F-FDG uptake at the malignant sites of lymphoma (*red arrow*) is compared with FDG activity in the background, blood pool (*black arrow*) and the liver (*blue arrow*). Thus, the normal tissues in the same patient at the same time point are used as comparators for grading the abnormal FDG avidity at the lesions. (*A–E*) Representative scores ranging from 1 to 5.

The Deauville criteria were adopted by the Lugano classification for interim and end-of-treatment response assessment, translating the five-point scale to the four conventional categories of response—complete metabolic response (CR), partial metabolic response (PR), stable metabolic disease (SD), and progressive metabolic disease (PD).[9]

DIAGNOSIS AND INITIAL STAGING

The combined whole-body structural and metabolic information gained from FDG-PET/CT is valuable in identifying patterns typical of lymphomatous involvement. These features in FDG-avid lymphomas include intensely hypermetabolic contiguous lymph nodes (typical of HL) or noncontiguous disseminated lymphadenopathy with/without extra-lymphatic involvement (typical of NHL). Involvement of the marrow, liver, and spleen is often characteristic. PET/CT features can suggest lymphoma as a major differential and guide toward an appropriate representative site for tissue sampling in patients with uncertain clinical diagnosis (**Fig. 2**).

After a tissue diagnosis has been established, imaging-guided staging of lymphoma provides important information about the disease extent, facilitating appropriate treatment selection, and disease prognostication and provides for a baseline reference for response assessment following treatment. The Ann Arbor classification and its subsequent modifications combined clinical, pathologic, and radiological assessment of the disease, classifying the disease extent into four stages, from involvement of limited sites to extensive involvement of lymph nodes and extranodal tissues.[10] This system of disease staging, while efficient in prognostication of patients with HL, did not correlate with survival outcomes in patients with NHL.[11] The advances in metabolic imaging, initially using FDG-PET (and later, hybrid PET/CT) led to the inclusion of functional imaging for assessment of disease at baseline and following treatment for response assessment. The current system for staging of lymphomas is based on the Lugano guidelines established in 2013.

Lugano Classification

FDG-PET/CT was established as a standard for initial staging and response assessment of the FDG-avid lymphomas which include the majority of histologies. The few histologies with low or variable FDG-avidity, where CT assumes the central role in staging and response assessment include small lymphocytic lymphomas (chronic lymphocytic leukemia), lymphoplasmacytic lymphoma (Waldenström's macroglobulinemia),

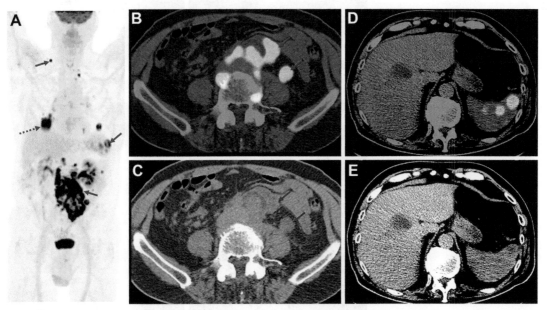

Fig. 2. ^{18}F-FDG-PET/CT in a 78-year-old man with a prior CT showing bilateral lung nodules concerning for metastatic disease. The FDG-PET/CT was requested for evaluation of a primary site. The images show extensive hypermetabolic lymphadenopathy above and below the diaphragm (*solid red arrows; A–C*), pulmonary lesions (*dotted red arrow; A*), involvement of the bone marrow (*thin red arrow; B*), and multifocal splenic involvement (*solid red arrows; D, E*). These findings raised the suspicion for a high-grade lymphoma. Subsequent biopsy from the pulmonary lesion (*dotted red arrow; A*) confirmed a diffuse large B-cell lymphoma.

cutaneous T-cell lymphomas, and marginal zone lymphoma (including lymphoma of the mucosa-associated lymphoid tissue) (**Fig. 3**).[9,12]

The Lugano classification (**Table 1**) described imaging criteria for disease involvement and incorporated the metabolic imaging-based assessment into the previous Ann Arbor classification. The Lugano classification also described patterns of disease involvement on FDG-PET/CT imaging. Unlike the CT-based criteria, the metabolic activity of the disease sites was prioritized over structural size for identification of disease sites. As an example, splenomegaly was not considered as a prerequisite for lymphomatous involvement and patterns on FDG-PET/CT such as diffuse increased uptake, focal nodules, or mass(es), even with a normal size spleen were considered as disease involvement (see **Fig. 2**). Similar patterns of involvement were described for the liver. It was also recognized that FDG-PET/CT is quite sensitive for detecting marrow involvement in the majority of patients with advanced lymphomas. It is now known that in patients with HL and aggressive NHLs, routine bone marrow biopsy does not provide any additional information compared with a positive FDG-PET/CT and hence may be omitted.[13,14] However, FDG-PET/CT is not sensitive for detecting low-volume marrow involvement and in certain histologies such as follicular lymphoma and indolent mantle cell lymphoma.[15] In addition, detection of marrow involvement becomes challenging in the setting of diffuse homogeneous or heterogeneous FDG avidity in the marrow, especially with recent administration of a bone marrow stimulating agent.[4]

Nuances in the Interpretation of ^{18}F-Fluorodeoxyglucose PET/CT

An accurate assessment of disease extent is useful for guiding treatment.[16] As an example, patients with limited stage diffuse large B-cell lymphomas are commonly treated with four cycles of R-CHOP, whereas those with advanced stage disease receive six cycles of R-CHOP-based treatment.[17] Similarly, the presence of bulky disease may require additional radiation therapy for adequate disease control. An accurate interpretation of the PET/CT findings is thus required to perform precise disease staging. The clinical interpretation of PET/CT may be confounded by the presence of synchronous malignancies, infective and inflammatory conditions that can have high uptake of ^{18}F-FDG.[18–21] In addition, it is important to recognize physiologic sites of ^{18}F-FDG uptake

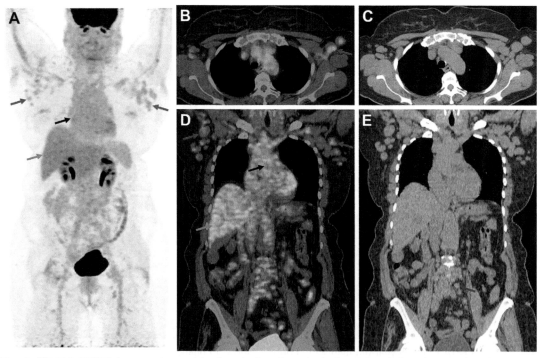

Fig. 3. ^{18}F-FDG-PET/CT in a patient with chronic lymphocytic leukemia/small lymphocytic lymphoma. The maximum intensity projection (*A*), transaxial (*B, C*) and coronal (*D, E*) images show the extensive lymphadenopathy above and below the diaphragm (*red arrows*), with FDG uptake slightly above blood pool (*black arrow*) and less than or similar to the liver (*blue arrow*). Contrast these with the FDG-avid histologies which typically show an FDG uptake markedly higher than that of the liver.

Table 1
Lugano classification for staging of lymphomas

Limited	Stage I	• Involvement of one node or a group of adjacent nodes[a] • Single extranodal lesion without nodal involvement[b]
	Stage II	• ≥2 nodal groups on the same side of the diaphragm • Limited contiguous extranodal involvement with stage I/II by nodal disease extent[b]
Advanced	Stage III	• Nodes on both sides of the diaphragm or nodes above the diaphragm with splenic involvement
	Stage IV	• Noncontiguous extralymphatic involvement

[a] Waldeyer's ring (adenoids, tubal, palatine, and lingual tonsils) and spleen are considered nodal tissue for the purposes of classification.
[b] A designation E is used to denote limited extranodal disease without nodal involvement (IE), or contiguous extranodal involvement with stage I/II nodal disease (IIE).

(Adapted from Cheson BD, Fisher RI, Barrington SF, et al. Recommendations for initial evaluation, staging, and response assessment of Hodgkin and non-Hodgkin lymphoma: the Lugano classification. J Clin Oncol. 2014;32:3059-3068).

such as Waldeyer's ring and brown fat that may mimic disease involvement (**Fig. 4**). FDG uptake in the bone marrow should also be interpreted with caution, as reactive marrow hyperplasia can show a mild diffuse or heterogeneous FDG uptake in the marrow versus an unifocal or multifocal ("patchy") pattern of uptake commonly seen with lymphomatous involvement. A caveat here is that patients with advanced lymphomas may have diffuse involvement of the marrow with markedly high FDG uptake. In these cases, it is important to correlate the imaging findings with laboratory values, medication history, and pathology findings.

Patients with a suspected primary central nervous system lymphoma often undergo FDG-PET/CT to evaluate for disease elsewhere and differentiate between a true primary central nervous system (CNS) lymphoma versus systemic lymphoma with additional CNS involvement.[22] In these cases, the field of view of PET/CT should include the whole brain and the intensity scale appropriately adjusted while interpretation to account for the high background FDG uptake in the normal brain parenchyma that may mask areas of lymphomatous involvement.

THERAPY MONITORING

The Lugano classification recommended assessment of response using the Deauville five-point scale (D5PS). Initially developed as a visual assessment method, further clarifications of the scale recommended the use of quantitative standardized uptake value (SUV) measurements for differentiating between the score of 4 and 5.[9] The D5PS involves comparing the FDG uptake at disease sites to that of the blood pool and the liver (see **Fig. 1**) and assigning a score from 1 (lowest) to 5 (highest) (**Table 2**). Similar to the previous section on initial staging, FDG-PET-derived D5PS for

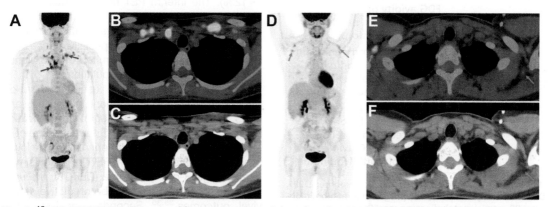

Fig. 4. ^{18}F-FDG-PET/CT in a 25-year-old woman with nodular sclerosing Hodgkin lymphoma. The baseline PET images (*A–C*) show involvement of lymph nodes above the diaphragm, including the supraclavicular, infraclavicular, and mediastinal stations (*red arrows*). Interim PET/CT performed at 2 months following two cycles of ABVD chemotherapy (adriamycin, bleomycin, vinblastine, dacarbazine) shows complete metabolic response (*D–F*). Note the physiologic FDG uptake in the brown fat (*blue arrows*) which should not be confused for malignant disease.

Table 2
Deauville five-point scale for FDG PET-based assessment of HL and NHL

Score	Interpretation (Based on ^{18}F-FDG Uptake)
1	Lesion uptake similar to or below background level
2	Lesion uptake $\leq$ mediastinal blood-pool
3	Lesion uptake > mediastinal blood-pool but $\leq$ liver
4	Lesion uptake moderately higher than that of liver
5	Markedly increased lesion uptake[a] and/or new sites of disease

[a] Suggested as uptake 2 to 3 times higher than the maximum SUV in the normal liver.
(Adapted from Meignan M, Gallamini A, Meignan M, Gallamini A, Haioun C. Report on the First International Workshop on Interim-PET-Scan in Lymphoma. Leuk Lymphoma. 2009;50:1257-1260.)

Table 3
Response assessment based on the Deauville five-point scale

Category	Definition
CR	D5PS 1–3, with no FDG-avid marrow lesions and no new lesions.
PR	D5PS 4 or 5 with reduction in FDG avidity of lesions compared with baseline, and no new lesions.
SD	D5PS 4 or 5 with no significant change in FDG avidity of lesions compared with baseline, and no new lesions
PD	D5PS 4 or 5 with increasing FDG avidity of lesions compared with baseline, and/or new FDG-avid lesions compatible with lymphoma

Abbreviations: CR, complete metabolic response; D5PS, Deauville five-point scale; PD, progressive metabolic disease; PR, partial metabolic response; SD, stable metabolic disease.
(Adapted from Cheson BD, Fisher RI, Barrington SF, et al. Recommendations for initial evaluation, staging, and response assessment of Hodgkin and non-Hodgkin lymphoma: the Lugano classification. J Clin Oncol. 2014;32:3059-3068.)

response assessment should be used only for the FDG-avid lymphomas.

The Lugano classification recommends the use of D5PS for response assessment at interim and end-of-treatment time points. The D5PS is assigned based on the FDG PET interpretation and is subsequently used to determine the response category (**Table 3**).

The interim PET for performing an early assessment of treatment response supports the measurement of a key response parameter "time-to-response." The degree of response is commonly captured as one of the response categories, for example, CR or PR; However, the time-to-response is an equally important measure that reflects the inherent tumor biology and the effectiveness of a particular treatment. This is emphatically described in terms of the tumor killing rate, where an interim PET can differentiate between patients with high tumor killing rate, manifesting as a complete response after two to three cycles of therapy, versus those with an insufficient tumor killing rate and a persistent positive interim PET.[4,23] The interim PET thus has a high prognostic value (see **Fig. 4**).[24]

The PETAL trial, a prospective randomized study of interim PET-guided therapy in patients with aggressive NHL, showed that while interim PET predicted survival in patients treated with R-CHOP, PET-based intensification of treatment did not lead to improved survival.[25] The trial also showed that the percentage change in maximum SUV (δSUVmax) with 66% as the cutoff was a better predictor of outcome than D5PS for the interim PET. The use of D5PS for interpreting interim PET led to a higher number of positive scans ($\sim$45.5%) when compared with the δSUVmax method ($\sim$12%). The interim PET has consistently been shown to have a high negative predictive value in HL and NHL.[26–31] However, its positive predictive value in patients with NHL, especially diffuse large B-cell lymphoma has been limited due to significant false positives in this population.[32–34]

FDG-PET/CT is routinely used for end-of-treatment response assessment in both HL and NHL. As with interim PET, Lugano classification recommends the use of D5PS for assessment of response at the end of treatment. Unlike the lower prognostic value of interim PET in patients with diffuse large B-cell lymphoma (DLBCL), the end-of-treatment PET is noted to be predictive of survival outcomes.[35,36] Secondary analysis of a phase 3 trial comparing standard-of-care R-CHOP with obinutuzumab with Cyclophosphamide, Hyrdoxydaunorubicin (Doxorubicin), Vincristine, Prednisone (CHOP) in patients with DLBCL showed that CR at the end-of-treatment PET using the Lugano classification was highly prognostic of both progression-free and overall survival.[36] The prognostic role of FDG-PET/CT has been described for assessment of patients, after completion of salvage chemotherapy and before autologous hematopoietic stem cell transplantation.[37]

FDG-PET/CT is also used for assessment of response to immunotherapy, especially with immune checkpoint inhibitors. As these agents act by activation of the immune system to induce cell-killing versus direct cytotoxic effects of conventional chemotherapy, there are distinct imaging patterns of response with the former agents. Of note, these patients may have pseudo-progression—a distinct phenomenon where the preexisting lesions seem more prominent (size and/or FDG uptake), with/without appearance of new lesions in a clinically improving patient.[4,38,39] This is a transient phenomenon due to changes in the tumor microenvironment and typically resolves on subsequent follow-up imaging. Separate response assessment criteria have been described to counter this issue of differentiating pseudo-progression versus true progression. The Lymphoma response to immunomodulatory therapy criteria introduced a separate category of indeterminate response and recommended a follow-up imaging at 12 weeks to either rule-in or exclude pseudo-progression.[40] The response evaluation criteria in lymphoma, expanded from

response evaluation criteria in solid tumours (RECIST) and primarily focused on structural imaging, were introduced in 2017 and included an additional category of minor response for patients who had a reduction in the sum of longest diameter of up to three target lesions, between ≥10% and less than 30%.[41] FDG-PET/CT has been used for assessment of response to radioimmunotherapy in patients with NHL.[42] Radioimmunotherapy that involves treatment with antibodies labeled to a therapeutic radionuclide has been shown to cause significant early decline in SUVs on FDG-PET.[42,43] FDG-PET/CT has also been shown to have prognostic value in patients undergoing chimeric antigen receptor T-cell (CART-cell) therapy. Although the initial response rate with these therapies is high, many patients eventually relapse posttreatment.[44] Given the high economic burden of these therapies, noninvasive tools are the need of the hour that can predict outcomes and optimize patient selection. A retrospective study of 171 patients undergoing CART-cell therapy showed that early PET/CT performed at 1 month was predictive of treatment failure.[44]

FDG-PET/CT is used for evaluation of lymphoma recurrence, although its utility in routine surveillance is limited.[45–48] Several studies have shown that the routine use of FDG-PET/CT in patients with lymphoma does not lead to improved outcomes and is not cost-effective.[46–48] However, detection of high-grade transformation of an

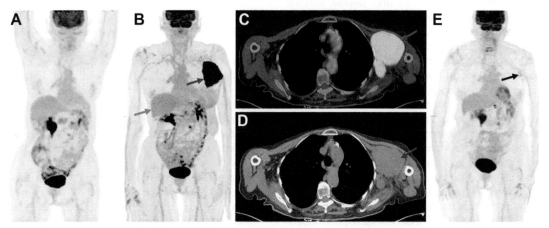

Fig. 5. ^{18}F-FDG-PET/CT in an 86-year-old woman with incidentally detected follicular lymphoma around 20 years back who was under observation. Her baseline ^{18}F-FDG PET/CT 1 year back did not show any evidence of disease (A). She developed an enlarging swelling in her left axilla which was suspicious for disease recurrence. Her FDG PET/CT showed a new markedly hypermetabolic left axillary nodal mass (*red arrow; B–D*) which had a markedly higher FDG uptake compared with the liver (*blue arrow*). This finding was suspicious for transformation of follicular lymphoma to an aggressive histology. Subsequent biopsy from the axillary nodal mass showed diffuse large B-cell lymphoma with a Ki-67 of 80%. The patient was treated with six cycles of R-miniCHOP (rituximab, cyclophosphamide, doxorubicin, vincristine, prednisone) and the posttreatment PET/CT (*E*) showed complete metabolic response to treatment, black arrow denotes the site of the treated lesion, which now has an FDG uptake similar to that of the blood pool..

otherwise indolent disease is a recognized indication of FDG-PET/CT (**Fig. 5**).[49] Richter's transformation refers to a transformation of an indolent lymphoma, such as chronic lymphocytic leukemia (CLL) to an aggressive variant, commonly DLBCL. FDG-PET/CT has a high sensitivity and specificity at detecting these sites of transformation and guiding toward an appropriate site for biopsy. Transformed lymphoma has a higher FDG uptake compared with the relatively lower uptake of disease elsewhere, which is typical for indolent lymphomas such as CLL.[50] SUV cutoffs of ≥ 5 and ≥ 10 have been proposed to detect sites of transformation on an FDG-PET/CT.[50,51]

SUMMARY AND FUTURE DIRECTIONS

The use of quantitative metrics, such as metabolic tumor volume (MTV), and total lesion glycolysis (TLG) in a research setting in several lymphoid and solid tumors has shown promise.[52–54] MTV is the metabolically active volume of the lesion, based on a predetermined SUV threshold. The TLG is derived as a product of the MTV and the mean SUV of the lesion. The MTV of lesions throughout the body can be summed to give a total body MTV (TMTV), which is representative of the global metabolically active disease burden. A retrospective study of 185 patients with follicular lymphoma who were receiving combination immune-chemotherapy showed that TMTV calculated on baseline PET was highly prognostic for both progression-free survival (PFS) and overall survival (OS).[55] However, there are challenges with these measurements, including lack of standardization (SUV threshold to be used for segmenting), suboptimal reproducibility of cutoff values and time required to perform these measurements in a clinical setting.[56] Although artificial intelligence-based tools are attempting to solve several of these limitations. The development and validation of artificial intelligence and radiomics-based tools has shown promise in disease prognostication.[57] It is anticipated that the use of quantitative metrics and radiomic analyses will grow significantly, especially with the advent of reliable automatic segmentation methods that can be deployed in busy clinical practices.[58] The development of new radiopharmaceuticals such as those targeting specific cellular/subcellular structures in the tumor microenvironment that can aid in both diagnosis and therapy is an area of active research.[59,60] We have come a long way in the integration of PET/CT in management of lymphomas, and with the new developments in radiopharmacy and physics, there will be additional avenues for imaging to aid in the management of these patients.

CLINICS CARE POINTS

- Presence of residual masses with no metabolic activity on FDG PET does not negate complete response in most lymphomas.
- Interim PET/CT helps in determining rate of response in addition to the degree of response. This has prognostic and predictive implications.
- Selection of a representative hypermetabolic lesion in patients with suspected high-grade transformation of a low-grade lymphoma is vital to an accurate diagnosis.
- Gross bone-marrow involvement at initial staging of non-Hodgkin lymphoma on FDG PET/CT often obviates the requirement of an additional bone marrow biopsy for staging.

REFERENCES

1. Alaggio R, Amador C, Anagnostopoulos I, et al. The 5th edition of the world health organization classification of haematolymphoid tumours: lymphoid neoplasms. Leukemia 2022;36:1720–48.
2. Lee IS, Kim SH, Song HG, et al. The molecular basis for the generation of Hodgkin and Reed-Sternberg cells in Hodgkin's lymphoma. Int J Hematol 2003; 77:330–5.
3. Cunningham J, Iyengar S, Sharma B. Evolution of lymphoma staging and response evaluation: current limitations and future directions. Nat Rev Clin Oncol 2017;14:631–45.
4. Parihar AS, Dehdashti F, Wahl RL. FDG PET/CT-based response assessment in malignancies. Radiographics 2023;43:e220122.
5. Cheson BD, Horning SJ, Coiffier B, et al. Report of an international workshop to standardize response criteria for Non-Hodgkin's Lymphomas. J Clin Oncol 1999;17:1244–53.
6. Cheson BD, Pfistner B, Juweid ME, et al. Revised response criteria for malignant lymphoma. J Clin Oncol 2007;25:579–86.
7. Juweid ME, Stroobants S, Hoekstra OS, et al. Use of positron emission tomography for response assessment of lymphoma: consensus of the imaging subcommittee of international harmonization project in lymphoma. J Clin Oncol 2007;25:571–8.
8. Meignan M, Gallamini A, Meignan M, et al. Report on the first international workshop on interim-pet-scan in lymphoma. Leuk Lymphoma 2009;50:1257–60.
9. Cheson BD, Fisher RI, Barrington SF, et al. Recommendations for initial evaluation, staging, and response assessment of Hodgkin and non-Hodgkin lymphoma: the Lugano classification. J Clin Oncol 2014;32:3059–68.

10. Lister TA, Crowther D, Sutcliffe SB, et al. Report of a committee convened to discuss the evaluation and staging of patients with Hodgkin's disease: cotswolds meeting. J Clin Oncol 1989;7:1630–6.

11. Rosenberg SA. Validity of the Ann Arbor staging classification for the non-Hodgkin's lymphomas. Cancer Treat Rep 1977;61:1023–7.

12. Weiler-Sagie M, Bushelev O, Epelbaum R, et al. 18) F-FDG avidity in lymphoma readdressed: a study of 766 patients. J Nucl Med 2010;51:25–30.

13. Kaddu-Mulindwa D, Altmann B, Held G, et al. FDG PET/CT to detect bone marrow involvement in the initial staging of patients with aggressive non-Hodgkin lymphoma: results from the prospective, multicenter PETAL and OPTIMAL>60 trials. Eur J Nucl Med Mol Imag 2021;48:3550–9.

14. Weiler-Sagie M, Kagna O, Dann EJ, et al. Characterizing bone marrow involvement in Hodgkin's lymphoma by FDG-PET/CT. Eur J Nucl Med Mol Imag 2014;41:1133–40.

15. Nakajima R, Moskowitz AJ, Michaud L, et al. Baseline FDG-PET/CT detects bone marrow involvement in follicular lymphoma and provides relevant prognostic information. Blood Adv 2020; 4:1812–23.

16. Vadi SK, Parihar AS, Mittal BR, et al. F-18 fluorodeoxyglucose positron-emission tomography-computed tomography in a case of extensive multi-organal extranodal lymphoma with cardiac involvement mimicking apical hypertrophic obstructive cardiomyopathy: staging and response evaluation. Indian J Nucl Med 2018;33:370–3.

17. Ngu H, Takiar R, Phillips T, et al. Revising the treatment pathways in lymphoma: new standards of care-how do we choose? Am Soc Clin Oncol Educ Book 2022;42:1–14.

18. Sood A, Mittal BR, Modi M, et al. 18F-FDG PET/CT in tuberculosis: can interim PET/CT predict the clinical outcome of the patients? Clin Nucl Med 2020;45: 276–82.

19. Vadi SK, Kumar R, Mittal BR, et al. 18F-FDG PET/CT in an atypical case of relapsed IgG4-related disease presenting as inflammatory pseudotumor in gall bladder fossa with extensive disease involvement. Clin Nucl Med 2018;43:e357–9.

20. Parihar AS, Singh H, Kumar R, et al. Pancreatic malignancy or not?: role of 18F-FDG PET/CT in solving the diagnostic dilemma and evaluating treatment response. Clin Nucl Med 2018;43: e115–7.

21. Parihar AS, Mittal BR, Vadi SK, et al. Groove pancreatitis masquerading as pancreatic carcinoma-Detected on (18)F-FDG PET/CT. Nucl Med Mol Imaging 2018;52:473–4.

22. Mohile NA, Deangelis LM, Abrey LE. The utility of body FDG PET in staging primary central nervous system lymphoma. Neuro Oncol 2008;10:223–8.

23. Wahl RL, Jacene H, Kasamon Y, et al. From RECIST to PERCIST: evolving Considerations for PET response criteria in solid tumors. J Nucl Med 2009; 50(Suppl 1):122S–50S.

24. Hutchings M, Barrington SF. PET/CT for therapy response assessment in lymphoma. J Nucl Med 2009;50(Suppl 1):21S–30S.

25. Dührsen U, Müller S, Hertenstein B, et al. Positron emission tomography-guided therapy of Aggressive Non-Hodgkin Lymphomas (PETAL): a multicenter, randomized phase III trial. J Clin Oncol 2018;36: 2024–34.

26. Straus DJ, Jung SH, Pitcher B, et al. Calgb 50604: risk-adapted treatment of nonbulky early-stage Hodgkin lymphoma based on interim PET. Blood 2018;132:1013–21.

27. Radford J, Illidge T, Counsell N, et al. Results of a trial of PET-directed therapy for early-stage Hodgkin's lymphoma. N Engl J Med 2015;372: 1598–607.

28. Kreissl S, Goergen H, Buehnen I, et al. PET-guided eBEACOPP treatment of advanced-stage Hodgkin lymphoma (HD18): follow-up analysis of an international, open-label, randomised, phase 3 trial. Lancet Haematol 2021;8:e398–409.

29. Casasnovas RO, Bouabdallah R, Brice P, et al. Positron emission tomography-driven strategy in advanced Hodgkin lymphoma: prolonged follow-up of the AHL2011 Phase III Lymphoma Study Association Study. J Clin Oncol 2022;40:1091–101.

30. Press OW, Li H, Schoder H, et al. US intergroup trial of response-adapted therapy for stage III to IV Hodgkin lymphoma using early interim fluorodeoxyglucose-positron emission tomography imaging: southwest Oncology group S0816. J Clin Oncol 2016;34:2020–7.

31. Johnson P, Federico M, Kirkwood A, et al. Adapted treatment guided by interim PET-CT scan in advanced Hodgkin's lymphoma. N Engl J Med 2016;374:2419–29.

32. Zeman MN, Akin EA, Merryman RW, et al. Interim FDG-PET/CT for response assessment of lymphoma. Semin Nucl Med 2023;53:371–88.

33. Eertink JJ, Burggraaff CN, Heymans MW, et al. Optimal timing and criteria of interim PET in DLBCL: a comparative study of 1692 patients. Blood Adv 2021;5:2375–84.

34. Burggraaff CN, de Jong A, Hoekstra OS, et al. Predictive value of interim positron emission tomography in diffuse large B-cell lymphoma: a systematic review and meta-analysis. Eur J Nucl Med Mol Imag 2019;46:65–79.

35. Cox MC, Ambrogi V, Lanni V, et al. Use of interim [18F]fluorodeoxyglucose-positron emission tomography is not justified in diffuse large B-cell lymphoma during first-line immunochemotherapy. Leuk Lymphoma 2012;53:263–9.

36. Kostakoglu L, Martelli M, Sehn LH, et al. End-of-treatment PET/CT predicts PFS and OS in DLBCL after first-line treatment: results from GOYA. Blood Adv 2021;5:1283–90.

37. Jacene HA. FDG PET for assessment of autologous stem cell transplantation. Semin Nucl Med 2021;51:380–91.

38. Lopci E, Meignan M. Current evidence on PET response assessment to immunotherapy in lymphomas. Pet Clin 2020;15:23–34.

39. Parihar AS, Haq A, Wahl RL, et al. Progression or response: new liver lesions in a patient with responding hodgkin lymphoma. J Nucl Med 2023;64:500.

40. Cheson BD, Ansell S, Schwartz L, et al. Refinement of the Lugano Classification lymphoma response criteria in the era of immunomodulatory therapy. Blood 2016;128:2489–96.

41. Younes A, Hilden P, Coiffier B, et al. International Working Group consensus response evaluation criteria in lymphoma (RECIL 2017). Ann Oncol 2017;28:1436–47.

42. Jacene HA, Filice R, Kasecamp W, et al. 18F-FDG PET/CT for monitoring the response of lymphoma to radioimmunotherapy. J Nucl Med 2009;50:8–17.

43. Parihar AS, Jacene HA, Tirumani SH, et al. Radionuclide therapy of lymphomas. In: Volterrani D, Erba PA, Strauss HW, et al, editors. Nuclear Oncology: from pathophysiology to clinical applications. Cham: Springer International Publishing; 2020. p. 1–18.

44. Kuhnl A, Roddie C, Kirkwood AA, et al. Early FDG-PET response predicts CAR-T failure in large B-cell lymphoma. Blood Adv 2022;6:321–6.

45. Sood A, Parihar AS, Malhotra P, et al. Pulmonary recurrence of lymphomatoid granulomatosis diagnosed on F-18 FDG PET/CT. Indian J Nucl Med 2020;35:167–9.

46. Thompson CA, Ghesquieres H, Maurer MJ, et al. Utility of routine post-therapy surveillance imaging in diffuse large B-cell lymphoma. J Clin Oncol 2014;32:3506–12.

47. El-Galaly TC, Jakobsen LH, Hutchings M, et al. Routine imaging for diffuse large B-cell lymphoma in first complete remission does not improve post-treatment survival: a Danish–Swedish population-based study. J Clin Oncol 2015;33:3993–8.

48. Huntington SF, Svoboda J, Doshi JA. Cost-effectiveness analysis of routine surveillance imaging of patients with diffuse large B-cell lymphoma in first remission. J Clin Oncol 2015;33:1467–74.

49. Sood A, Parihar AS, Lad D, et al. An unusual presentation of Richter's transformation of chronic lymphocytic leukemia in liver and lung on (18)F-labeled fluoro-2-deoxyglucose positron emission tomography/computed tomography. Indian J Nucl Med 2020;35:70–1.

50. Bruzzi JF, Macapinlac H, Tsimberidou AM, et al. Detection of Richter's transformation of chronic lymphocytic leukemia by PET/CT. J Nucl Med 2006;47:1267–73.

51. Michallet AS, Sesques P, Rabe KG, et al. An 18F-FDG-PET maximum standardized uptake value > 10 represents a novel valid marker for discerning Richter's Syndrome. Leuk Lymphoma 2016;57:1474–7.

52. Mikhaeel NG, Heymans MW, Eertink JJ, et al. Proposed new dynamic prognostic index for diffuse large b-cell lymphoma: international metabolic prognostic index. J Clin Oncol 2022;40:2352–60.

53. Akhtari M, Milgrom SA, Pinnix CC, et al. Reclassifying patients with early-stage Hodgkin lymphoma based on functional radiographic markers at presentation. Blood 2018;131:84–94.

54. Mettler J, Muller H, Voltin CA, et al. Metabolic tumour volume for response prediction in advanced-stage hodgkin Lymphoma. J Nucl Med 2018;60:207–11.

55. Meignan M, Cottereau AS, Versari A, et al. Baseline metabolic tumor volume predicts outcome in high-tumor-burden follicular lymphoma: a pooled analysis of three multicenter studies. J Clin Oncol 2016;34:3618–26.

56. Schoder H, Moskowitz C. Metabolic tumor volume in lymphoma: hype or hope? J Clin Oncol 2016;34:3591–4.

57. Driessen J, Zwezerijnen GJC, Schoder H, et al. Prognostic model using 18F-FDG PET radiomics predicts progression-free survival in relapsed/refractory Hodgkin lymphoma. Blood Adv 2023;7:6732–43.

58. Blanc-Durand P, Jegou S, Kanoun S, et al. Fully automatic segmentation of diffuse large B cell lymphoma lesions on 3D FDG-PET/CT for total metabolic tumour volume prediction using a convolutional neural network. Eur J Nucl Med Mol Imag 2021;48:1362–70.

59. Rizvi SN, Visser OJ, Vosjan MJ, et al. Biodistribution, radiation dosimetry and scouting of 90Y-ibritumomab tiuxetan therapy in patients with relapsed B-cell non-Hodgkin's lymphoma using 89Zr-ibritumomab tiuxetan and PET. Eur J Nucl Med Mol Imag 2012;39:512–20.

60. Wester HJ, Keller U, Schottelius M, et al. Disclosing the CXCR4 expression in lymphoproliferative diseases by targeted molecular imaging. Theranostics 2015;5:618–30.

PET/Computed Tomography Transformation of Oncology Immunotherapy Assessment

Alireza Ghodsi, MD[a], Rodney J. Hicks, MD, FRACP[b,c,d], Amir Iravani, MD, FRACP[a,*]

KEYWORDS

- Molecular imaging • Immunotherapy • ^{18}F-FDG PET/CT • Radiopharmaceuticals
- Immune response

KEY POINTS

- Although immunotherapeutic strategies have substantially changed the treatment landscape of various cancers, selecting patients is still challenging, and more accurate prognostic and predictive biomarkers are required.
- Atypical response patterns posed challenges for the conventional response criteria based on structural imaging and molecular imaging with 2-deoxy-2-[^{18}F]fluoro-D-glucose positron emission tomography/computed tomography (^{18}F-FDG PET/CT), while the overall rate of these responses remains low. Multiple immune-related response criteria for ^{18}F-FDG PET/CT have been developed but large imaging repositories or multicenter prospective studies are needed for validation.
- ^{18}F-FDG PET/CT holds promise for guiding treatment-related decisions through baseline prognostication and response monitoring during the course of immunotherapy with potential added value of detection of immune-related adverse events.
- Novel immuno-PET radiopharmaceuticals present the potential for non-invasive and longitudinal characterization of individual tumors' immune tumor microenvironment by targeting the mechanisms involved in the immunotherapeutic strategies.

INTRODUCTION

Therapeutically modulating the immune microenvironment for the management of cancer has caused a paradigm shift in oncology.[1] Agents that increase anti-tumor responses through downregulating immunosuppressive targets, including monoclonal antibodies acting as immune checkpoint inhibitors (ICIs), specifically anticytotoxic T-lymphocyte antigen 4 (anti-CTLA-4), anti-programmed cell death receptor 1 (anti-PD-1), and anti-programmed death ligand 1 (anti-PD-L1), are the most common approach and represent examples of passive immunotherapy.[1]

Despite having demonstrated impressive disease control in some patients and documented benefits for overall survival in several cancers, the effectiveness of all these treatment options is constrained by the relatively small number of patients who achieve a durable objective response due to primary or secondary therapeutic resistance, or whose treatment is complicated by potentially life-threatening immunotherapy-related adverse events (irAEs).[2] Therefore, it is necessary to identify novel response

[a] Department of Radiology, University of Washington, 1144 Eastlake Avenue East, Seattle, WA 98109, USA; [b] Department of Medicine, St Vincent's Hospital, The University of Melbourne, Australia; [c] Department of Medicine, Central Clinical School, The Alfred Hospital, Monash University, Melbourne, Australia; [d] The Melbourne Theranostic Innovation Centre, North Melbourne, Australia
* Corresponding author.
E-mail address: airavani@uw.edu

PET Clin 19 (2024) 291–306
https://doi.org/10.1016/j.cpet.2023.12.012
1556-8598/24/© 2023 Elsevier Inc. All rights reserved.

predictors and resistance mechanisms. Evidence from large-scale clinical trials of current immunotherapeutic approaches using morphologic imaging demonstrated the limitations of previous response criteria based on computed tomography (CT) and MRI leading to an immune-based version of response evaluation criteria in solid tumors (iRECIST) with the concept of an indeterminate response or unconfirmed progressing disease, necessitating follow-up imaging confirmation.[3] Non-invasive monitoring of the immune system's response during treatment is made possible by molecular imaging. In recent years, it has been demonstrated that 2-deoxy-2-[^{18}F]fluoro-D-glucose positron emission tomography/CT(^{18}F-FDG PET/CT) can be used for immunotherapy to investigate response patterns, determine treatment responses, image irAEs, and provide knowledge regarding the prognosis of patients.[4]

This article aims to comprehensively review the current concepts of tumoral and systemic immune response assessment following immunotherapy, with a focus on ^{18}F-FDG PET/CT. Furthermore, it aims to provide an overview of novel immuno-PET tracers.

CHALLENGES IN DEFINING EARLY RESPONSE TO IMMUNOTHERAPY ON CONVENTIONAL IMAGING

Pseudoprogression has been recognized as an important confounder in assessing response to immune checkpoint therapy on CT or MRI. This phenomenon is defined as the initial increase in tumor burden caused by a rise in the size of the lesion or the occurrence of new lesions, followed by an eventual decrease in tumor burden at the subsequent imaging follow-up.[5] It was first objectively evaluated in a phase II clinical trial that included 227 patients with advanced melanoma which found 4 distinctive patterns of response following treatment with ipilimumab (anti-CTLA-4). These patterns were stable disease; reduction of the initial lesion without the occurrence of new lesions; responses following an initial increase in total tumor burden; and responses in the presence of newly formed lesions.[6] The last 2 responses, which the authors defined as pseudoprogression, accounted for about 10% of the cohort and had substantially greater survival rates compared to nonresponders. These findings promoted the idea of treating patients beyond what would generally be considered conventional morphologic progression.[6]

Subsequent reports of therapeutic response to anti-PD-1/PD-L1 have reported a lower rate of pseudoprogression than anti-CTLA-4, demonstrating that the type of immune checkpoint inhibitors (ICI) may impact the incidence of pseudoprogression. The rate of pseudoprogression was 7.3% in a subgroup of KEYNOTE-001 patients with advanced melanoma who receive pembrolizumab (anti-PD-1), and this was lower than the reported rate in the setting of ipilimumab using the same criteria.[7] In a retrospective study that evaluated over 800 patients with different malignancies using atezolizumab (anti-PD-L1), there was a greater rate of pseudoprogression in melanoma compared to non-small cell lung cancer (NSCLC) (7.3% vs 2.3%–2.8%, respectively),[8] suggesting that the type of cancer may also influence the incidence of pseudoprogression.

THE CASE FOR METABOLIC IMAGING USING FDG PET/CT

Metabolic imaging with FDG PET has increasingly been adopted in evaluation of therapeutic response to chemotherapy, radiotherapy, and various targeted therapies and can provide information earlier and that is not uncommonly discordant compared with anatomic imaging responses. It is, therefore, not surprising that it has also been evaluated for evaluating response to immunotherapy therapy response.

The first ^{18}F-FDG PET/CT-based assessment criteria incorporating metabolic response for oncological disease monitoring were developed by the European Organisation for Research and Treatment of Cancer (EORTC).[9] The EORTC criteria were eventually supplemented by the PET Response Criteria in Solid Tumors (PERCIST), which was developed by Wahl and colleagues.[10] Preliminary results in a small number of NSCLC patients found that ^{18}F-FDG PET/CT response using either EORTC or PERCIST criteria following 2 or 3 immunotherapy sessions correlated with a subsequent radiologic complete or partial response.[9–11]

However, due to subsequent demonstration of limitations of EORTC and PERCIST criteria in patients receiving immunotherapy, modified response evaluation criteria have been proposed.[12,13] In a study of 20 advanced melanoma patients receiving ICI, various response criteria were compared to assess ^{18}F-FDG PET/CT scans as an early predictor of response to ICIs. For predicting the best overall response, RECIST 1.1[14] was more accurate than PERCIST at the end of 1 month. As a result, new criteria were created by combining PERCIST and RECIST 1.1 and named the PET/CT Criteria for Early Prediction of Response to Immune Checkpoint Inhibitor Therapy (PECRIT), which showed a sensitivity of 100%, a specificity of 93%, and an accuracy of 95% in anticipating tumor response. Based on PECRIT response evaluation, patients with an early increase of greater than 15.5% in ^{18}F-FDG uptake and stable disease (by RECIST 1.1) commonly demonstrated eventual clinical benefit.[13] This study was, however, limited by a small sample cohort and *post hoc* definition of response criteria.

Further new response criteria, known as the PET Response Evaluation Criteria for Immunotherapy (PERCIMT), were created to consider the number and size of the new lesions on ^{18}F-FDG PET/CT. These demonstrated considerably greater sensitivity for predicting lack of clinical benefit compared to the EORTC on early ^{18}F-FDG PET/CT in patients with melanoma receiving ipilimumab. Moreover, they reported that there were no significant changes between responders and non-responders in ^{18}F-FDG uptake intensity in response to treatment.[15] In another study with a similar population treated with ipilimumab and vemurafenib, PERCIMT was substantiated on late ^{18}F-FDG PET/CT.[16] Further, when using PERCIMT after 2 cycles of ipilimumab to predict the best clinical response in patients with metastatic melanoma, the accuracy was 87.8% compared to 70.7% for conventional EORTC PET response criteria.[17] Again, these studies were relatively small and included a non-standard definition of response that involved clinical benefit rather than survival and objective response.

Further novel response criteria as a modification of the PERCIST criteria, known as the immunotherapy-modified PERCIST5 (imPERCIST5), employed the sum of ^{18}F-FDG uptake of up to 5 lesions, and unlike the PERCIMT criteria, the presence of new lesions was not routinely assumed to represent progressing disease.[18] In this study, a substantial difference in overall survival at 2 years was observed, with 66% for responders and 29% for non-responders, demonstrating the ability of imPERCIST5 for forecasting prognosis.[18]

Two studies of patients with Hodgkin lymphoma raised attention to the significance of tumor types for evaluating immunotherapy response in non-solid tumors.[19,20] The lymphoma response to immunomodulatory treatment criteria (LYRIC), a modification of the Lugano criteria,[21] were used in both studies about 3 months following the initiation of anti-PD-1 treatment.[22] The difference between the LYRIC and other response criteria for progression is the addition of the category of an indeterminate response, necessitating either a biopsy or further follow-up imaging to confirm or rule out pseudoprogression or progressive disease.[22] Chen and colleagues[20] evaluated 45 patients with Hodgkin lymphoma, and all of the patients with an indeterminate response showed progression after 3 months. Both the Lugano criteria and LYRIC indicated a precise prognostic classification of those with progression in comparison to patients without progression.

A molecular imaging approach, similar to the iRECIST criteria developed for anatomic imaging,[3] has been devised due to the prevalence of indeterminate responses in immunotherapy patients, known as immune PERCIST (iPERCIST). In a retrospective study of 28 patients with NSCLC treated with anti-PD-1 ICI (nivolumab), 13 patients had unconfirmed progressive disease; 4 of them underwent confirmatory studies 4 weeks later; and the other 9 patients discontinued immunotherapy due to clinical deterioration.[23]

Similar to iRECIST, the clinical state of the patient and metabolic response are taken into consideration when choosing whether to pursue immunotherapy between the first and second imaging follow-ups.[3,23]

A summary of the modified response criteria for interpretation of FDG PET/CT for ICI therapeutic response assessment is included in **Table 1**. While the research investigations underpinning the development of these criteria have improved our knowledge of the challenges that are associated with ^{18}F-FDG PET/CT response evaluation, most of the available information comes from single-center analyses with a small number of patients, variable timing after initiation of treatment, *post hoc* analyses defining diagnostic cut-offs, and non-standardized outcome measures. As a result, none of these criteria could be considered to have been validated as either prognostic or predictive biomarkers and require further assessment across the growing number of immunooncology treatment indications and approaches.

DIFFERENTIATING PSEUDOPROGRESSION FROM HYPERPROGRESSION

With further experience with use of imaging to evaluate response, additional patterns of response have been identified. These include hyperprogression, which is characterized by an unexpected acceleration of tumor progress following the initiation of immunotherapy. It is still unclear what biological mechanism ultimately causes hyperprogression.[24]

Patients who have hyperprogression have an extremely poor survival rate.[25] Therefore, it is crucial for physicians to detect hyperprogression and differentiate it from pseudoprogression as early as possible since there is a limited window of time in which to transition to another effective treatment. Currently, there are no specific evidence-based variables for ^{18}F-FDG PET/CT that might indicate hyperprogression. Nevertheless, it has been demonstrated that baseline metabolic tumor volume (MTV) and total lesion glycolysis (TLG) were all considerably greater in patients with melanoma who had hyperprogression.[26] In a similar study, 50

Table 1
A summary of immune-modified ^{18}F-FDG PET/CT response criteria

Criteria	Tumor Type	N	ICI	Modality	PR	CR	SD	PD	Confirmation of PD	Advantages
PECRIT[13]	Melanoma	20	Anti-CTLA-4	CT + ^{18}F-FDG PET/CT	Per RECIST 1.1 [14]	Per RECIST 1.1	Per RECIST 1.1 (Neither PR/CR, nor PD) Clinical benefit: >15.5% change in SUL$_{peak}$ per PERCIST[10] No clinical benefit: ≤15.5% change in SUL$_{peak}$ per PERCIST	Per RECIST 1.1 (≥20% increase in TL diameter (minimum 5 mm); new lesions)	No confirmation required.	• First effort in modifying ^{18}F-FDG PET/CT response criteria for ICIs. • Combining the metabolic characteristics of PERCIST with the morphologic aspects of RECIST. • 100% sensitivity, 93% specificity. • Higher accuracy (95%) rather than PERCIST (70%) or RECIST 1.1 (75%) alone.
PERCIST[10]	-	-	-	^{18}F-FDG PET/CT	• ≥30% reduction in SUL$_{peak}$ of hottest lesion. • Minimum of 0.8 units absolute decrease in SUL$_{peak}$ of hottest lesion	• Complete resolution of ^{18}F-FDG uptake in measurable TL. • Disappearance of other lesions to the level of background blood pool.	Neither PR/CR, nor PD	• >30% increase in SUL$_{peak}$ of ^{18}F-FDG uptake (minimum of 0.8 unit absolute increase of SUL$_{peak}$) • Appearance of new ^{18}F-FDG-avid lesions • 75% increase in total lesion glycolysis	N. A	Develop basic recommendations for ^{18}F-FDG PET/CT response criteria, such as • Standardizing the protocol for imaging • Establishing a 30% cut-off for changes indicating PD or PR. • Using SUL$_{peak}$

PERCIMT[15]	Melanoma	41	Anti-CTLA-4	CT + 18F-FDG PET/CT	• Decrease in number or size of lesions on brain MRI and 18F-FDG PET/CT. • Decrease or no increase in LDH. • No new lesion.	• Resolution of lesions on brain MRI and 18F-FDG PET/CT. • No new lesion • Decrease or no increase in LDH.	Neither PR/CR, nor PD	New lesions predict no clinical benefit: ≥ 2 lesions more than 1.5 cm, or ≥ 3 lesions more than 1 cm, or ≥ 4 lesions <1 cm.	No confirmation required.	• Clinical benefits were incorporated into the response criteria.
LYRIC[19,22]	Hodgkin's lymphoma	16	Anti-PD-1	CT + 18F-FDG PET/CT	Per Lugano classification[21]	Per Lugano classification	Neither PR/CR, nor PD	Per Lugano classification, except: IR1: ≥ 50% increase in SPD in first 12 wk. IR2a: < 50% increase in SPD with new lesion. IR2b: < 50% increase in SPD with ≥50% increase in PPD of a lesion IR3: increase in 18F-FDG uptake without PD-defining increase in lesion size New lesion: IR2a	Confirmatory PD up to 12 wk	• Using the idea of IR as long as subsequent imaging or biposy reveals either true progression or pseudoprogression. • Confirmatory imaging is important since IRs were recorded in 13% of instances that were all delayed for more than 12 months.

(continued on next page)

Table 1
(continued)

Criteria	Tumor Type	N	ICI	Modality	PR	CR	SD	PD	Confirmation of PD	Advantages
imPERCIST[18]	Melanoma	60	Anti-CTLA-4	18F-FDG PET/CT	Per PERCIST in 5 lesions	Per PERCIST in 5 lesions	Per PERCIST in 5 lesions	• Change in sum of SUL$_{peak}$ in 5 lesions >30% • The total sum incorporates any new lesions.	No confirmation required.	• Incorporating new lesions into the sum of the metabolic activity of lesions and not instantly declaring PD. • Compared to PERCIST, imPERCIST had a greater overall concordance with survival (HR 3.85, p: 0.005).
iPERCIST[23]	NSCLC	28	Anti-PD-1	18F-FDG PET/CT	Per PERCIST	Per PERCIST	Per PERCIST	Similar to PERCIST considering UPMD at first evaluation.	A repeat 18F-FDG PET/CT at 4–8 wk is required to classify UPMD as CPMD.	• Introducing UPMD with clinical stability. • Allowing continuation of the treatment.

Abbreviations: 18F-FDG PET/CT, 2-deoxy-2-[18F]fluoro-D-glucose positron emission tomography/computed tomography; CPMD, confirmed progressive metabolic disease; CR, complete response; CTLA-4, cytotoxic T lymphocyte antigen-4; HL, Hodgkin's lymphoma; HR, hazard ratio; ICI, immune checkpoint inhibitor; imPERCIST, immunotherapy-modified PERCIST; iPERCIST, immune PERCIST; IR, indeterminate response; LDH, lactate dehydrogenase; LYRIC, lymphoma response to immunotherapy criteria; MRI, magnetic resonance imaging; NSCLC, non-small cell lung cancer; PD, progressive disease; PD-1, programmed cell death protein 1; PECRIT, PET/CT criteria for early prediction of response to immune checkpoint inhibitor therapy; PERCIMT, PET response evaluation criteria for immunotherapy; PERCIST, PET response criteria in solid tumors; PPD, product of perpendicular diameters; PR, partial response; RECIST, response evaluation criteria in solid tumors; SD, stable disease; SPD, sum of the product of the perpendicular diameters; SUL$_{peak}$, peak standardized uptake value corrected for lean body mass; TL, total lesion; TLG, total lesion glycolysis; UPMD, unconfirmed progressive metabolic disease.

patients with NSCLC treated with anti-PD-1 ICI who had greater MTV and higher plasma neutrophil-to-lymphocyte ratios were shown to be at an elevated risk for hyperprogression, indicating that the development of a multiparameter model might enhance the prediction of tumor response.[27]

DISSOCIATED RESPONSE

Another pattern of response on morphologic imaging is termed "dissociated response," also known as "mixed response," which is the combination of non-responding (progressive disease or stable disease) and responding (partial response or complete response) based on RECIST 1.1 within the same patient.[28,29] An immune-dissociated response has also been described in ^{18}F-FDG PET/CT studies as an immunologic response in some lesions associated with evasion in others.[30]

Dissociated responses in patients receiving ICIs ranged from 3.3% to 9.2% of cases, and they had better overall survival compared to patients with progression.[4,30] This phenomenon can be explained by various physiopathological concepts, including differences in the tumor microenvironment (TME) throughout the various metastatic locations and genomic tumor heterogeneity.[29,31] The lack of information in this situation might be caused by the difficulty in identifying this phenomenon using the standard RECIST evaluation. In this context, ^{18}F-FDG PET/CT could be useful by determining persistent metabolic activity in residual anatomic abnormalities on CT in terms of metabolic response at additional disease spots, specifically when responsive to local salvage therapy.

In addition, radiologists need to be cautious about several notable differential diagnosis of dissociated response, including side effects of treatment (such as sarcoid-like reactions), pseudoprogression of 1 metastatic site, synchronous cancers, and inflammation-induced tracer uptake on ^{18}F-FDG PET/CT.[32] Nevertheless, in cancer patients receiving ICIs, there was no relationship between dissociated response and the site of metastases, but liver metastases were often less responsive to immunotherapy compared to metastatic lymph nodes and lung metastases.[28]

^{18}F-FDG PET/COMPUTED TOMOGRAPHY PROGNOSTICATION

MTV and tTLG, 2 quantitative FDG PET/CT measurements, have the potential to serve as indicators of prognosis in melanoma patients on immunotherapy. In a study of 122 melanoma patients treated with nivolumab and ipilimumab, baseline MTV on ^{18}F-FDG PET/CT was an independent prognostic indicator, regardless of treatment line.[33] Similarly, a systematic review of 24 studies involving patients with metastatic melanoma found that the baseline TLG and MTV parameters are potential predictors of the final response to immunotherapy[12] (Fig. 1).

Early ^{18}F-FDG PET/CT scan, which serves as non-invasive method to assess the effectiveness of immunotherapy, could be beneficial for anticipating the clinical benefit as well as modifying treatment regimens.[12,33] Early detection of patients that are not expected to respond to immunotherapy may cause treatment discontinuation, which could mitigate the risk of irAEs, reduce the high costs of immunotherapy, and allow the implementation of a new therapeutic regimen.[12,13]

Tan and colleagues evaluated the role of ^{18}F-FDG PET/CT in the potential timing of therapy discontinuation in 104 melanoma patients receiving immunotherapy. This study demonstrated that patients with a complete metabolic response on FDG PET/CT scans at 12 months had a continuing response to treatment. Interestingly, pseudoprogression was excluded by response on the 12-month FDG PET/CT scan. They also reported that complete metabolic response was noted in 68% of patients with partial response on CT indicating deepening of response over time[34] (Fig. 2). In another study, all patients experienced changes in the response category from progressive metabolic disease to stable metabolic disease, partial metabolic response, or complete metabolic response before 12 months indicating the temporal variability of pseudoprogression.[33] As a result, it might be proposed that therapy can be discontinued after 12 months of consolidative treatment following a complete metabolic response, incorporating a more individualized strategy as opposed to the generally used 2-year cut-off point for cessation of therapy.

^{18}F-FDG PET/COMPUTED TOMORAPHY, SYSTEMIC IMMUNE RESPONSE, AND IMMUNOTHERAPY-RELATED ADVERSE EVENTS

Following checkpoint inhibition, cytotoxic T lymphocytes first expand and recruit in the lymph nodes, where they can be found as new ^{18}F-FDG-avid lymph nodes throughout the body or in the nearby draining nodal stations.[35] All patients who had newly detected mediastinal or hilar nodal uptake on ^{18}F-FDG PET/CT in the context of ipilimumab for melanoma revealed evident clinical benefit following therapy.[36]

Preclinical and clinical investigations revealed dynamic alterations in the immune cell composition in both the bone marrow and spleen that

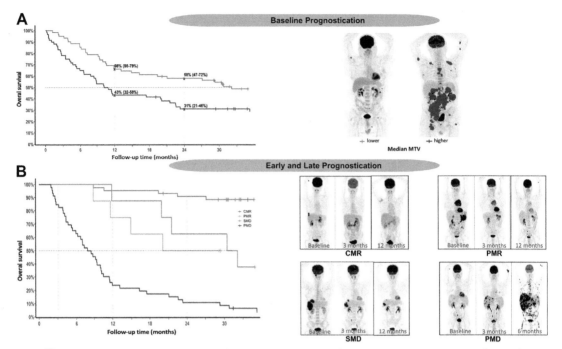

Fig. 1. ^{18}F-FDG PET/CT in prognostication and response monitoring. (*A*) Baseline prognostication, the Kaplan Meier curves show better survival of the patients with lower metabolic tumor volume (contoured in *red*). (*B*) The Kaplan Meier curves show better survival of the patients based on metabolic response at 3 months(early) and at 12 or 24 months(late) during immunotherapy. Representative cases of various metabolic responses are shown. CMR, complete metabolic response; MTV, metabolic tumor volume; PMD, progressive metabolic disease; PMR, partial metabolic response; SMD, stable metabolic disease.

resulted in the bone marrow's enhanced metabolic activity as detected on ^{18}F-FDG PET/CT.[37] These alterations can be seen either before or after the course of therapy and could be helpful in determining whether ICIs can be considered effective or not.[37] In a retrospective study of 55 patients with metastatic melanoma who underwent anti-PD1 immunotherapy, an initial rise in bone marrow metabolism on ^{18}F-FDG PET/CT was correlated with shorter survival. Furthermore, enhanced metabolism of bone marrow was significantly correlated with transcriptomic profiles such as regulatory T-cell markers.[38] To investigate the application of these findings in the therapeutic settings, further clinical and translational studies are needed.

Immune system reactivation that occurs with the administration of immunotherapeutic medications not only has anti-tumor effects but may also have adverse effects on healthy tissue, and these irAEs can affect any tissue or organ and manifest with a wide range of symptoms.[39]

The normal length of time for the onset of irAEs is 2 to 16 weeks; however, irAEs can also happen within days or persist for more than a year after treatment is completed.[39] Since the majority of these irAEs are managed with systemic immunosuppression, early

detection of irAEs might enhance the clinical outcome.[40] On the other hand, the occurrence of irAEs can have prognostic importance and sometimes be accompanied by good outcomes, considering the hypothesis that immune activation that causes the toxicity can similarly exert a cytotoxic impact on tumors.[39,41] In addition to clinical manifestations and biological indicators, conventional CT and MRI are crucial in detecting and monitoring irAEs. However, ^{18}F-FDG PET/CT could potentially provide a distinctive perspective regarding the process of inflammatory reactions (**Fig. 3**, **Table 2**).

The 2 most common abdominal irAEs are colitis and diarrhea, both of which have a significant probability of association with anti-CTLA-4 therapy alone or combination therapy (up to 22% and up to 50%, respectively).[42–44] Several studies characterized segmental, diffuse, and isolated rectosigmoid patterns of ^{18}F-FDG uptake; one of them reported a substantial association between increased ^{18}F-FDG uptake and severe diarrhea in patients with melanoma receiving ipilimumab.[45–47] Additionally, it has been demonstrated that ^{18}F-FDG uptake is correlated with less frequent immune-related upper gastrointestinal toxicities, including duodenitis, gastritis, and esophagitis.[32,48] Hepatic irAEs are reported in up to 19% of cases that are mostly

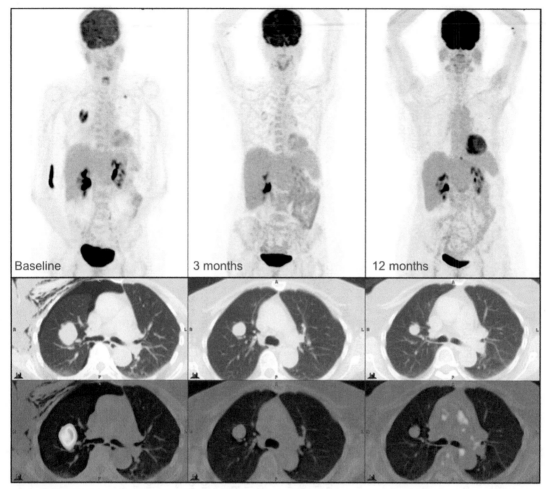

Fig. 2. ^{18}F-FDG PET/CT in a patient with partial anatomic response but with complete metabolic response at 12 months post treatment with immune checkpoint inhibitor as seen on PET (*top*), CT (*middle*), and PET/CT (*bottom*) images.

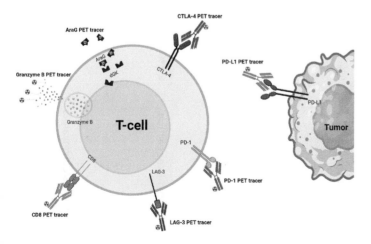

Fig. 3. ^{18}F-FDG PET manifestations of immune-related adverse events.

Table 2
irAEs and associated ^{18}F-FDG PET/CT findings

irAEs	Incidence[39]	Clinical Presentations	ICI	^{18}F-FDG PET/CT Findings
Pneumonitis	1%–3%	Dry cough, dyspnea, chest pain, and occasionally fever	Frequently common with anti-PD-(L)1 agents	Various uptake appearances, including focal organizing pattern or diffuse (hypersensitivity, ground-glass opacity patterns), and interstitial patterns, must be taken into account in the setting of findings on the CT component.[49,50,66]
Colitis	0.3%–22%	Abdominal pain, diarrhea	Frequently common with anti-CTLA-4 agents	Increased uptake with segmental or diffuse pattern.[45–47]
Thyroiditis	6%–22%	Typically, asymptomatic Thyroiditis followed by hypothyroidism, necessitating hormone replacement treatment.	Frequently common with anti-PD-(L)1 agents	Diffuse uptake.[50,66]
Hepatitis	5%–10%	Abnormal liver function tests, commonly just an increase in transaminases, and rarely liver failure	Equally common with anti-PD-(L)1 and anti-CTLA-4 agents	Increased uptake with diffuse pattern.[49]
Hypophysitis	1%–8%	May be asymptomatic Visual change, headache, fatigue, polyuria, polydipsia	Frequently common with anti-CTLA-4 agents	Increased focal uptake that might be challenging to detect because of background uptake in adjacent cortex.[50,66]
Sarcoid-like reaction	< 1%–6%	May be asymptomatic Dyspnea, fever, fatigue Skin could be affected such as Lofgren syndrome	Frequently common with anti-CTLA-4 agents	Increased bilateral uptake in the mediastinal and/or hilar lymph nodes. On rare occasions, liver or spleen diffuse or multifocal uptake. Extrathoracic node involvement is rare.[56]
Arthritis/polymyalgia rheumatica	1%	Stiffness, joint pain	Frequently common with anti-PD-(L)1 agents	Diffuse uptake in one or more affected joints

Abbreviations: CTLA-4, cytotoxic T lymphocyte antigen-4; irAE, immune-related adverse event; PD-1, programmed cell death protein 1.

asymptomatic and commonly detected with trasaminase increases, but diffuse ^{18}F-FDG uptake in the parenchyma of the liver has been noticed.[49]

Thyroiditis is reported in up to 22% of patients and is usually asymptomatic; however, it can present with diffuse ^{18}F-FDG uptake, leading to a hypothyroid situation necessitating hormone replacement.[50] Eshghi and colleagues[51] revealed that ^{18}F-FDG PET/CT has the ability to detect irAE thyroiditis prior to hormonal abnormalities. Thus, identifying an increase in thyroid gland activity on ^{18}F-FDG PET/CT could caution physicians to monitor for hypothyroidism symptoms. Although hypophysitis is a rare irAE, receiving anti-CTLA-4 has been associated with hypophysitis in up to 8% of cases. Increased focal ^{18}F-FDG uptake in the hypophysis is documented; however, because of the background uptake in the brain, it can be missed without thorough evaluation.[39]

Musculoskeletal adverse events are relatively common in patients receiving ICIs, including myalgia (up to 21%) and arthralgia (up to 43%).[52] Arthritis and myositis are less common irAEs, but have been documented in the setting of ^{18}F-FDG PET/CT with diffuse joint or muscle uptake, respectively.[53] There are preliminary data suggesting that rheumatic irAEs may be associated with more favorable outcomes.[54] Vasculitis and fasciitis are 2 further connective tissue inflammations that are associated with ICIs, which are uncommon but have been documented.[55]

Pneumonitis is an uncommon but potentially fatal irAE with an incidence of 1% to 10%, and contrary to other irAEs, it is more frequently reported with anti-PD-1 agents and combination treatment.[43,44] Sarcoid-like reactions are mostly asymptomatic and could be misdiagnosed with progression by mimicking lymphadenopathy of the hilar and mediastinal lymph nodes with increased ^{18}F-FDG uptake. Sarcoid-like reactions are not limited to thoracic manifestations and it can rarely involve extrathoracic lymph nodes as well as organomegaly, so multifocal or diffuse uptake in the liver or spleen should be taken into account.[56] Although there is a significant amount of literature reporting and documenting the detection of irAEs on ^{18}F-FDG PET/CT, no systematic research or validated screening methods for their evaluation are available.

Since irAEs may first become clinically manifest or even occur following discontinuation of ICIs, a potential function for ^{18}F-FDG PET/CT in predicting irAEs is noteworthy and obviously requires further investigation. Therefore, it is important that any possible irAEs be detected and documented during ^{18}F-FDG PET/CT evaluations of immunotherapy patients.

NOVEL PET TRACERS

Novel molecular radiotracers that target precisely the main molecules of immune checkpoint pathways and immunologic responses are developing in addition to morphologic and metabolic-based imaging[57] (**Fig. 4**). As intact monoclonal antibodies represent the majority of the current ICIs, using a rather long-lived radionuclide is required because of the kinetics of blood clearance. As a result, many of them can be labeled with ^{64}Cu or [89]Zr.[58] Anti-PD-1 agents are able to be labeled with ^{64}Cu or [89]Zr and could be used for imaging PD-1-expressing tumor-infiltrating lymphocytes in vivo, which may be considered a promising method for the non-invasive detection and evaluation of PD-1 expression.[57]

In a first-in-human study utilizing the radiolabeled anti-PD-1 monoclonal antibody [89]Zr-nivolumab in NSCLC patients, there was a significant [89]Zr-nivolumab tumor uptake, which was greater in those with immunohistochemically confirmed

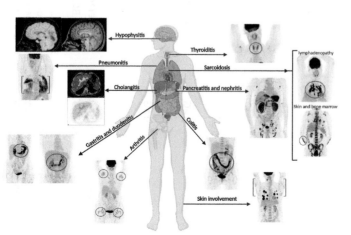

Fig. 4. Schematic mechanisms of the most promising novel Immuno-PET agents.

Table 3
Overview of PET tracers under evaluation for immune targets in cancer

	Target	Tumor	Radioisotope	NCT Number	Primary Objective
PD-1	Pembrolizumab	NSCLC	^{89}Zr	NCT03065764	Evaluating the safety, irAEs, and tumor uptake
	Nivolumab	Melanoma	^{89}Zr	NCT05289193	Assessing major pathologic responses
PD-L1	Atezolizumab	Renal cell carcinoma	^{89}Zr	NCT04006522	Examining whether ^{89}Zr-DFO-Atezolizumab uptake across metastatic sites of renal cell carcinoma correlates with PD-L1 expression as well as response to ICIs.
	Atezolizumab	Rectal and esophageal cancer	^{89}Zr	NCT04564482	Using ^{89}Zr-atezolizumab PET to evaluate intramural changes of PD-L1 expression induced by neoadjuvant CRT or SCPRT (at baseline and between day 10–14)
	BMS-986192	Oral squamous cell carcinoma	^{18}F	NCT03843515	In this phase 1 trial of neoadjuvant nivolumab, BMS-986192 and ^{18}F-FDG PET will be employed for response prediction.
	Avelumab	NSCLC	^{89}Zr	NCT03514719	Evaluating tumor and systemic tissue uptake, as well as the potential to predict response
	Envafolimab	PD-L1 positive advanced solid tumors	^{89}Zr	NCT03638804	Determine regions of interest, radiation dosimetry, and target lesion uptake
Granzyme B	hGZP	Solid tumors, lymphoma	^{68}Ga	NCT04169321	Evaluating the safety, effectiveness, irAEs, and tumor uptake
AraG	F-AraG	NSCLC	^{18}F	NCT04726215	Measuring ^{18}F F-AraG uptake pre- and post-treatment, and its correlation with radiographic response.
	F-AraG	Healthy volunteers and NSCLC	^{18}F	NCT04678440	Uptake and pharmacokinetics in tumor and healthy tissue
	F-AraG	Solid tumors	^{18}F	NCT03142204	Biodistribution of the PET tracer pre- and post-immunotherapy
CTLA-4	Ipilimumab	Melanoma	^{89}Zr	NCT03313323	Evaluating tumor uptake and biodistribution
LAG-3	REGN3767	DLBCL	^{89}Zr	NCT04566978	Evaluating tumor uptake and its correlation with LAG-3 expression

Abbreviations: ^{18}F-FDG PET, 2-deoxy-2-[18F]fluoro-D-glucose positron emission tomography; AraG, arabinofuranosyl guanine; CTLA-4, cytotoxic T lymphocyte antigen-4; DLBCL, diffuse large B cell lymphoma; ICI, immune checkpoint inhibitor; irAE, Immune-related adverse event; LAG-3, lymphocyte activation gene-3; NSCLC, non-small cell lung cancer; PD-1, programmed cell death protein 1; PD-L1, programmed death-ligand 1.

PD-1 positive tumor-infiltrating immune cells in comparison to those with PD-1 negative tumors.[59] Furthermore, PD-1 and PD-L1 PET/CT revealed heterogeneous tumor uptake between patients and also divergent uptake between various tumor lesions intraindividually.[59,60]

PD-L1 tracers for PET/CT that are accessible in clinical settings demonstrated an association with PD-L1 status evaluated by immunohistochemistry. Examining PD-L1 expression on PET/CT is conducted through the utilization of PD-L1 tracers, including ^{18}F-labeled anti-PD-L1 adnectin (^{18}F-BMS-986192) and ^{68}Ga-labeled adnectin (^{68}Ga-BMS-98619). Notably, a stronger association of the tumor response to ICI treatment was discovered on PET/CT utilizing [89]Zr-atezolizumab in comparison to immunohistochemical analysis of the expression of PD-L1.[61] In addition, [89]Zr-durvulumab has been examined in the PINCH trial (NCT03829007), a prospective clinical and imaging trial in patients with metastatic or recurrent head and neck cancer who are receiving durvalumab.[62] Although the safety of [89]Zr-durvulumab could be demonstrated, its uptake did not correspond to the durvalumab treatment response.[62] In addition to employing PET to image PD-L1, a number of novel biomarkers were added to molecular imaging in preclinical models, like interferon-γ immuno-PET (Zr-anti-IFN-γ), which facilitated imaging of active lymphocytes inside tumor lesions.[63]

The challenge of evaluating tumor response in patients treated with ICIs led to the creation of new radiotracers, including [89]Zr-Df-IAB22M2C ([89]Zr-Df-Crefmirlimab), which target CD8-positive T cells as well as ^{18}F-arabinofuranosyl guanine (^{18}F-AraG) and ^{68}Ga-NOTA-GZP that target activated CD8+ T cells. An ongoing clinical trial called the iPREDICT trial intends to assess the safety of repeated doses of [89]Zr-Df-IAB22M2C in patients with metastatic solid tumors as well as the correlation between [89]Zr-Df-IAB22M2C uptake and CD8+ immunohistochemistry. The protease granzyme B (GZP) is a novel target that is produced throughout immune-induced, caspase-dependent apoptosis by cytotoxic CD8+. Targeting imaging using ^{68}Ga-NOTA-GZP enabled highly accurate preclinical model predictions of immunotherapy response.[64] The ^{18}F-AraG's ability to image the activation of T cells and, consequently, propose early indications of adaptive response to immunotherapies is being studied in several phase II trials.[65] **Table 3** provides an overview of the PET tracers currently under investigation in human studies for immunologic targets. These optimistic attempts highlight the need for more research into immuno-PET and its thorough translation into clinical use in order to further enhance patient selection in pretreatment, response evaluation, and clinical management.

SUMMARY

Although many of the studies that have been published thus far lack high-level evidence validating the role of ^{18}F-FDG PET/CT criteria for response assessment, these preliminary data support the ability of this investigation to provide incremental information of potential clinical and prognostic benefit beyond that routinely available from CT. Its main benefit seems to be in providing earlier assessment of treatment benefit than anatomic imaging but remains challenged by the phenomena of pseudoprogression, hyperprogression, and dissociated response. Novel immuno-PET tracers may have a role in these situations by more directly assessing the immune microenvironment. Detection of important irAEs on ^{18}F-FDG PET/CT could also minimize their associated morbidity and, in some cases, mortality. Incorporation of ^{18}F-FDG PET/CT into clinical trials with consistent protocols and outcome measures will help to provide a clearer understanding of the clinical value of this technique in monitoring rapidly evolving treatment immunotherapy paradigms that are increasingly used in combination with chemotherapy and radiotherapy as well as targeted agents, and to assess its impact on modifying patient care.

CLINICS CARE POINTS

- Although atypical response patterns in patients receiving immunotherapy pose challenges for covential imaging response criteria, the overal rate of psueodprogression remains low and and decision to continue immunotherapy beyond progression should be taken with caution.

- Whole body tumor burden on baseline ^{18}F-FDG PET/CT is a promising metabolic parameter that provide prognostic information.

- ^{18}F-FDG PET/CT is a promsing modality for response monitroing in patients receiving immunotherapy.

- ^{18}F-FDG PET/CT performed for response monitoring should be interrogated for manifestations of immune-related adverse events.

- Multiple novel immuno-PET radiopharmaceuticals are currently under investigations and may hold promise in improving the understanding of the complex interplay of tumor and systemic immune response to immunotherapeutic strategies.

DISCLOSURE

The authors declare no relevant disclosure.

REFERENCES

1. Decazes P, Bohn P. Immunotherapy by immune checkpoint inhibitors and nuclear medicine imaging: current and future applications. Cancers 2020;12(2): 371.
2. Unterrainer M, Ruzicka M, Fabritius MP, et al. PET/CT imaging for tumour response assessment to immunotherapy: current status and future directions. Eur Radiol Exp 2020;4:1–13.
3. Seymour L, Bogaerts J, Perrone A, et al. iRECIST: guidelines for response criteria for use in trials testing immunotherapeutics. Lancet Oncol 2017; 18(3):e143–52.
4. Berz AM, Dromain C, Vietti-Violi N, et al. Tumor response assessment on imaging following immunotherapy. Front Oncol 2022;12:982983.
5. Borcoman E, Nandikolla A, Long G, et al. Patterns of response and progression to immunotherapy. Am Soc Clin Oncol Educ Book 2018;38:169–78.
6. Wolchok JD, Hoos A, O'Day S, et al. Guidelines for the evaluation of immune therapy activity in solid tumors: immune-related response criteria. Clin Cancer Res 2009;15(23):7412–20.
7. Hodi FS, Hwu WJ, Kefford R, et al. Evaluation of immune-related response criteria and RECIST v1.1 in patients with advanced melanoma treated with pembrolizumab. J Clin Oncol 2016;34(13):1510.
8. Hodi FS, Ballinger M, Lyons B, et al. Immune-modified response evaluation criteria in solid tumors (imRECIST): refining guidelines to assess the clinical benefit of cancer immunotherapy. J Clin Oncol 2018;36(9):850–8.
9. Young H, Baum R, Cremerius U, et al. Measurement of clinical and subclinical tumour response using [18F]-fluorodeoxyglucose and positron emission tomography: review and 1999 EORTC recommendations. Eur J Cancer 1999;35(13):1773–82.
10. Wahl RL, Jacene H, Kasamon Y, et al. From RECIST to PERCIST: evolving considerations for PET response criteria in solid tumors. J Nucl Med 2009; 50(Suppl 1):122S–50S.
11. Park S, Lee Y, Kim TS, et al. Response evaluation after immunotherapy in NSCLC: early response assessment using FDG PET/CT. Medicine (Baltimore) 2020;99(51):e23815.
12. Ayati N, Sadeghi R, Kiamanesh Z, et al. The value of 18 F-FDG PET/CT for predicting or monitoring immunotherapy response in patients with metastatic melanoma: a systematic review and meta-analysis. Eur J Nucl Med Mol Imaging 2021;48:428–48.
13. Cho SY, Lipson EJ, Im HJ, et al. Prediction of response to immune checkpoint inhibitor therapy using early-time-point 18F-FDG PET/CT imaging in patients with advanced melanoma. J Nucl Med 2017;58(9):1421–8.
14. Eisenhauer EA, Therasse P, Bogaerts J, et al. New response evaluation criteria in solid tumours: revised RECIST guideline (version 1.1). Eur J Cancer 2009; 45(2):228–47.
15. Anwar H, Sachpekidis C, Winkler J, et al. Absolute number of new lesions on 18 F-FDG PET/CT is more predictive of clinical response than SUV changes in metastatic melanoma patients receiving ipilimumab. Eur J Nucl Med Mol Imaging 2018;45: 376–83.
16. Sachpekidis C, Kopp-Schneider A, Hakim-Meibodi L, et al. 18F-FDG PET/CT longitudinal studies in patients with advanced metastatic melanoma for response evaluation of combination treatment with vemurafenib and ipilimumab. Melanoma Res 2019;29(2):178–86.
17. Sachpekidis C, Anwar H, Winkler J, et al. The role of interim 18 F-FDG PET/CT in prediction of response to ipilimumab treatment in metastatic melanoma. Eur J Nucl Med Mol Imaging 2018;45:1289–96.
18. Ito K, Teng R, Schöder H, et al. 18F-FDG PET/CT for monitoring of ipilimumab therapy in patients with metastatic melanoma. J Nucl Med 2019;60(3):335–41.
19. Dercle L, Seban RD, Lazarovici J, et al. 18F-FDG PET and CT scans detect new imaging patterns of response and progression in patients with Hodgkin lymphoma treated by anti–programmed death 1 immune checkpoint inhibitor. J Nucl Med 2018;59(1): 15–24.
20. Chen A, Mokrane FZ, Schwartz LH, et al. Early 18F-FDG PET/CT response predicts survival in relapsed or refractory Hodgkin lymphoma treated with nivolumab. J Nucl Med 2020;61(5):649–54.
21. Cheson BD, Fisher RI, Barrington SF, Alliance, Australasian Leukaemia and Lymphoma GroupEastern Cooperative Oncology GroupEuropean Mantle cell lymphoma Consortium, et al. Recommendations for initial evaluation, staging, and response assessment of Hodgkin and non-Hodgkin lymphoma: the Lugano classification. J Clin Oncol. 2014;32(27): 3059-3068.
22. Cheson BD, Ansell S, Schwartz L, et al. Refinement of the Lugano Classification lymphoma response criteria in the era of immunomodulatory therapy. Blood J Am Soc Hematol 2016;128(21):2489–96.
23. Goldfarb L, Duchemann B, Chouahnia K, et al. Monitoring anti-PD-1-based immunotherapy in non-small cell lung cancer with FDG PET: introduction of iPERCIST. EJNMMI Res 2019;9(1):1–10.
24. Adashek JJ, Subbiah IM, Matos I, et al. Hyperprogression and immunotherapy: fact, fiction, or alternative fact? Trends Cancer 2020;6(3):181–91.
25. Ferrara R, Mezquita L, Texier M, et al. Hyperprogressive disease in patients with advanced non–small

cell lung cancer treated with PD-1/PD-L1 inhibitors or with single-agent chemotherapy. JAMA Oncol 2018;4(11):1543–52.

26. Nakamoto R, C Zaba L, Rosenberg J, et al. Imaging characteristics and diagnostic performance of 2-deoxy-2-[18 F] fluoro-D-glucose PET/CT for melanoma patients who demonstrate hyperprogressive disease when treated with immunotherapy. Mol Imaging Biol 2021;23:139–47.

27. Castello A, Rossi S, Mazziotti E, et al. Hyperprogressive disease in patients with non–small cell lung cancer treated with checkpoint inhibitors: the role of 18F-FDG PET/CT. J Nucl Med 2020;61(6):821–6.

28. Vaflard P, Paoletti X, Servois V, et al. Dissociated responses in patients with metastatic solid tumors treated with immunotherapy. Drugs R 2021;21:399–406.

29. Humbert O, Chardin D. Dissociated response in metastatic cancer: an atypical pattern brought into the spotlight with immunotherapy. Front Oncol 2020;10:566297.

30. Tazdait M, Mezquita L, Lahmar J, et al. Patterns of responses in metastatic NSCLC during PD-1 or PDL-1 inhibitor therapy: comparison of RECIST 1.1, irRECIST and iRECIST criteria. Eur J Cancer 2018;88:38–47.

31. Dong ZY, Zhai HR, Hou QY, et al. Mixed responses to systemic therapy revealed potential genetic heterogeneity and poor survival in patients with non-small cell lung cancer. Oncol 2017;22(1):61–9.

32. Iravani A, Hicks RJ. Pitfalls and Immune-Related Adverse Events. In: Lopci E, Fanti S, editors. *Atlas of response to Immunotherapy*. Springer International Publishing; 2020. p. 101–15.

33. Iravani A, Wallace R, Lo SN, et al. FDG PET/CT prognostic markers in patients with advanced melanoma treated with ipilimumab and nivolumab. Radiology 2023;307(3):e221180.

34. Tan AC, Emmett L, Lo S, et al. FDG-PET response and outcome from anti-PD-1 therapy in metastatic melanoma. Ann Oncol 2018;29(10):2115–20.

35. Tsai KK, Pampaloni MH, Hope C, et al. Increased FDG avidity in lymphoid tissue associated with response to combined immune checkpoint blockade. J Immunother Cancer 2016;4(1):1–5.

36. Sachpekidis C, Larribère L, Kopp-Schneider A, et al. Can benign lymphoid tissue changes in 18 F-FDG PET/CT predict response to immunotherapy in metastatic melanoma? Cancer Immunol Immunother 2019;68:297–303.

37. Schwenck J, Schörg B, Fiz F, et al. Cancer immunotherapy is accompanied by distinct metabolic patterns in primary and secondary lymphoid organs observed by non-invasive in vivo 18F-FDG-PET. Theranostics 2020;10(2):925.

38. Seban RD, Nemer JS, Marabelle A, et al. Prognostic and theranostic 18F-FDG PET biomarkers for anti-PD1 immunotherapy in metastatic melanoma: association with outcome and transcriptomics. Eur J Nucl Med Mol Imaging 2019;46:2298–310.

39. Ramos-Casals M, Brahmer JR, Callahan MK, et al. Immune-related adverse events of checkpoint inhibitors. Nat Rev Dis Primer 2020;6(1):38.

40. Fujii T, Colen RR, Bilen MA, et al. Incidence of immune-related adverse events and its association with treatment outcomes: the MD Anderson Cancer Center experience. Invest New Drugs 2018;36:638–46.

41. Nobashi T, Baratto L, Reddy SA, et al. Predicting response to immunotherapy by evaluating tumors, lymphoid cell-rich organs, and immune-related adverse events using FDG-PET/CT. Clin Nucl Med 2019;44(4):e272–9.

42. Sosa A, Lopez Cadena E, Simon Olive C, et al. Clinical assessment of immune-related adverse events. Ther Adv Med Oncol 2018;10. 1758835918764628.

43. Chan KK, Bass AR. Autoimmune complications of immunotherapy: pathophysiology and management. BMJ 2020;369:m736.

44. Kottschade LA. Incidence and management of immune-related adverse events in patients undergoing treatment with immune checkpoint inhibitors. Curr Oncol Rep 2018;20:1–8.

45. Martins F, Sofiya L, Sykiotis GP, et al. Adverse effects of immune-checkpoint inhibitors: epidemiology, management and surveillance. Nat Rev Clin Oncol 2019;16(9):563–80.

46. Lang D, Wahl G, Poier N, et al. Impact of PET/CT for assessing response to immunotherapy—a clinical perspective. J Clin Med 2020;9(11):3483.

47. Barina AR, Bashir MR, Howard BA, et al. Isolated recto-sigmoid colitis: a new imaging pattern of ipilimumab-associated colitis. Abdom Radiol 2016;41:207–14.

48. Hughes DJ, Subesinghe M, Taylor B, et al. 18F FDG PET/CT and novel molecular imaging for directing immunotherapy in cancer. Radiology 2022;304(2):246–64.

49. Raad RA, Pavlick A, Kannan R, et al. Ipilimumab-induced hepatitis on 18F-FDG PET/CT in a patient with malignant melanoma. Clin Nucl Med 2015;40(3):258–9.

50. Iravani A, Galligan A, Lasocki A, et al. FDG PET in the evaluation of immune-related hypophysitis and thyroiditis following combination ipilimumab and nivolumab in advanced melanoma. J Nucl Med 2020;61(supplement 1):482.

51. Eshghi N, Garland LL, Nia E, et al. 18F-FDG PET/CT can predict development of thyroiditis due to immunotherapy for lung cancer. J Nucl Med Technol 2018;46(3):260–4.

52. Cappelli LC, Gutierrez AK, Bingham CO III, et al. Rheumatic and musculoskeletal immune-related adverse events due to immune checkpoint inhibitors:

a systematic review of the literature. Arthritis Care Res 2017;69(11):1751–63.

53. Calabrese LH, Calabrese C, Cappelli LC. Rheumatic immune-related adverse events from cancer immunotherapy. Nat Rev Rheumatol 2018;14(10):569–79.

54. Mitchell EL, Lau PKH, Khoo C, et al. Rheumatic immune-related adverse events secondary to anti–programmed death-1 antibodies and preliminary analysis on the impact of corticosteroids on anti-tumour response: a case series. Eur J Cancer 2018;105:88–102.

55. Henderson D, Eslamian G, Poon D, et al. Immune checkpoint inhibitor induced large vessel vasculitis. BMJ Case Rep CP 2020;13(5):e233496.

56. Gkiozos I, Kopitopoulou A, Kalkanis A, et al. Sarcoidosis-like reactions induced by checkpoint inhibitors. J Thorac Oncol 2018;13(8):1076–82.

57. Natarajan A, Mayer AT, Reeves RE, et al. Development of novel immunoPET tracers to image human PD-1 checkpoint expression on tumor-infiltrating lymphocytes in a humanized mouse model. Mol Imaging Biol 2017;19:903–14.

58. Wierstra P, Sandker G, Aarntzen E, et al. Tracers for non-invasive radionuclide imaging of immune checkpoint expression in cancer. EJNMMI Radiopharm Chem 2019;4(1):1–20.

59. Niemeijer AN, Leung D, Huisman MC, et al. Whole body PD-1 and PD-L1 positron emission tomography in patients with non-small-cell lung cancer. Nat Commun 2018;9(1):4664.

60. Verhoeff SR, van den Heuvel MM, van Herpen CM, et al. Programmed cell death-1/ligand-1 PET imaging: a novel tool to optimize immunotherapy? Pet Clin 2020;15(1):35–43.

61. Bensch F, van der Veen EL, Lub-de Hooge MN, et al. 89Zr-atezolizumab imaging as a non-invasive approach to assess clinical response to PD-L1 blockade in cancer. Nat Med 2018;24(12):1852–8.

62. Verhoeff SR, van de Donk PP, Aarntzen EH, et al. 89Zr-DFO-Durvalumab PET/CT before durvalumab treatment in patients with recurrent or metastatic head and neck cancer. J Nucl Med 2022;63(10):1523–30.

63. Gibson HM, McKnight BN, Malysa A, et al. IFNγ PET imaging as a predictive tool for monitoring response to tumor immunotherapy. Cancer Res 2018;78(19):5706–17.

64. Larimer BM, Wehrenberg-Klee E, Dubois F, et al. Granzyme B PET imaging as a predictive biomarker of immunotherapy response. Cancer Res 2017;77(9):2318–27.

65. Levi J, Song H. The other immuno-PET: metabolic tracers in evaluation of immune responses to immune checkpoint inhibitor therapy for solid tumors. Front Immunol 2023;13:1113924.

66. Gandy N, Arshad MA, Wallitt KL, et al. Immunotherapy-related adverse effects on 18F-FDG PET/CT imaging. Br J Radiol 2020;93(1111):20190832.

Moving?

Make sure your subscription moves with you!

To notify us of your new address, find your **Clinics Account Number** (located on your mailing label above your name), and contact customer service at:

Email: journalscustomerservice-usa@elsevier.com

800-654-2452 (subscribers in the U.S. & Canada)
314-447-8871 (subscribers outside of the U.S. & Canada)

Fax number: 314-447-8029

Elsevier Health Sciences Division
Subscription Customer Service
3251 Riverport Lane
Maryland Heights, MO 63043

Printed and bound by CPI Group (UK) Ltd, Croydon, CR0 4YY

03/10/2024

01040365-0018